W0043579

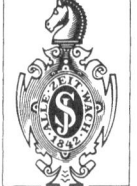

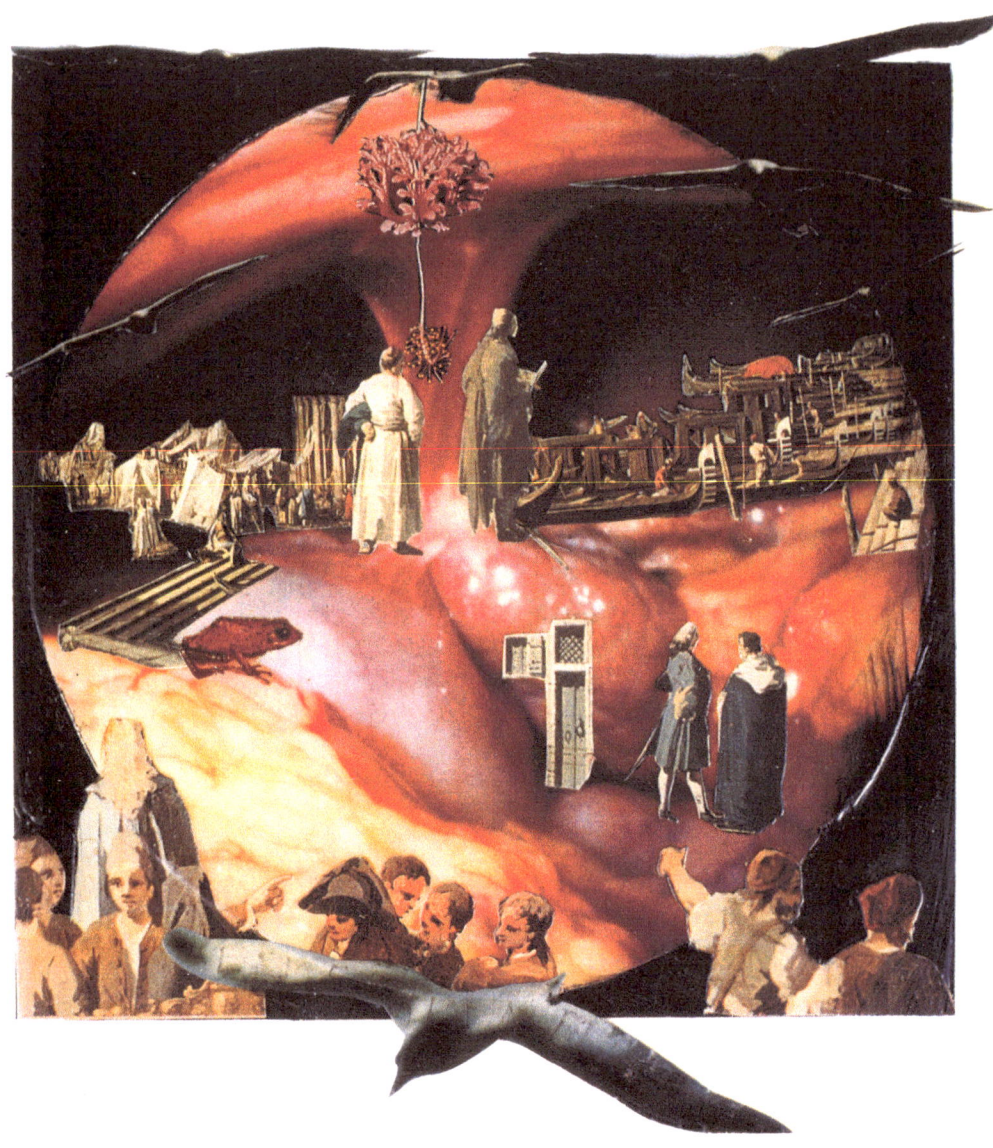

Esmeralda Ruspoli: Laparoscopic "capriccio", 1976
(Collage made on a laparoscopic photograph. 20 × 20 cm)

Giorgio Dagnini

Laparoscopy
and Imaging Techniques

Translated by Sara Pearcey

With a Foreword by F. Vilardell

With 187 Figures, 145 in Color

Springer-Verlag Berlin Heidelberg GmbH

Prof. Dr. Giorgio Dagnini
Via del Vescovado 24
I-35141 Padova

ISBN 978-3-642-74647-5   ISBN 978-3-642-74645-1 (eBook)
DOI 10.1007/978-3-642-74645-1

Library of Congress Cataloging-in-Publication Data. Dagnini, Giorgio. Laparoscopy and imaging techniques / G. Dagnini; translated by Sara Pearcey. p. cm. ISBN-13: 978-3-642-74647-5 (U.S.: alk. paper) 1. Laparoscopy. 2. Abdomen – Imaging. I. Title. [DNLM: 1. Peritoneoscopy – methods. WI 575 D127L] RC944.D34 1989 617.5'507545 – dc20 DNLM/DLC 89-26250

© Springer-Verlag Berlin Heidelberg 1990
Softcover reprint of the hardcover 1st edition 1990

The use of registered names, trademarks, etc. in this publication does not imply, even in the absence of a specific statement, that such names are exempt from the relevant protective laws and regulations and therefore free for general use.

Product liability: The publisher can give no guarantee for information about drug dosage and application thereof contained in this book. In every individual case the respective user must check its accuracy by consulting other pharmaceutical literature.

Typesetting: Best-set Typesetter Ltd., Hong Kong

2121/3130-543210 - Printed on acid-free paper

Foreword

Laparoscopy has been used in Europe since the turn of the century. The interest of gastroenterologists in laparoscopy was greatly expanded in the 1930s by the work of Kalk in Germany and Ruddock in the United States. Since then, laparoscopy has been widely employed all over the world.

Opinions concerning the indications of laparoscopy vary a great deal. More than 50 years ago Korbsch, a well-known German gastroenterologist and endoscopist, recommended that "Laparoscopy should be used if the diagnosis cannot be established by other means and there is a good chance of visualizing the lesion"; this is still valid. However, as Professor Dagnini states, the advent of newer imaging techniques have doubtless changed these indications, narrowing them in some areas but expanding them in others. These examination methods have by no means negated the use or value of laparoscopy. We believe, with Professor Dagnini, that laparoscopy should be employed in the diagnosis of obscure abdominal disease if other tests fail to give a definite answer, as is often the case with imaging techniques, when laparotomy, for one reason or another, should be avoided.

Gynecologists' wide utilization of laparoscopy to perform surgical procedures is now being matched by abdominal surgeons who are now performing laparoscopic appendectomies and particularly cholecystectomies. In some countries, such as France, the latter are being done in several centers and extensive experience has been accumulated.

This magnificent book by Professor Giorgio Dagnini, one of the foremost representatives of laparoscopic techniques in Europe, is timely and courageous. It addresses several important points: (1) the comparison with imaging techniques and the emergence of new indications secondary to imaging discoveries; (2) The progress in technology, such as fine needles for pneumoperitoneum, laparoscopy with flexible instruments, the use of the bio-plug, and echolaparoscopy; (3) Laparoscopy of the pancreas, and biopsy of the pancreas and spleen for the staging of lymphomas, an indication for laparoscopy with which the school of Professor Dagnini has very wide experience.

There follows a series of chapters on the traditional indications for laparoscopy, including the diagnosis of ascites, splenomegaly, hepatomegaly, and abdominal masses and the role of combined sonography and laparoscopy in their final assessment. The chapter on liver diseases shows clearly that laparoscopy retains a major role in diagnosis, as imaging methods are usually only able to demonstrate pronounced changes, not early disease.

Laparoscopy has an important role in the staging of tumors and also in abdominal emergencies, although in the latter, imaging techniques have narrowed its use.

The book is illustrated by many outstanding colour photographs, which are well known to be one of Professor Dagnini's strengths. It presents the current status of laparoscopy objectively and dispassionately: there are large numbers of references in several languages supporting the discussions, and the text is clear and to the point, probably a consequence of the great experience of Professor Dagnini as a teacher and clinician.

All laparoscopists and also gastroenterologists and surgeons should read this book. It will be an invaluable source of references, and will be helpful in many ways to the beginner as well as to the seasoned endoscopist. This superb monograph is a joy to read and a great achievement.

Professor Francisco Vilardell
President, World Organisation
of Gastroenterology (OMGE)

Preface

Since laparoscopy has become a less frequent topic of discussion, it might seem anachronistic to write a book on it. Far from this being the case, however, a review such as this is the natural outcome of the revolution in the diagnosis of abdominal diseases brought about by the increasingly wide spread use of imaging techniques. We are all aware of the extraordinary diagnostic potential of the "new" noninvasive techniques, and it is therefore logical to ask ourselves why the "old" laparoscope, which is invasive and more risky, should still be even considered.

In recent years, people have sometimes asked me in an ironic tone whether I still believe in laparoscopy and continue to perform it. The question gives me the unpleasant sensation of being a "has been." I can only give a decent answer to it after, on the one hand, considering the state of the art of laparoscopy with respect to new technical and methodological advances and, on the other, ascertaining systematically whether sonography or other noninvasive techniques can really replace laparoscopy in all cases.

The aim of this book is to answer these question along two lines. The first part describes the most recent developments, progress that has greatly enhanced the efficacy and reduced the risks of laparoscopy. The second part deals with the complex issue of the present indications for this technique.

We have used echography and laparoscopy in combination for several years, with the same operator performing both techniques. This qualifies us to make an impartial assessment of them. Now, when faced with a particular diagnostic problem we can directly evaluate and compare the advantages, potential, gaps, and drawbacks of each technique and then consider the clues in order to work out the quickest and most advantageous way of reaching a satisfactory diagnosis in a given case. We have greatly modified and updated the entire protocol for the indications for laparoscopy. Some have been abandoned in favor of sonography while others must still be considered valid. Lastly, new indications have emerged.

This book is based on direct observation from my own experience, and it follows the scheme of teaching in daily practice. I did not intend to write a treatise, but preferred to deal with the innovations made in laparoscopy since these innovations are the window of opportunity for laparoscopy itself. Because of this, most references are to works published from 1980 onwards.

This book has, of course, been written for laparoscopists and sonographists. But it is, above all, for clinicians, internal physicians, surgeons, gastroenterologists, and oncologists. I trust that it provides them with a clear picture of the value of laparoscopy and that it helps them decide if and when it is opportune to use this glorious technique to resolve a particular diagnostic problem.

Giorgio Dagnini

Contents

The **reference list** appear at the end of each chapter

Introduction

It is obvious that with the now widespread use of non-invasive imaging techniques with high diagnostic efficacy, the indications for laparoscopy have greatly changed. Yet it is difficult to make a reliable critical appraisal of the present status of laparoscopy in the diagnosis of abdominal diseases.

To make this evaluation we must (a) specify the contribution made by imaging techniques to our knowledge and to the diagnosis of various abdominal diseases and work out any effect it may have on the use of laparoscopy and (b) bear in mind recent improvements made in laparoscopy itself.

The systematic use of the CT scan and ultrasonography (US) has meant that less interest is now shown in laparoscopy, and so it appears to be indicated in fewer cases. However, in 1988, Boyd [1] stated that "in several pockets of resistance, a large number of laparoscopies were still done, so that critical evaluation of laparoscopy in the diagnosis of liver and other abdominal disease continued."

These observations suggest that the phenomenon is more complex than it appears to be at first sight. Gandolfi and co-workers [2] looked at the changes in the indications for laparoscopy after the advent of sonography by comparing the laparoscopic diagnoses made in two groups of patients respectively in the 2-year periods 1973–1974 and 1980–1981 (Table 1). The results can be summarized as follows: (a) There has been a marked reduction in the number of laparoscopies performed for certain indications (obstructive jaundice, abdominal masses, and liver metastases). (b) There has been a slight increase in the indications for laparoscopy in diffuse diseases of the liver (e.g., chronic hepatitis, steatosis, cirrhosis, and intrahepatic cholestasis). (c) There has been a significant increase in the diagnosis of

Table 1. Indications for laparoscopy before and after the introduction of sonography (from Gandolfi et al. [2])

	Before (1973–1974)		After (1980–1981)	
	No. of cases	%	No. of cases	%
Chronic hepatitis	44	6.6	30	4.2
Cirrhosis	260	39.0	306	42.6
Fatty liver	94	14.1	130	18.1
Cholestasis				
Intrahepatic	14	2.1	21	2.9
Extrahepatic	24	3.6	6	0.8*
Cysts of the liver	8	1.2	2	0.3
Primary liver tumors				
Benign	4	0.6	26	3.6*
Malignant	20	3.0	28	3.9
Metastatic liver tumors	80	12.0	46	6.4*
Malignant tumors of the gallbladder	2	0.3	8	1.1
Abdominal masses	21	3.1	8	1.1**
Peritoneal diseases	42	6.3	32	4.4
Miscellaneous	54	8.1	76	10.6

* $P < 0.1$
** $P < 0.5$

benign liver tumors. (d) The total number of laparoscopies performed after the advent of sonography has not diminished, but rather increased.

Buscarini and co-workers [3] compared the results of 100 laparoscopies done before with those of another 100 done after the advent of both ultrasound and fine-needle biopsy in abdominal diagnostics (Table 2) and found that there has been (a) a marked reduction in the number of laparoscopies performed to diagnose liver metastases, (b) a considerable increase in the number of laparoscopies performed to diagnose chronic liver disease, (c) a slight increase in diagnosis of liver carcinoma via laparoscopy.

Our findings are in agreement with the above. We compared the laparoscopic diagnoses made in 1976 with those made in 1986 and discovered that (a) in cases of "hepatomegaly" (liver metastases, primary tumors, cysts, collections, etc.) the percentage of cases in which laparoscopy is performed has fallen from 10.8% to 4.8%, and in jaundice from 4% to 1.04%; (b) in cases of diffuse liver disease any variations in the percentages have been slight; and (c) there has been a reduction in the total number of laparoscopies performed, from 851 to 768.

These data from large series allow us to make some interesting general conclusions along three lines. First, laparoscopy has now lost some of its traditional indications. This was to be expected: In cases of hepatomegaly due to a primary or metastatic liver tumor, or to cysts, angiomas, or collections, laparoscopy is no longer indicated. The example shown in Fig. 1 now belongs to the annals of the history of laparoscopy and should not appear in any up-to-date work on laparoscopy, because such cases are diagnosed with sonography (Fig. 2), aided, where necessary, by fine-needle biopsy (Fig. 3).

Second, although there has been a considerable reduction in the number of indications for laparoscopy during a year at any endoscopy center, laparoscopy itself is performed more often than might be expected. The above figures demonstrate that in spite of imaging techniques, the number of laparoscopies performed per year has not really changed. This observation might appear contradictory, but it is borne out by the data. Moreover, it is universally accepted that laparoscopy is still valid for some indications: diffuse liver disease (non-cirrhotic hepatopathy, cirrhosis, primary biliary cirrhosis), peritoneal disease, or acute abdomen [4]. In diffuse hepatopathy the

indications for laparoscopy appear to have increased [3]. There also appears to have been an increase in the percentage of laparoscopies performed in cases of benign focal liver lesions. This is a direct consequence of the widespread use of sonography, both for screening and in cases where an abdominal disease is suspected, which has led to an enormous increase in the number of unexpected findings in the liver. Often the diagnosis can be made on the basis of echographic images alone, or with the help of fine-needle biopsy. In some cases, however, the diagnosis is uncertain, and other diagnostic techniques are required. For this reason, there has been an increase in the number of laparoscopic diagnoses of benign liver tumors. In the presonographic era, such tumors were often found expectedly during laparoscopy performed for other reasons. Here mention must be made of liver angioma, because it frequently gives rise to diagnostic doubts. An angioma can easily be detected with US, but it often gives misleading pictures. Fine-needle biopsy is often not performed because accidents are feared and the findings may be inconclusive; nor can it reliably rule out a malignancy. This also applies to other benign liver formations such as adenoma and focal nodular hyperplasia, because cytology and microhistology do not necessarily indicate whether a particular lesion is benign. In the cirrhotic liver, sonography can indicate a tumor, but only with laparoscopy can the diagnosis be guaranteed (Figs. 4 and 5).

Thus, imaging techniques obviate a number of laparoscopies, but imaging techniques themselves give rise to an enormous number of indications for laparoscopy. We therefore agree with Lightdale, who is of the opinion that sonography and CT "are making more extraordinary diagnoses but are also producing some vague findings that require visual clarification" [5]. This also explains why laparoscopy is indicated more often than it once was in the diagnosis of hepatocarcinoma with cirrhosis: sonography unexpectedly detects asymptomatic formations, but as it fails to clarify them, laparoscopy is called for. It is therefore misleading to say that US has brought about a decrease in the indications for laparoscopy; rather, the indications have been modified because our diagnostic approach has changed.

Third, we must bear in mind that in recent years some new indications have emerged, and these have in turn given rise to new diagnostic needs. The number of laparoscopies performed in the

Table 2. Distribution of indications for two series of laparoscopies performed before (series I) and after (series II) introduction of fine-needle biopsy (from Buscarini et al. [3])

	Series I (% of 100 LPs)	Series II (% of 100 LPs)
Chronic hepatopathies	42	63*
Hepatocellular carcinoma	5	11
Hepatic metastases	27	8**
Staging of lymphomas	13	9
Various	13	9

* $P < 0.005$
** $P < 0.001$
LP, Laparoscopy

Fig. 1. Multinodular liver metastases from carcinoma of the large intestine. Round ligament and part of right and left lobes of the liver are enlarged and greatly altered by gross, elevated, whitish-pink, shiny, discrete or confluent nodes, some of which have a crater-like depression. (From [14])

Fig. 2. Oblique subcostal echographic scan, showing enormous roundish subdiaphragmatic formations which are hyperechogenic and form a large network with clear borders

Fig. 3. Metastasis from carcinoma of the kidney; material collected by echo-guided fine-needle biopsy. Atypical cellular elements

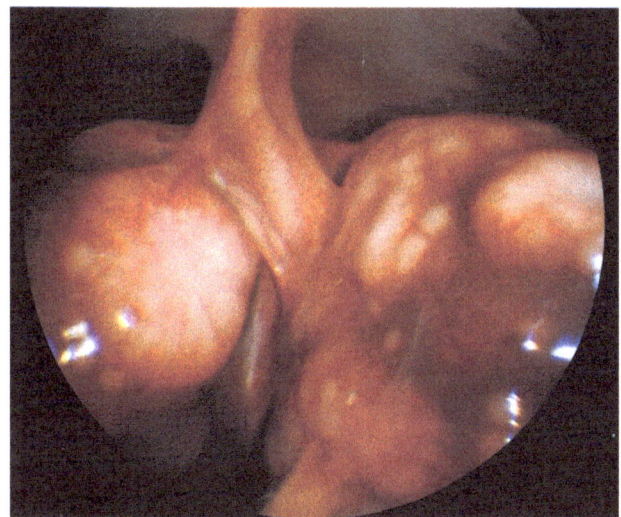

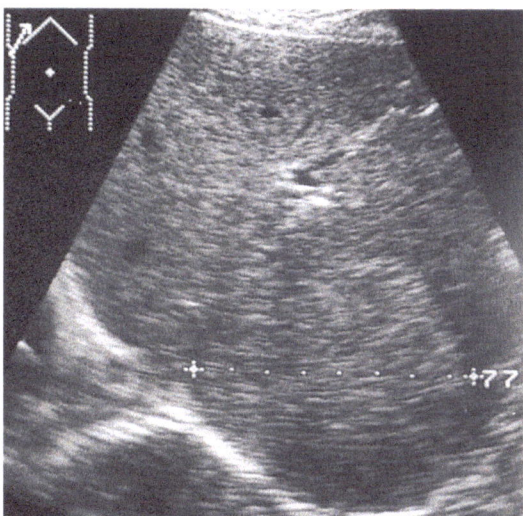

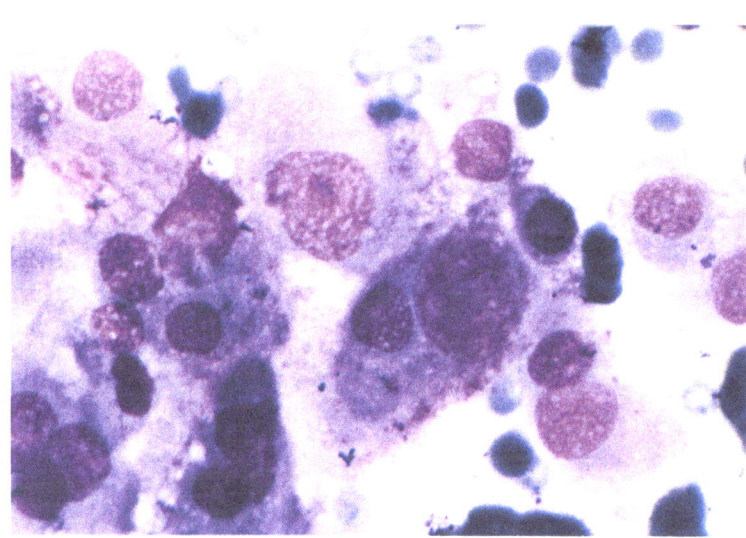

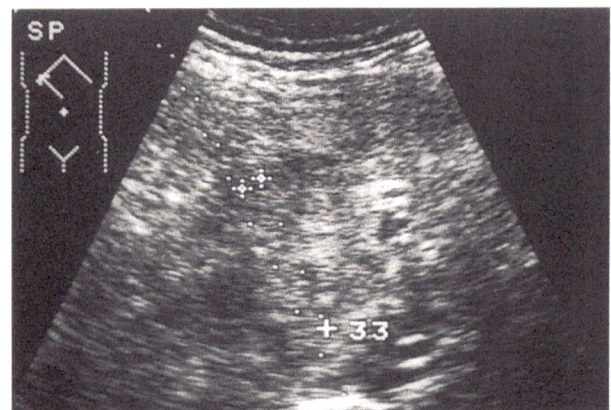

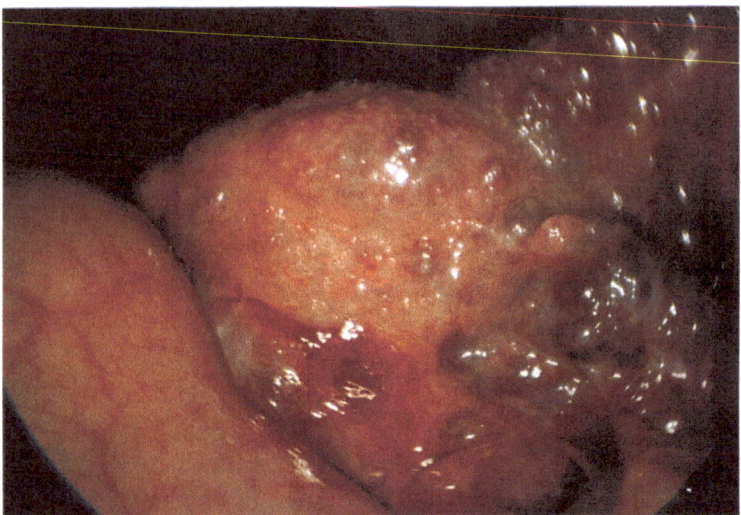

Fig. 4. Oblique subcostal echographic scan. Liver has a markedly inhomogeneous and hyperechogenic structure; between segments V and VII is a spherical nodule which is slightly less echogenic (diameter 3.3 cm). Echoguided biopsy: liver cells without atypia

Fig. 5. Same case as Fig. 4: Medium cirrhotic nodules with flat, pinkish areas and features that suggest carcinoma of the liver. Biopsy demonstrated common cirrhosis of the liver

staging and follow-up of some malignant tumors has increased enormously and in this field imaging techniques do not always provide the oncologist with reliable findings.

To accurately evaluate the present status of laparoscopy we must carefully evaluate the improvements made in this technique. Laparoscopy has now been used in clinical diagnostics for over 60 years. The changes it has undergone are not all obvious and are therefore not well known, but they are of great importance. New instruments are now available and continual improvements have been made in the technique and the method of exploration.

Laparoscopy has maintained its traditional features, but it is no longer the technique of 60 years ago. Its diagnostic potential has greatly increased and its risk has been reduced to a minimum. The difference between the percentage of accidents reported by Brühl in 1966 [6] and that reported by Henning in 1985 [7] speaks for itself. Among 63 845 cases considered by Brühl, there were major complications in 0.30% and deaths in 0.03%, whereas among the 11 017 cases reported by Henning, major complications occurred in 0.027% and deaths in 0.009%. In our experience, with the technical safeguards we recently, proposed, there have been no deaths since 1980 and the major complications have all been controlled endoscopically, without surgery being necessary.

Last and of great importance is the concept that sonography and laparoscopy are two complementary techniques: when used together, they are of extraordinary diagnostic utility.

These are the most important considerations for a critical appraisal of the use of laparoscopy today, in the era of imaging techniques. It is known to have great diagnostic potential; it is only slightly invasive and has a good cost-benefit ratio. In the United States great interest is now being shown in this technique, following a long period of underutilization [8–13]. The "anabiosis" of laparoscopy [1] is being discussed, and it is said [5] that "it would be a shame if the enthusiasm for scan-guided biopsy by radiologists led to a generation of gastroenterologists unable to perform this endoscopic procedure. Every major gastrointestinal teaching program and referral centre should maintain expertise in laparoscopy or a lot more unnecessary laparotomies are going to be done."

References

1. Boyd WP (1988) The anabiosis of laparoscopy? Gastrointest Endosc 3:280–281
2. Gandolfi L, Rossi A, Leo P, Solmi L, Muratori R (1985) Indications for laparoscopy before and after the introduction of ultrasonography. Gastrointest Endosc 31(1):1–3
3. Buscarini L, Sbolli G, Civardi G, Di Stasi M, Fermi S, Buscarini E, Cavanna L, Fornari F (1987) La biopsie percutanée guidée sous echographie modifie-t-elle les indications de la laparoscopie en hépatologie? Acta Endosc 2:85–88
4. Mörl M (1987) Laparoscopy. Present situation and prospects. Endoscopy 19:167–168
5. Lightdale CJ (1985) Laparoscopy in the age of imaging. Gastrointest Endosc 1:47–48
6. Brühl W (1966) Zwischenfälle und Komplikationen bei der Laparoskopie und gezielten Leberpunktion. Dtsch Med Wochenschr 91:2297–2999
7. Henning H (1985) The Dallas report on laparoscopic complications (letter). Gastrointest Endosc 31:104–105
8. Phillips R, Reddy KR, Jeffers LJ, Schiff ER (1987) Experience with diagnostic laparoscopy in a hepatology training program. Gastrointest Endosc 6:417–420
9. Brady PG, Goldschmid S, Chappel G, Slone FL, Boyd P A Comparison of biopsy techniques in suspected focal liver disease. Gastrointest Endosc 33:289–292
10. Jeffers L, Spieglman G, Reddy R, Dubow R, Nadji M, Ganjei P, Schiff ER (1988) Laparoscopically directed fine-needle aspiration for the diagnosis of hepatocellular carcinoma: a safe and accurate technique. Gastrointest Endosc 3:235–237
11. Sturmann MF (1988) Pelvic examination versus fiberoptic laparoscopy (Editorial). J. Clin Gastroenterol 6:612–613
12. Anonymous (1988) The role of laparoscopy in the diagnosis and management of gastrointestinal disease. Guidelines for clinical application. Gastrointest Endosc 3(Suppl):30 S–31 S (editorial)
13. Boyce HW (1988) Reassessment of laparoscopy in 1988: is it a useful test? Acta Post-graduate course, American Society of Gastroenterology and Endoscopy, New Orleans
14. Dagnini G (1980) Clinical laparoscopy Piccin Medical, Padua

I Progress in Laparoscopy

1 New Instruments

1.1 Fine Needles for Pneumoperitoneum

The first step in laparoscopy is pneumoperitoneum, the technique for which is well known: a needle is inserted in the abdominal cavity and gas is introduced through it. The abdominal cavity, which is normally virtual, is thus transformed into a real cavity that can be entered by the trocar and then by the laparoscope. This initial step is very important because only if it is successful can good laparoscopic results be obtained. It should be pointed out here that from a technical viewpoint it is difficult to perform pneumoperitoneum, and unsuccessful or unsatisfactory results depend in most cases upon particular conditions, above all the presence of extensive adhesions. Sometimes, however, even the most skilled operator can encounter difficulty in apparently simple cases.

Moreover, this first step in laparoscopy does carry some risks. The various accidents, sometimes severe, that can occur are due to introduction of the needle and to the effects of introduction of gas into the abdomen.

Accidents due to needle introduction are (a) hemorrhages due to laceration of vessels of the abdominal wall and of the omental tissue or to lesions of organs (above all the spleen in cases of splenomegaly) or pathological masses, and (b) perforations of the intestine, of the stomach, and of other hollow organs or pathological cavities.

The main accidents caused by gas introduction are (a) emphysema (cutaneous and subcutaneous, e.g., of the omental fat, of the mediastinum), the severity of which depends on the site and the entity, and (b) phenomena secondary to the increased abdominal pressure, which range from important or negligible subjective complaints (feeling of tension and suffocation, pain to vagal shock that can be very serious.

It is very important to carefully choose the most suitable point in the abdominal wall for puncture if accidents due to needle positioning are to be

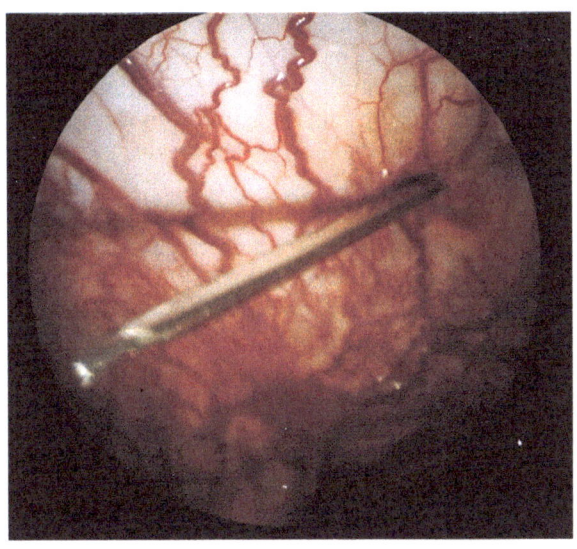

Fig. 1.1. Veress needle inserted in cavity. On the abdominal wall can be seen a dense network of fine, turgid veins (collateral circulation from portal hypertension), indicating risk of hemorrhage

avoided; the type of instrument used is also important. Now, thanks to "echography for laparoscopy," the criteria governing the choice of the point at which to sink the needle in order to minimize any risk are much more reliable and accurate than they once were (see Sect. 2.2). Echography can be performed to find out whether any dilated vessels, organs, and hollow formations have an atypical position which would contraindicate insertion at a particular point. It cannot, however, indicate arteries with a small caliber or a dense network of fine turgid venous capillaries that may be present in, for example, portal hypertension (Fig. 1.1). In such cases, the risk of damaging the formation and a consequent hemorrhage cannot be predicted, and the safety of the operation can be improved upon only by using needles that can reduce to a minimum the chance of damaging these small vessels.

1.1.1 Veress Needle

The Veress needle is the classical instrument for pneumoperitoneum and is used by the majority of laparoscopists. It consists of a cannula with a 2-mm diameter and a safety device – a hollow stylet with a hole for air; its rounded tip projects out up to 2 mm from the needle tip, and when it comes into contact with resistance from the different strata of the abdominal wall, the stylet is retracted by a spring, allowing the exposed tip to perforate the tissues. However, once in the cavity, the stylet returns to its original position, its rounded tip protecting the organs from the needle.

Notwithstanding these safety devices, accidents do occur, and some are serious enough to warrant surgical intervention. Henning made an exhaustive review of the data that appeared in the literature from 1954 to 1981, from a total of 46 364 laparoscopies (1), and found that important accidents due to damage from the needle for pneumoperitoneum were as follows:

1. Bleeding from lesions to small arteries or veins of the abdominal wall with hematoma of the wall or hemoperitoneum: 46 cases, five of which required surgery
2. Bleeding from lesions to vessels of the mesentery or to the omentum: 43 cases
3. Puncturing of the abdominal aorta: two cases
4. Lesions of the spleen: seven cases, three of which required surgery
5. Perforation of the stomach: 5 cases
6. Perforation of the small intestine: 14 cases, four of which required surgery

It is evident that the most common accident is hemorrhage from lesions to the small vessels. The characteristics of the Veress needle, with its fairly large caliber, and the way in which its needle penetrates the tissue through a cutting action make this risk quite serious. In our experience with 14 000 laparoscopies [2] up to 1986, hemorrhage occurred in 30 cases and surgery was necessary in five of them. A high proportion of the accidents reported in the literature are lesions to organs and perforations that the device should theoretically prevent. But if the needle penetrates a parenchymatous organ or a solid mass, it encounters a resistance greater than that of the spring; the blunt trocar is then retracted and the exposed needle tip damages the tissue.

The intestinal loops usually offer no resistance and are therefore only moved by the blunt trocar,

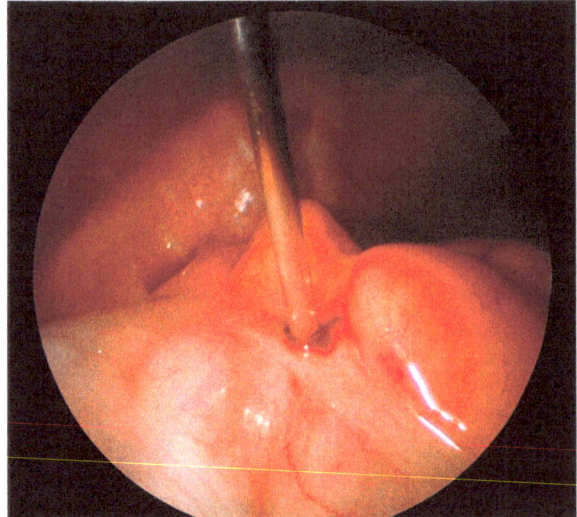

Fig. 1.2. Despite the safety device, the Veress needle has penetrated near a small intestine loop

but if the stomach or the intestinal loops have adhesions the safety trocar may encounter resistance and be retracted, thus allowing the exposed needle to perforate the wall (Fig. 1.2).

1.1.2 Fine Needle

In order to reduce the risks incurred when the needle is introduced for pneumoperitoneum, we designed a fine needle (Fig. 1.3) and have used it since 1986. It consists of a cannula with a Luer-lock connector and an inner stylet. The cannula tip is 1.5 mm long; it has a blunt edge and is beveled with a semicircular transverse cut. The maximum outer diameter of the cannula is 1.2 mm; its length ranges from 50 to 80 mm. The stylet, a solid steel cylinder, projects 2 mm from the cannula tip; its point is like that of a hypodermic needle (Fig. 1.4).

The technique for using the needle is simple: a local anesthetic is applied and a tiny skin incision made. The patient is then asked to contract the abdominal muscles and the needle is introduced into the cavity by applying pressure from the index finger on the stylet and by firmly pressing the needle between the thumb and the middle finger at the juncture. The stylet is then removed and the position of the needle checked in the usual ways. It is advisable to introduce 20–30 cc of gas with a springe; if the needle is correctly positioned this enters the cavity without any resistance. The needle is then connected to the gas insufflator.

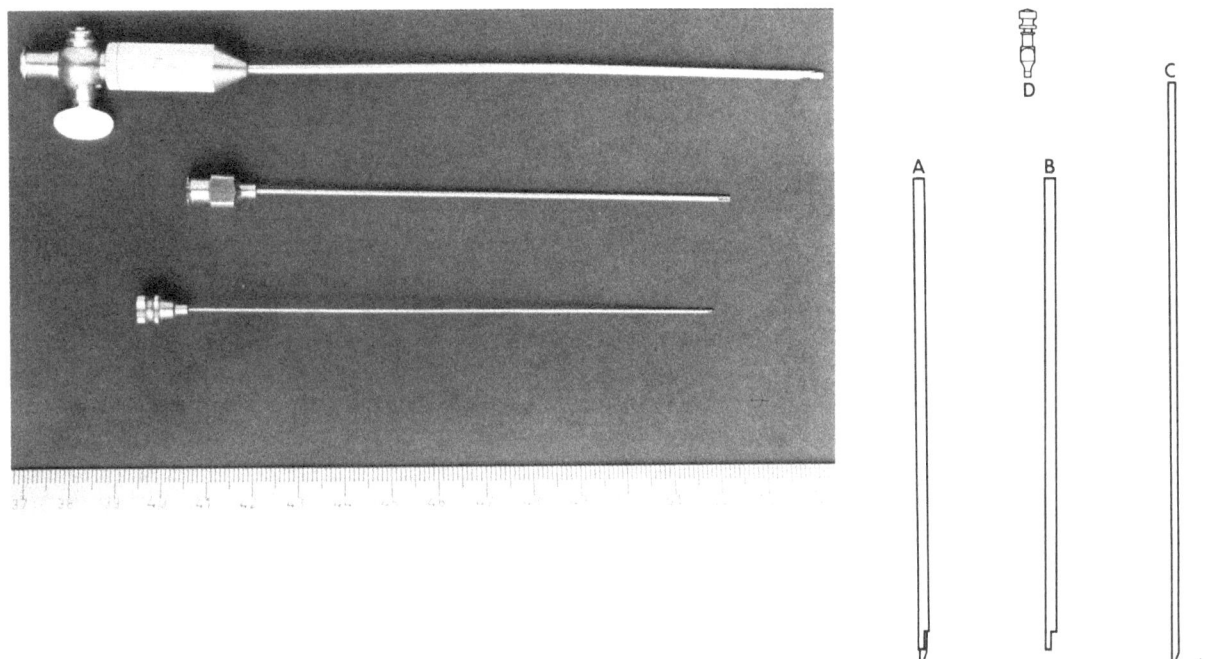

1.3

1.4

Fig. 1.3. *Top*: Veress needle. *Bottom*: the fine needle (1.2 mm); casing and stylet

Fig. 1.4. Parts of the fine needle: entire needle (*a*), casing (*b*), stylet (*c*), Luer-lock connector (*d*)

The fine needle has been routinely used in our Padua center since 1986 (941 cases), and the only complication observed was a small hematoma of the wall, which occurred in two cases. It has also been used at the Institute of Hepatology of Miami [3] for patients with abdominal scars and suspected adhesions (30 cases, no complications).

The small caliber and the shape of the tip of this needle allow it to penetrate the tissues by separating rather than cutting them, thereby reducing the risk of lacerating the abdominal wall or the intra-abdominal vessels, which slide away from the needle. Moreover, the needle is so fine that even if there are lesions to the parenchyma or perforations of the wall of a hollow organ, the consequences are usually negligible.

As the caliber of the instrument is small, the flow of gas is reduced and pneumoperitoneum therefore takes longer to perform. This is not a disadvantage, because the abdomen is given more time to adjust to the gas and disturbances due to tension are reduced, as are the frequency and severity of post pneumo peritoneum shock.

1.1.3 Conclusions

1. The fine needle for pneumoperitoneum (1.2 mm) is an interesting innovation of considerable practical importance.

2. When it is used systematically, all the risks of pneumoperitoneum, such as hemorrhages and perforations, are greatly reduced.

1.2 Laparoscopy with Flexible Instruments

Laparoscopic exploration with the traditional rigid instrument can be performed in all quadrants of the abdominal cavity distended by pneumoperitoneum. The laparoscope can be pushed forward or retracted in order to bring the image closer, and if the point corresponding to the introduction hole is kept as a flucrum, the instrument can be moved and oriented in all directions.

However, some areas are inaccessible to the laparoscope. For example, the upper parietal peritoneum adjacent to the point of laparoscope introduction is never visible because it is situated above the instrument itself. This also applies to the lateral and upper surface of the right lobe of the liver, to the borders at the diaphragm, and to some peritoneal recesses. Visualization is also hindered by adhesions, which, if numerous, can even totally preclude satisfactory endoscopy. The rigid laparoscope with oblique optics does allow a wider visual field in the lateral sectors, but the visual angle of this instrument is never over 45°.

1.2.1 Fiberscope Used as a Laparoscope

To obviate the above difficulty, a fiberscope instead of the rigid instrument was proposed [4, 5]. The Olympus G.I.F. P2 fiberscope was therefore designed. With its diameter of 10 mm it can be introduced through the trocar, and it therefore appeared the most suitable instrument. The results obtained by performing laparoscopy first with a rigid telescope and then with the fiberscope have been promising; no complications have been observed and the field of exploration is wider than that provided by traditional laparoscopy, thanks to the lateral movements and to a penetration of up to 45 cm.

The exploration of the dome of the liver, in particular, is possible through the right supradia-phragmatic space and through the peritoneum of the lower abdominal quadrants [2]. The main advantage of this technique is that is enables us to detect adhesions that are too lateral to be visualized with the rigid laparoscope. Above all, the flexible instrument allows us to circumvent adhesions and thus visualize sectors that would otherwise be completely hidden [5]. Of course, biopsies can be taken at the sites visualized: peritoneal samples are obtained using flexible pincers inserted in the laparoscopic channel, while samples from the liver are obtained with the usual needles, but through the second hole.

When used as a laparoscope, however, the Olympus fiber-scope has shortcomings: it is very long and therefore difficult to maneuver and its luminous band is weak, the illumination often being inadequate, even if a CLX light source is used [5].

Although many aspects of the experience with flexible instruments to data have been encouraging, the proposal to use these instruments for laparoscopy has not been taken up.

1.2.2 Rigid Laparoscope with a Mobile Head

We believe that the rigid telescope is the best available instrument. It has several advantages, not the least of which is its relaibility. Yet in certain situations it is of vital diagnostic importance to use an instrument with a degree of mobility so that obstacles can be overcome and the largest possible exploration field obtained.

We therefore asked the Olympus company to make a special instrument that would provide the maneuverability of a traditional rigid laparoscope and also have, whenever required, the prerogatives and advantages of a flexible endoscope. Thus, the "mobile head" laparoscope (Olympus prototype A 3635) was made (Fig. 1.5). The instrument, which is 50 cm long, consists of a telescope with a diameter of 10 cm; the entire shaft, the part that enters the body, is 33.5 cm long and consists of a rigid segment measuring 22 cm that is continued distally by a flexible segment measuring 11.5 cm. The flexible end can be bent up to 100° (Fig. 1.6); if the instrument is rotated on its axis the same angulation is reached for the entire arc of 360°. As with gastroscopes, movements of the head are made by rotating a knob on the handle of the instrument, which also has a lever enabling us to immobilize the flexible part. The laparoscope can thus be transformed into an instrument that is almost completely rigid. The prototype has an operative channel through which special instruments such as probes, needles, or pincers can be introduced to perform the usual maneuvers. It is also equipped with a camera for taking endoscopic pictures.

We have used this prototype since 1983, and results have been promising. It has all the advantages of totally flexible instruments, allowing us to explore areas to the rigid laparoscope, such as the lateral portion of the right lobe of the liver, particularly the more distant parts proximal to the diaphragm. The head movements render accessible tiny recesses in the peritoneum, and in certain cases the exploration of such areas is of crucial importance. But the "mobile head" is above all of great value where there are large adhesions that either preclude or hinder exploration. First, as mentioned above, the adhesion can be circumvented. Moreover, this instrument makes it easier to by pass adhesions by traveling through natural or artificially created openings (see Sect. 3.2.2). If the axis of the adhesion is perpendicular to the laparoscope a rigid instrument can easily be in-

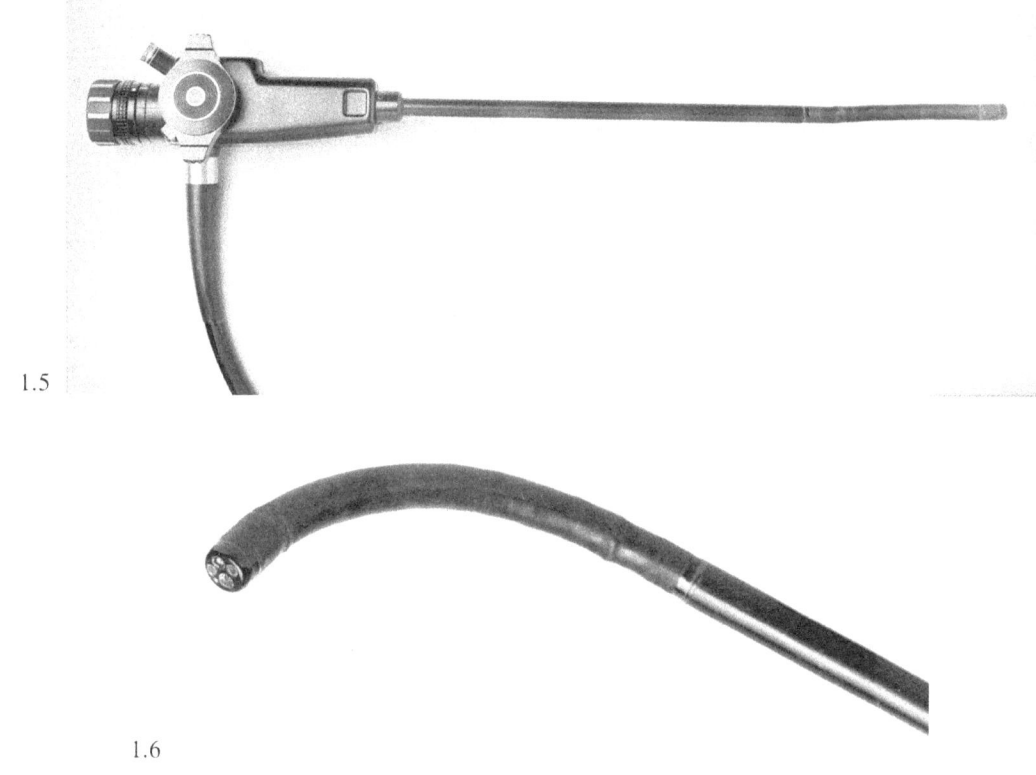

1.5

1.6

Fig. 1.5. The "mobile-head" laparoscope (Olympus prototype A 3635)

Fig. 1.6. Detail of the mobile head

serted. However, the more oblique the adhesional plane, the more difficult the maneuver, and the maneuver cannot be made at all if the plane is parallel to the axis of the telescope. In such cases the problem can be overcome only if the laparoscope head is bent until it is perpendicular to the adhesion plane and then introduced through the aperture. Finally, when the instrument can be brought beyond the adhesions covering a particular part of the abdomen, the field for exploration that is obtained with the laparoscope with a mobile head is always wider than that obtained with a rigid instrument.

Our experience therefore confirms that a mobile instrument is very useful in some situations. The Olympus prototype has the following advantages: (a) It is much shorter than the normal fiberscope and can therefore be maneuvered more easily without the exploration being compromised because it can penetrate to a depth of 45 cm. (b) The

device that stops the movement of the distal portion allows us to transform the instrument into a "quasi-rigid" telescope. This useful mechanism facilitates penetration into the abdomen through the trocar and allows us to make some of the maneuvers made with a rigid laparoscope; for example, the liver lobes can be raised to examine the lower surface of the liver.

The examination is always performed using the rigid laparoscope first. If some parts of the abdomen that appear to be of particular diagnostic importance cannot be explored and it is thought that a laparoscope with a mobile head might complete the examination, the rigid instrument can be retracted and a laparoscope with a mobile tip inserted.

We have used this instrument in about 4% of all the laparoscopies performed at our center, but it is difficult to quantify the results: being able to explore "blind" areas has not always resulted in a diagnosis. It must be borne in mind, however, that a wider exploration, even if negative, enhances the reliability of the results of the entire examination and, particularly in staging and follow-up, where the results depend upon the thoroughness of the exploration, reduces that risk of false negatives.

As the instrument can be used in patients with adhesions, it is of particular value in the staging and follow-up of carcinoma of the ovary. In such cases a peritoneal exploration is essential; it should be made over the largest possible surface. Moreover, in a high percentage of cases laparoscopy is performed on operated patients, who often have extensive, thick adhesions, and the mobile head can overcome these barriers. This is the most commonly cited indication: in daily practice cases very considerably, there being several in wich this type of laparoscope can be of particular diagnostic value.

1.2.3 Conclusions

1. The classical rigid laparoscope is still the most suitable instrument available for performing laparoscopy.

2. There are, however, cases in which a flexible instrument can be of great utility in the exploration of parts of the abdomen that are otherwise inaccessible.

3. In such cases the traditional fiberscope does not provide the necessary maneuverability, while a rigid laparoscope with a mobile head does.

4. This particular laparoscope should be used at the end of a laparoscopic examination performed with a traditional telescope to observe structures that otherwise cannot be visualized.

5. This instrument enables us to widen the field of exploration and in some cases to explore sectors hidden by adhesions.

1.3 Bio-Plug

It is well known that target biopsy performed during laparoscopic examination is less dangerous than transcutaneous biopsy and gives more satisfactory results (see Sect. 3.4): under direct vision the most suitable point for puncturing can be chosen and any highly vascularized areas or hollow organs can thus be avoided. Moreover, under laparoscopic control any accidents can be dealt with more satisfactorily: if there is bleeding coagulation can be facilitated and accelerated by using the probe to apply pressure underneath the biopsy

hole and by instilling coagulants. It is also possible to perform diathermocoagulation.

In spite of these measures, organ biopsy is a risky procedure and is the most frequent cause of accidents in connection with laparoscopy, sometimes fatal ones. It can cause heavy bleeding, e.g., if a large parenchymal vessel is damaged. In such cases the hemorrhage cannot be stopped by the usual maneuvers and a surgical suture is required (this does not always save the patient), or the bleeding stops and the accident appears to have been resolved, but a few hours later the apparently safe clot detaches and bleeding resumes. Such situations are particularly dangerous because hemoperitoneum has an insidious onset and therefore therapeutic measures are often taken too late.

It should also be borne in mind that while hemorrhaging is the most widely known complication, liver puncture can also cause bile leakage which, if not resolved, causes choleperitoneum, with serious consequences. This complication is to be feared, mainly because it can occur even in patients with no appreciable cholestasis, i.e. patients without any detectable contraindication to the biopsy, and the cholorrhea cannot be arrested by the traditional means available to the laparoscopist, but always requires surgery, which in turn is not always effective. The percentages of accidents during laparoscopic biopsy reported in the literature are well known, and data recently reported from larger series attest to a risk that cannot be ignored. In a survey made in the main centers of the Federal Republic of Germany, there were 81 liver biopsy accidents that were considered important; hemorrhages occurred in 35 patients, two of whom died, while 46 had cholorrhea [6]. Among 3000 examinations at the medical and surgical centers of Modena [7, 8], four patients had fatal hemorrhages and in a further ten patients the bleeding was checked by medical treatment. In our series of 8321 liver biopsies performed from 1967 to 1981 [9] there were nine cases of severe hemorrhage that were resolved laparoscopically and three in which surgery was called for; one of the patients died 4 days later (biopsy was performed for liver carcinoma with cirrhosis). Another death was due to late hemorrhage. The biopsy was made for liver metastases, and a clot had formed as usual after normal bleeding, which had given no cause for concern. Later, however, the clot detached.

In our series there were also two cases of severe cholorrhea after liver biopsy without any signs of biliary stasis; in one case the complication was resolved surgically, but the other patient died.

The complications are fairly rare, but they can be extremely serious. Therefore, in an attempt to reduce to a minimum the risk from organ biopsies during laparoscopy, we decided to try and permanently stop any hemorrhage or cholorrhea by plugging the biopsy hole during laparoscopy. We devised and had manufactured a simple instrument that enabled us to make this maneuver; the instrument proved satisfactory and has been used by us clinically since 1981 [9]. In an article published in 1984 [10], the practicability of this idea was confirmed by experimental results obtained in dogs. The "bovine collagen fleece" was introduced as a semi-rigid plug and used successfully in surgery as a hemostatic in cases of laceration of the liver. The duration of bleeding was markedly shorter in the treated dogs than in the untreated ones. During a follow-up of 3 months no complications were observed.

1.3.1 Instrument and Technique

The Bio-Plug we designed [9, 11] consists of a 47-cm-long 14-gauge cannula needle with a caliber equal to that of the biopsy needle. The cannula has no point; in the lumen of the distal end is a 2-cm-long cylindrical fibrin cartridge. The cannula has a stylet fixed to the handle of the instrument. When freed from its hinge, the stylet can be slid forward

2 cm, like a piston, to drive the cartridge out of the cannula (Fig. 1.7).

The instrument is simple to use: By means of the biopsy needle, a physiological serum is used to wash any blood from the organ surface so that the hole to be plugged can be visualized. Then the Bio-Plug is passed along the operating laparoscopic channel; it is directed toward the biopsy hole and the rounded point is introduced a few millimeters inside the hole. Under endoscopic control the stylet is freed from its lock and is made to slide forward as far as it can go; the stylet thus pushes the cartridge into the hole. The instrument is withdrawn, and for a few minutes the effect of the plugging is observed: the sponge should become soaked and dilate slightly so as to leave the wound perfectly closed (Fig. 1.8). The bleeding, or the bile leakage, stops immediately (Fig. 1.9, 1.10). If the situation remains stable, the complication can be considered resolved.

No accidents have been reported following fibrin sponge plugging using the above-described technique; the fibrin is spontaneously reabsorbed.

Of course, the Bio-Plug cannula is disposable: the cartridge which is introduced into the paren-

Fig. 1.7. Bio-Plug. **A** Proximal extremity: *a*, hilt; *b*, piston and mandrel; **B** distal extremity; **B₁** detail with cannula sleeve (*c*), mandrel (*d*), and fibrin (*e*). **C** Plugging with Bio-Plug: mandrel moved forward (*d*) to insert the fibrin cartridge in the biopsy hole (*f*); *g*, liver tissue

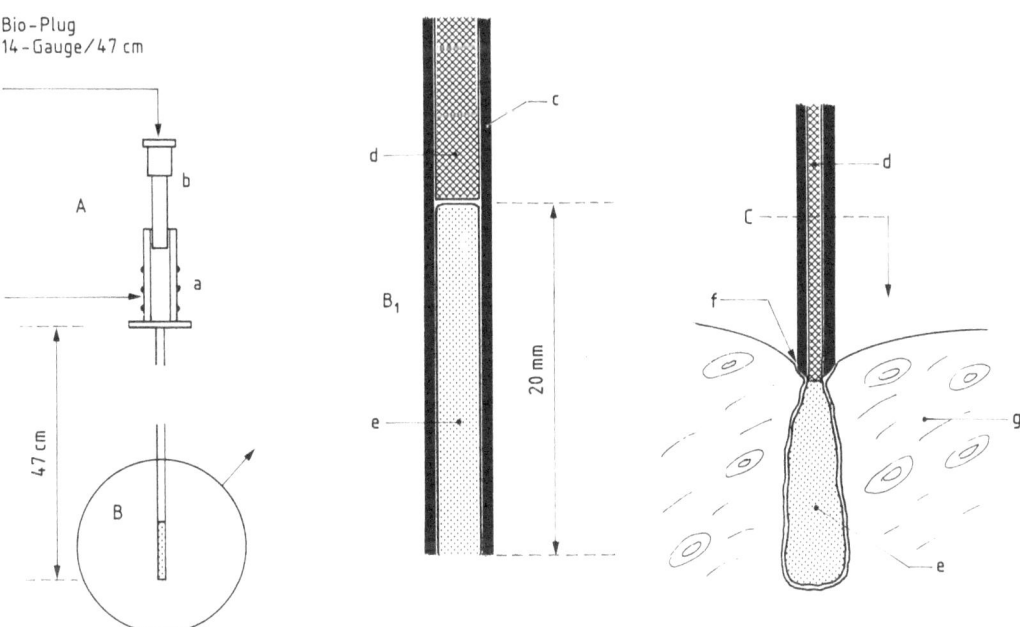

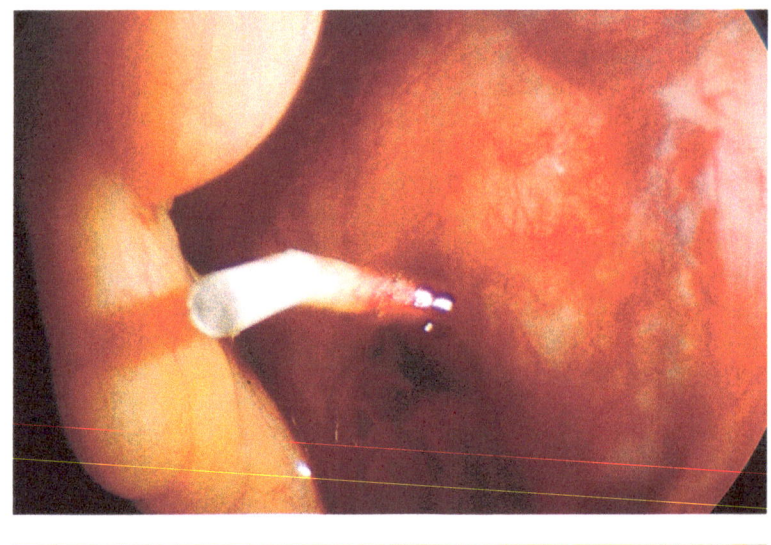

1.8

1.9

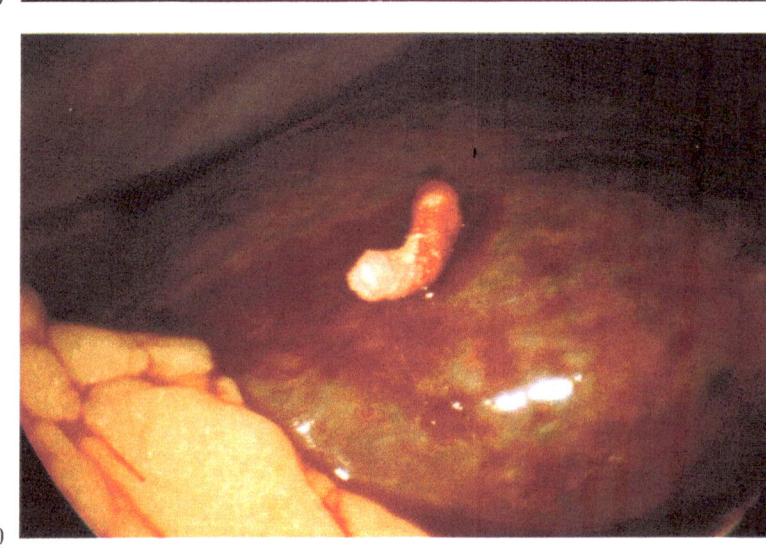

1.10

chyma must be absolutely sterile; otherwise it would be a dangerous source of infection. Friedrich and Henning [12] recently proposed the use of a stell, nondisposable instrument for cartridge insertion.

1.3.2 Results

From 1981, when the Bio-Plug was first used systematically at the Padua center, until now, no accidents following either liver biopsies or other types of biopsy (spleen, masses, etc.) have been observed. In particular, in the series of 3347 liver and 453 spleen biopsies performed from 1981 to 1985 [11], the Bio-Plug was used in 30 of the liver biopsies (to stop severe hemorrhage in 23 and cholorrhea in seven) and in ten of the spleen biopsies.

The Bio-Plug is required in only a small number of cases; it has been used only in patients with serious hemorrhage which cannot be stopped by pressure from the probe. Our experience, however, indicates that the Bio-Plug should be used more freely, above all to control hemorrhages that appear to be minor but cannot be stopped; it should also be used to prevent any late bleeding from clot detachment. In particular, in biopsies from liver carcinoma with cirrhosis, where there is a high risk of hemorrhage, it is advisable to use fibrin-sponge plugging almost systematically. In patients with cholorrhea a Bio-Plug is mandatory, because only rarely does the bile leakage stop spontaneously and it is usually difficult to ascertain endoscopically whether it has definitely stopped or not.

The results obtained with the Bio-Plug can therefore be considered optimal. Now that we use it systematically, other precautions are no longer necessary, such as the instillation of coagulants or diathermocoagulation. When the hemorrhage is really severe and cannot be stopped, such tech-

niques hardly ever resolve the condition, and they are totally ineffective in cases of cholorrhea.

The Bio-Plug is now being used successfully in many centers, both in Italy and abroad. In Germany, Henning has used it successfully in 52 cases of severe hemorrhage among 464 laparoscopies; he stated that the Bio-Plug is a valuable new technique in cases of bleeding or bile see page following liver biopsy [12]. The Bio-Plug is also used in pediatric laparoscopy [13].

1.3.3 Conclusions

1. It is now possible to introduce a hemostatic fibrin plug laparoscopically into the biopsy hole to almost totally arrest any hemorrhage following organ biopsies or any bile leakage from liver biopsies.

2. In fact, the Bio-Plug has enabled us to reduce any risk from laparoscopic biopsy to almost nil.

3. Moreover, liver and spleen biopsies can be done without any danger of hemorrhaging, even in patients with coagulation problems. Biopsies can also be taken in highly vascularized parenchymas and from livers compromised by severe cholestasis without a risk of choleperitoneum.

4. Not only has the Bio-Plug provided greater safety; it has also enhanced the diagnostic efficacy of laparoscopy, because biopsies of organs can now done in conditions that were once considered preclusive.

Fig. 1.8. Fibrin plug inserted in biopsy hole to arrest hemorrhage from a highly vascularized primary liver cancer

Fig. 1.9. Biopsy hole in liver with marked cholestasis: cholorrhea (bile seepage)

Fig. 1.10. Fibrin plug inserted in hole; cholorrhea arrested

References

1. Henning H, Look D (1985) Laparoskopie. Thieme, Stuttgart, pp 33–36
2. Dagnini G, Bergamo S, Caldironi MW, Marin G, Papaleo E, Patella M (1980) Incidenti della laparoscopia: rapporto su 7870 casi. G Gastroenterol Endosc 3:9–14
3. Piccigallo E, Jeffers LJ, Reddy KR, Marin G, Schiff ER (1988) Experience with a 1.2-mm pneumoperitoneum needle for laparoscopy. Gastrointest Endosc 34:471–473
4. Partika EK, Kozarek RA, Sanowaski RA (1980) Evaluation of a flexible endoscope for laparoscopy. Gastrointest Endosc 26:74
5. Sanowski RA, Kozarek RA (1982) Laparoscopy using a flexible endoscope. Acta Endosc 12(1):61–66

 6. Henning H, Look D, Paradisi Barrios CE (1978) Laparoscopie. Ses possibilitées et ses limites. Acta Endosc 8:329–344
 7. Manenti A, Manenti F, Villa E, Ferrari A, Malagoli M, Cortesi M, (1980) Complications de la laparoscopie: expérience sur 6563 observations. Acta Endosc 10:373–379
 8. Manenti A, Ferrari A, Gibertini G Jr, Borruto A, Manenti F, Cortesi N (1983) Biopsie hépatique sous contrôle laparoscopique. Expérience de 3000 cas. Acta Endosc 13:21–27
 9. Dagnini G, Caldironi MW, Marin G, Patella M (1981) Tamponamento per via laparoscopica con spugna di fibrina negli incidenti da biopsia d'organo. G Ital Endosc Dig 4:339–344
10. Protell RL, Kogan FJ, Chvapil M (1984) Collagen plugs: a new hemostatic modality for experimental laparoscopic liver biopsy sites. Gastrointest Endosc 2:148
11. Dagnini G, Caldironi MW, Marin G, Patella M (1985) Fibrin sponge plugging of hemorrhage from laparoscopic biopsy. Gastrointest Endosc 1:35–36
12. Friedrich K, Henning H (1987) Laparoscopische Blutstillung nach Leberbiopsie durch Instillation eines Gelatine-Zylinders. Z Gastroenterol 25:726–730
13. Esposito G, Porreca A (1986) La laparoscopia in età pediatrica. Aggiorn Med 2:122–131

2 Integration of Laparoscopy with Sonography

The clinical use of imaging techniques has radically changed the approach to diagnosis of abdominal diseases. It has also greatly increased the likelihood of making a sound, accurate diagnosis. As sonography is noninvasive, can be performed repeatedly, and is relatively inexpensive and highly effective, it has been developed well. This technique is indicated in the study of various abdominal conditions, for it yields information that is often decisive. Moreover, the use of fine-needle transcutaneous biopsies taken under echographic guidance has enhanced the value of this technique. Biopsies obtained in this way enable us to make a diagnosis on the basis of the disease itself by means of a cytological or histological examination of small tissue samples. In abdominal disease, sonography now must immediately follow the clinical and laboratory study of the patient; it must also precede any other instrumental investigation required.

These changes in the diagnostic approach have in turn radically affected both the use of and the indications for laparoscopy. Yet, although both laparoscopy and echography are valuable techniques, they both have shortcomings. Laparoscopy, for example, does not allow examination of the retroperitoneal organs and structures – any pathological formations of the retroperitoneal organs can be visualized only if they reached the abdominal cavity. Diseased endoperitoneal organs or formations that are hidden or made inaccessible by adhesions, or that are covered by normal structures or neoformations that cannot be shifted with the normal endoscopic maneuvers cannot be visualized, and lesions located within large organs like the liver and spleen cannot be detected. Alterations (e.g., irregular shapes, enlargements, tumefactions, or surface alterations) can be detected and a disease may therefore be suspected, but the diagnosis is difficult to make. Moreover, it is usually impossible to take a biopsy from a lesion that is not visualized and it is always risky to attempt one. Examination of the liver or spleen by laparoscopy is also difficult if the organ is covered by a thick or opaque capsule from a previous peri-hepatitis or peri-splenitis, because this precludes visualization of the underlying parenchyma.

Satisfactory echography, on the other hand, may be hindered by (a) the presence of gas in the hollow organs (stomach and intestine), for this masks the underlying organs; (b) the patient's constitution (obesity, etc.); and (c) lack of collaboration from the patient. Nor can lesions be visualized if they (a) are small (diameter less than 2 cm); (b) are smooth and thin (plaques on the surface of the parenchyma, the peritoneum, etc.); (c) are localized in particular areas, such as the liver margins, proximal to the gallbladder, at ligaments and adhesion attachments; or (d) have an echo-structure similar to that of the surrounding tissue, as is the case, for example, when focal lesions develop in a cirrhotic liver. The reliability of a diagnosis based upon sonographic findings also depends upon the experience of the examiner, on the attention he pays, and on the patience with which he performs the examination.

Notwithstanding the above shortcomings, ultrasound is now an extra-ordinarily valuable diagnostic tool. In many cases an accurate diagnosis is made with the help of US-guided biopsy using a fine needle. Guided biopsy is highly sensitive but not highly specific, while laparoscopy is less sensitive but more specific, and biopsies taken under laparoscopy have a greater diagnostic value.

It is therefore evident that ultrasound and laparoscopy should be considered two complementary techniques, each compensating for the shortcomings of the other. A close integration between sonography and laparoscopy has been achieved through *echolaparoscopy* and *sonography for laparoscopy*.

2.1 Echolaparoscopy

With the echolaparoscope, which has a small sonographic probe that can be introduced into the abdomen, the most complete integration between sonography and laparoscopy appeared to have been achieved. The probe is placed directly on the organs to be explored, and the abdominal wall, interpositioning of gas from the hollow organs, or any other hindrance to the transmission of echoes is thus avoided. As the probe is guided under direct vision it can be moved to the areas most important for a diagnosis and to those areas that may appear endoscopically suspect. Echolaparoscopy was first attempted by Yamakawa and Wagai [1]. In 1963, Wagai defined certain echographic findings that were typical of the gallbladder with A-mode scanning under laparoscopic guidance. However, this technique was invasive and the information it yielded was not of great value. It was therefore abandoned until The Olympus Optical Company of Tokyo made the first prototype of an echolaparoscope. In 1974 a further attempt to study the gallbladder was made in Germany [2]. The first clinical experience of echolaparoscopy, however, was reported in Dubrovnik in 1981, at the 4th Congress on Ultrasound in Medicine.

The idea of placing the echographic probe directly on the organ for exploration with a view to improving the accuracy of findings has in recent years resulted in the development of the following analogous techniques:

1. In the field of fiberendoscopy, *Endoscopic sonography of the digestive tract*, which has yielded interesting results, above all in the esophagogastric tract
2. In the field of surgery, *intraoperative sonography*, which is now becoming a widely used technique

It is important to point out here that echolaparoscopy is a technique based upon valid theoretical principles that are still at an experimental stage. It is therefore necessary to carefully evaluate all the negative and positive aspects of this technique that have so far been observed in its application, with a view to establishing its practical value.

2.1.1 Instruments

The only instruments that have been used to perform echolaparoscopy to date are *prototypes* that firms have supplied to certain centers for ex-

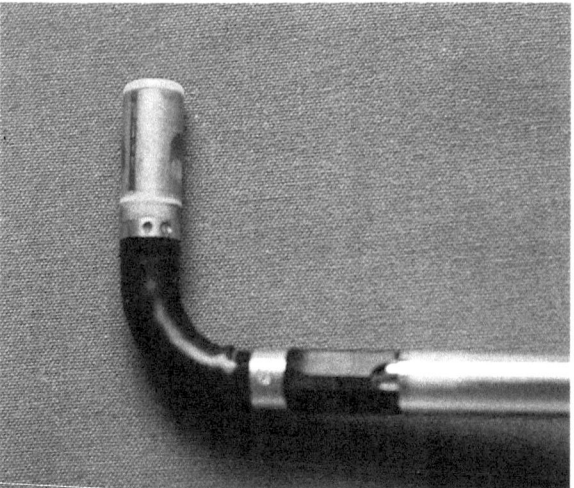

Fig. 2.1. Olympus echolaparoscope. Detail of the probe, which appears to be at a right angle

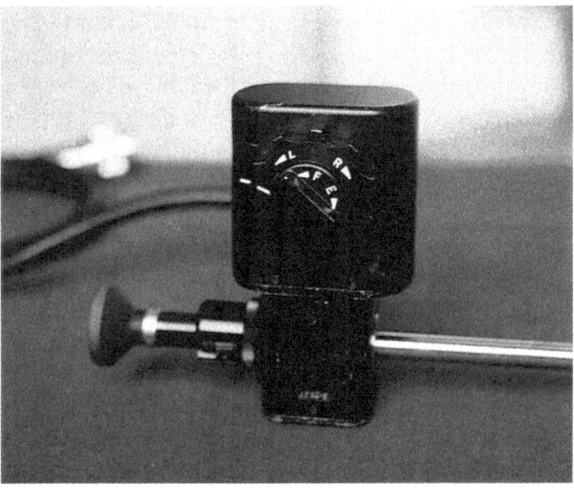

Fig. 2.2. Detail of the proximal part of the apparatus with the eyepiece of the small laparoscope

perimentation on patients. The apparatus consists of a laparoscope fitted with a US probe and a display unit. Two different echolaparoscope models are now made, one with a *sectorial* and one with a *linear* probe. The sectorial-probe laparoscope, manufactured by the Olympus Optical Co. of Tokyo, is the result of improvements made on two previous proto-types. The first model had a probe with a diameter of 12 mm, which was larger than that of the trocar used for the introduction of the usual laparoscope. The main shortcoming of this unit was that two laparoscopes were used in parallel to confirm the position of the haed of the

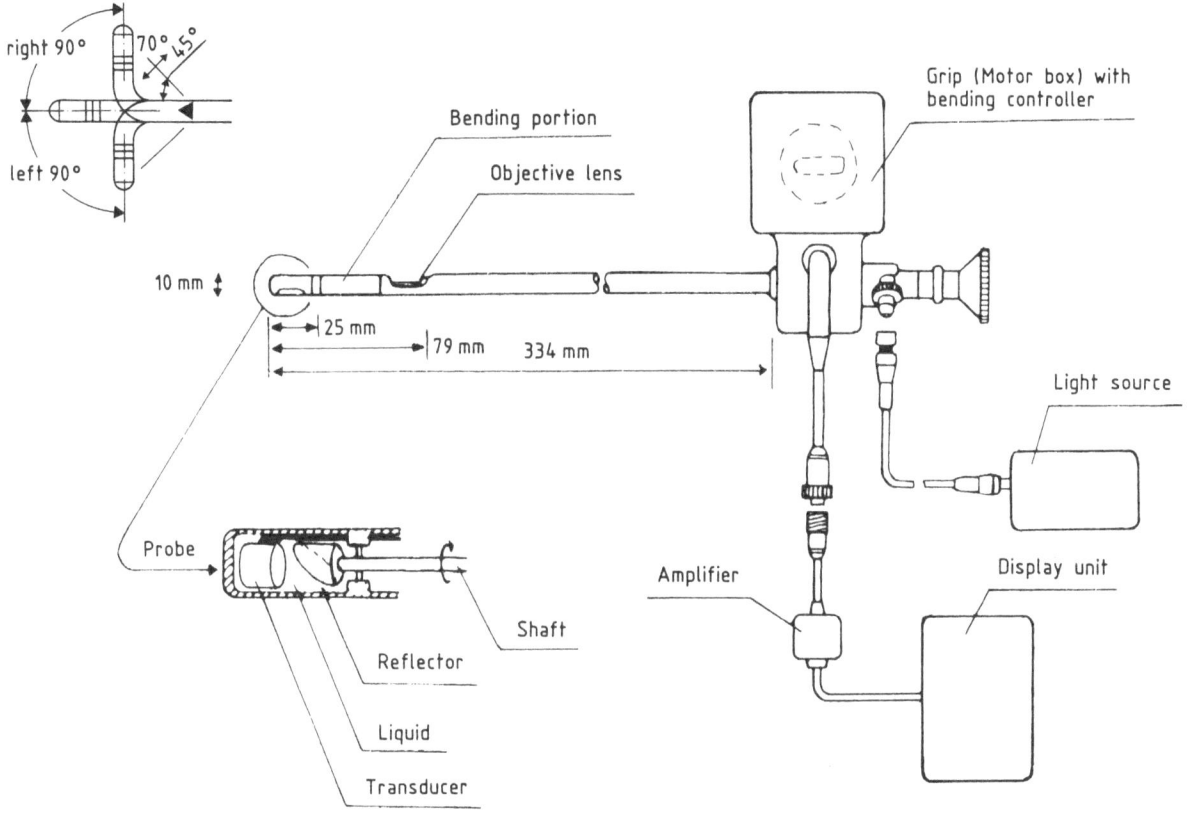

right 90° 70° 45°

left 90°

10 mm

25 mm

79 mm   334 mm

Bending portion

Objective lens

Grip (Motor box) with
bending controller

Light source

Probe

Amplifier

Display unit

Shaft

Reflector

Liquid

Transducer

echolaparoscope and avoid any danger of damage to the organs from the equipment. Another drawback was the limited scanning field of 90°.

The latest model consists of a rigid instrument, with a diameter of 10 mm that allows it to be used with regular laparoscopes. The probe is sectorial with a 7.5-MHz frequency and a diameter of 7 mm. The field of view, which corresponds to the perpendicular plane of the axis of the telescope, is 180° (Fig. 2.1). Probe placement and maneuvers are usually guided and controlled by means of a small laparoscope with lateral 45° vision incorporated in the instrument (Fig. 2.2). The echolaparoscope is connected to a display unit (Aloka, Tokyo) with a digital scan converter and produces 90°–180° dynamic sector images. Figure 2.3 shows the entire system.

The main advantages of this prototype are (a) the wide, 180° + 45° aperture, ensuring that the field of view is large enough to search for occult lesions; (b) the high sensitivity of the probe, producing excellent sonograms; and (c) the stability of the images – this is good because scanning is done by rotating a mirror directly in the unit's DC motor. The high frequency of the probe (7.5 MHz) gives accurate details of anatomical structures,

Fig. 2.3. Diagram of the Olympus echolaparoscope prototype

such as intraparenchymal vessels, and detects slight alterations in the architecture and structure of tissues, thanks to the system's high resolution power.

This power has been studied experimentally both with a phantom test and on the human liver, and it has been compared with the resolution of an electronic dynamic scanner with 3.5-MHz transducer elements of the U-Sonic model RT 2000 [3]. The phantom test consists of a series of numerous nylon threads stretched between two parallel wooden boards; this apparatus is immersed in water and then submitted to sonography. The value of the sonographic resolution has been defined as the minimum distance between the threads that can be discerned on the echogram.

A comparison made between the echolaparoscopic system and the control demonstrated that the lateral resolution is from 1 to 1.3 mm at a depth of 2.5 for the "system" and just 3 mm at a depth of 3 cm for the control. No differences were observed between the axial resolutions of the two scanners at a depth of 2.5 cm, but with the system a value of 3–8 cm was obtained, while a value of up to 5 cm was found in the control.

A study of the resolution in a human liver with a tumor (both at autopsy with a sample immersed in water and intraoperatively with the scanner held directly on the surface) clearly demonstrated the presence of the tumor, the irregular shape of the mass, and the clear margins. It also demonstrated that with scanning in series it is possible to obtain a three-dimensional image. As well as having a high resolution potential, the sectorial probe also appears particularly suitable because it requires only a small surface area on which to fix the probe. This facilitiates contact between the transducer and the tissue.

In Germany, an echolaparoscope with a linear probe has been made [4]. This instrument is 30 cm long and has a diameter of 10 mm and can therefore be introduced through the commonly used trocars. The linear array is fixed to the tip of the probe, and the frequency is 7 MHz. The laparoscope is not incorporated in the instrument: a 3-mm-diameter optic is introduced into the abdomen through a second hole. The sonographic display unit is the Siemens Sonoline 8000. The findings obtained with the two types of probe appear to be equivalent: the linear probe seems more suitable for the study of fields that are smooth and large enough for easy probe placement. The sectorial probe, on the other hand, can be particularly suitable for cases in which irregular and limited surfaces hinder contact between the probe and the organ.

2.1.2 Technique

Echolaparoscopic examination is done in cases where, after a clinical, laboratory, and instrumental study, laparoscopy is definitely indicated, i.e., when the diagnosis is still problematic or when persistent doubts must be clarified. The echolaparoscopic step is therefore always preceded by laparoscopy following the routine technique. The laparoscope is then withdrawn but the trocar is kept in place for introduction of the echographic probe. The preliminary findings from laparoscopy provide an important basis for the successive echographic study, even if they do not always solve the particular diagnostic problem. By means of the small laparoscope, the probe is directed and placed under visual guidance at the points considered most opportune; the sonographic findings are then collected and recorded.

The echographic probe can be fixed on all the areas accessible to the laparoscope:

1. One the entire surface of the liver, on the right and left lobes (Fig. 2.4)
2. On the gallbladder (Fig. 2.5) and in the area of the extrahepatic biliary ducts
3. Underneath the left lobe of the liver and on the entire gastric area, with pressure exerted to expel air, mainly to study the pancreas
4. On the median and upper surface of the spleen
5. On the deep planes of the abdomen, to explore the retroperitoneum – care is taken to shift the intestinal loops, both by changing the patient's position and by making the appropriate maneuvers
6. On the organs of the pelvis

Echolaparoscopy allows us to take biopsies of lesions that do not appear on the surface of an organ and that cannot be visualized laparoscopically, but that can be detected and localized using the sonographic probe [4].

For taking the biopsy, different techniques have been proposed. With the linear probe echolaparoscope Menghini's needle can be used; this is introduced vertically through the abdominal wall above the quadrate lobe of the liver. The probe is placed on the suspect area and the needle is introduced into the part of the liver to be explored with the probe. The needle tip can be seen on the echographic monitor and can be guided to the area with a different echogenicity.

In such cases [5], this can be considered the technique of choice for the more accurate selection of the point for biopsy. Fukuda and co-workers [6], who use the sectorial probe, advocate the injection of a carmine-indigo solution into the area adjacent to the mass detected with the probe. As this solution is only slightly echogenic, it is possible to recognize and follow the needle's course with sonolaparoscopy. If the direction and the depth are correct, biopsy is performed by pricking the area of the liver colored with carmine. This biopsy technique gave satisfactory results in four patients with tumors that were not visible on the organ surface and that were identified with echolaparoscopy [6]. Echolaparoscopy can also effectively guide biopsy of organs and retroperitoneal formations, such as the head of the pancreas, the pancreas itself, and the suprarenal glands.

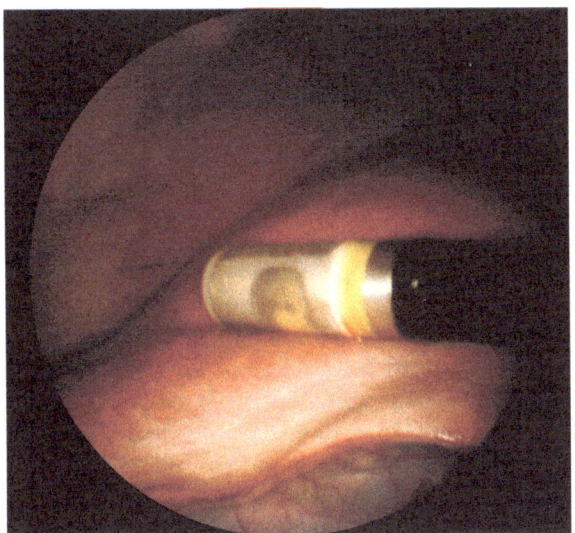
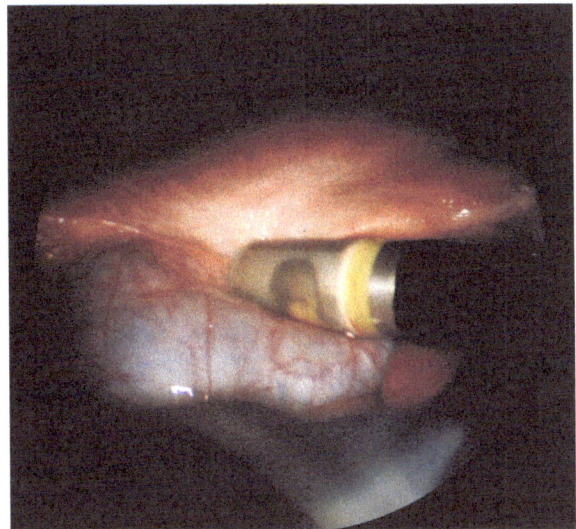

2.4

2.5

Fig. 2.4. Echographic probe for the upper surface of the right lobe of the liver

Fig. 2.5. Echographic probe placed directly on the gallbladder

2.1.3 Results

So far, experimental results with echolaparoscopy have demonstrated the high quality of the echographic images. This is because placement of the probe directly on the organ to be examined eliminates any interference. This allows the use of frequencies of 7.5–10 MHz, which are much higher than the 3.5 MHz routinely used for echography. With the endoscopic probe we can thus obtain a high resolution and remarkably fine detail without being hindered by deep penetration. The most significant results reported in the literature are:

1. Findings of hepatocarcinoma nodules on cirrhosis, or metastases too small to be detected echographically and discovered only with echolaparoscopy [3, 6]
2. Cases in which, thanks to the detail seen with the endoscopic probe, it was possible to establish the benign hemoangiomatous nature of a lesion of the liver which appeared echographically to be malignant [6]
3. Clarifications of several characteristics of the portal circulation in cases of cirrhosis
4. Accurate findings in the gallbladder (Fig. 2.6) and biliary ducts when studying the walls and detection of stones too small to be seen by routine echography
5. Diagnosis of lesions of the suprarenal capsules [4]

We studied a series of 27 patients using the Olympus prototype, and our results confirm the above findings [7]. In particular, a comparison with results of routine echography has demonstrated that echolaparoscopy provided diagnostically useful information in three cases. In one of these echolaparoscopy was decisive; the diagnosis was reached because it detected a tiny stone in the common bile duct that had not been seen previously.

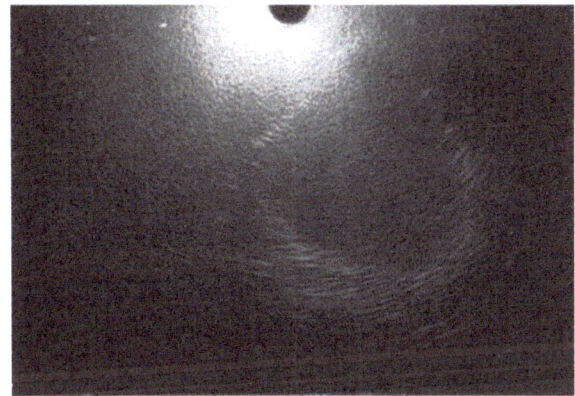

Fig. 2.6. Echolaparoscopic picture of the gallbladder wall

2.1.4 Clinical Applications

It appears that the combined use of sonography and laparoscopy can have advantages over the two techniques used separately [6], although the practical applications that might be suggested for echolaparoscopy are more limited than those for the two separate techniques.

Echolaparoscopy is in fact useful only when – after a complete clinical study that includes routine echography, and after laparoscopy – there are still diagnostic problems that may be resolved by placement of the probe directly on the organ.

The field for echolaparoscopic application is therefore limited. In the future, however, it may be indicated in the following conditions:

1. Cases in which a primary or secondary liver tumor is suspected, but both preliminary echography and laparoscopy give negative findings. This applies in particular to primary tumors of the liver in cirrhosis.
2. Hepatocarcinomas, above all of the cirrhotic liver, that according to routine echography and laparoscopy appear to consist of a single nodule and are therefore theoretically suitable for radical surgery. The echolaparoscopic examination may confirm that the lesion is single, or it may demonstrate other nodules, thereby indicating that surgery should be reconsidered.
3. Suspected but not confirmed neoplasms of the pancreas or, more generally, of the retroperitoneum.
4. Staging of malignant tumors and follow-up during therapy. Echolaparoscopy can reveal overlooked metastases, thus correcting echographic and laparoscopic false negatives.
5. Where disease of the gallbladder and the extrahepatic biliary ducts is suspected but echographic and laparoscopic findings are negative.

2.1.5 Practical Value

Although the claims here outlined are valid and the value of the findings reported undeniable, echolaparoscopy has not lived up to expectations. This technique was considered a window of opportunity. Yet no further prototypes have been made, and therefore no echolaparoscopes are commercially available.

We believe that the integration of sonography with laparoscopy is extraordinarily effective for the diagnosis of abdominal diseases, but we are also of the opinion that echolaparoscopy is not of great practical value, and there are several reasons for this.

In recent years, the years in which prototypes were manufactured for echolaparoscopy, great technological progress has been made in this field and the instruments for performing routine echography have been greatly improved upon. Now the shortcomings of sonographic exploration have been reduced to a minimum, so the need for direct placement of the probe on the organ rather than on the skin above it has also been greatly reduced.

Present echographs give images and findings that are as good as, if not better than, those provided by echolaparoscopes. For deep penetration, the high frequency of the endoscopic probe does not always appear to be adequately compensated for by the lack of echo interference from tissues or air. Where skin probes at a frequency of 3.5 MHz are used to examine deep-seated areas, the findings are even more satisfactory.

Echographic examination performed with an endoscopic probe also has the following technical shortcomings: Although it can be used to localize the areas for exploration, thanks to endoscopic findings and to reliable reference points found visually, the instrument can be difficult to maneuver, thus hindering probe placement on the areas chosen. As contact between the small probe and the organ surface is not always complete, the transducer to organ coupling may be unsatisfactory, resulting in poor-quality images and prolonging the examination. With the mechanical sectorial probe the conical image considerably reduces the resolution in the more superficial parts, and the limited field sometimes precludes any detection of the traditional echographic reference points.

It must also be borne in mind that endoscopic echography requires a laparoscopic examination, while the main advantage of echography lies in its ability to reduce to a minimum the need for an invasive examination. Moreover, examination with an endoscopic probe prolongs laparoscopy by several minutes and necessitates frequent changes in the patient's position and various endoscopic maneuvers (shifting the organs with the probe, traction on tissues) which are not well tolerated and increase the overall risk of the examination itself.

Finally, echo-guided biopsy is fairly easy to perform and accurate when traditional echography is used; considering the excellent results, we cannot assert that echolaparoscopy is any more advantageous. It is therefore apparent, also in view of the paucity of indications for echolaparoscopy, that this technique has only a slight practical value. Of course, there are cases in which the diagnosis made depends entirely upon echolaparoscopy, but these exceptional cases do not justify the systematic use of a technique that requires complex and expensive equipment and highly skilled staff. We are therefore of the opinion that as yet the results do not compensate for the costs.

2.1.6 Conclusions

1. The technique of echolaparoscopy is still at an experimental stage, and only prototypes are presently available.

2. These prototypes have high-frequency probes and therefore give good echograms for surface examinations, but they are less satisfactory for deep penetration. To effectively complete laparoscopy, which is limited to the external visualization of organs, lower-frequency probes are required for a satisfactory exploration of the deeper layers.

3. In recent years, traditional echographs have been so well developed technically that their short-comings have been remarkably reduced. They can therefore give a very high percentage of decisive results, and laparoscopy is thereby avoided.

4. There are, of course, cases that cannot be resolved with traditional echography, and in these cases an echolaparoscopic study can contribute findings that are diagnostically decisive; however, such cases are not very frequent.

5. Although there are certainly possible indications for echolaparoscopy, the number is small. We may therefore conclude that, at present, the practical application of this technique is limited.

2.2 Sonography for Laparoscopy

Sonography is the best available filter for the selection of patients to undergo laparoscopy. Here, however, we focus upon sonography for laparoscopy, which we first proposed in 1984 [8].

Sonography for laparoscopy is analogous to intraoperative sonography, where great progress has been made in recent years. Not only is sonography performed to improve upon the diagnosis; it is used mainly to overcome difficulties that are closely linked with surgery. Because this technique is used routinely it has consistently been improved upon, and now, particularly in the field of oncology, intraoperative sonography is an invaluable guide to the surgeon, helping him decide upon the most opportune strategy. Like intraoperative sonography, which is performed by the surgeon, *sonography for laparoscopy* must be performed by an expert who can correctly interpret the findings and utilize them to solve problems related to laparoscopy. One person, a laparoscopist cum echographist, must perform both techniques, and perform them well.

Sonography is thus performed by the laparoscopist himself, who uses traditional echography (Fig. 2.7) and then, in a second step, can perform the laparoscopy if necessary. (Fig. 2.8) If the two examinations are done by one person, the most satisfactory possible integration of the two techniques is attained and a more balanced basis for decision-making is achieved. Echography and laparoscopy thus become two steps in one examination.

Sonography for laparoscopy consists first of a complete echographic examination of the abdomen; this is performed as a preliminary step in all patients about to undergo laparoscopy *prior to pneumoperitoneum*. In certain cases, as we shall see later, a US examination must also be made *after pneumoperitoneum*. Finally, it is sometimes useful to perform a US examination *after laparoscopy*.

2.2.1 Sonography Before Pneumoperitoneum

This is the most important step in the examination: the exploration must be made carefully, with the entire abdomen examined and particular attention paid to organs and sites where a disease is suspected.

The main aim of the US exploration is to *check indications*. In the past, any indication was "confirmed" on the basis of the clinical, laboratory, and instrumental findings. With modern sonography, however, we can both (a) confirm any previous findings and therefore check reliably the indication for laparoscopy and (b) obtain a different picture – the change may depend either on

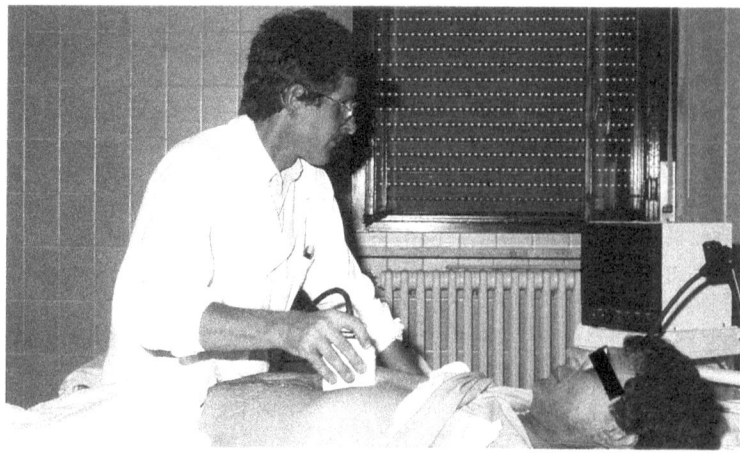

2.7

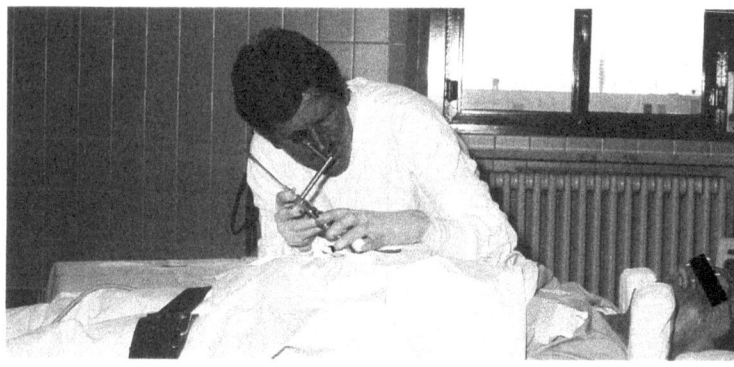

2.8

Fig. 2.7. Sonography for laparoscopy: first step, sonography

Fig. 2.8. Sonography for laparoscopy: second step, laparoscopy

the fact that, during the interval between the two examinations, signs that were undetectable have become detectable, or on the fact that lesions that were detected but not diagnosed may have assumed more specific morphological features that at last allow a diagnosis to be made. Moreover, it must be borne in mind that the first sonographic findings may not be correct. In such cases the indication for laparoscopy must be considered on the basis of the new US findings. When the sonographic examination demonstrates focal lesions before laparoscopy is performed, it is necessary to take an extemporaneous US-guided biopsy using a fine needle and to await the results.

Prelaparoscopic sonography not only clarifies the indications; it also enables us to predict whether or not the laparoscopy will be effective. It can show us whether the organ or the diseased structure to be examined can be explored endoscopically or not, and it can show whether the part to be examined lies in the abdominal cavity and is therefore accessible, or whether it is seated in the retroperitoneum or is covered by other formations which make it inaccessible to laparoscopy. In such cases laparoscopy might be indicated, but it can be avoided because it will not yield useful information.

In focal lesions of the liver or spleen, preliminary echography can also accurately indicate if lesions will be visible and if so, whether the laparoscopy can be performed. An example of this is given in Fig. 2.9, which shows a round hypoechogenic area at the left lobe of the liver; this was difficult to interpret. Guided biopsy with a fine needle did not give satisfactory data and the nature of the lesion remained uncertain. In a case like this, laparoscopy is certainly indicated because it is the means to a diagnosis.

Sonography enables us to predict whether in this case the endoscopic examination will solve the diagnostic difficulty: the nodule appears to protrude from the margin of the left lobe; it is free and uncovered, and therefore will be easily visualized

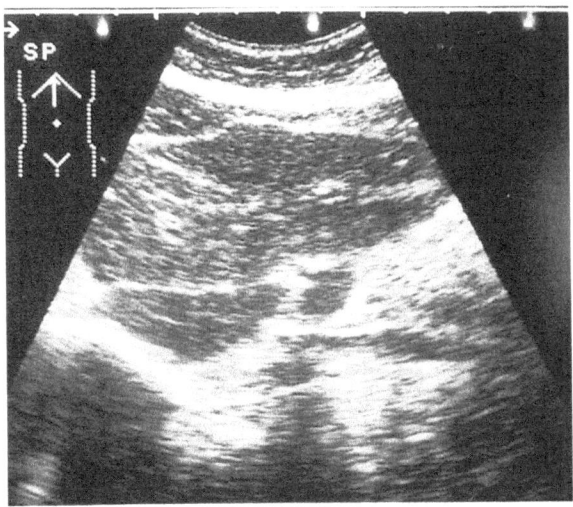

Fig. 2.9. Staging for carcinoma of the ovary. Prelaparoscopic sonography, transverse epigastric scan. Shape, size, and echostructure of left lobe of the liver are normal. At segment III a hypoechogenic nodule (diameter 1.9 cm) protrudes from the margin. Findings of echo-guided fine-needle biopsy were not significant

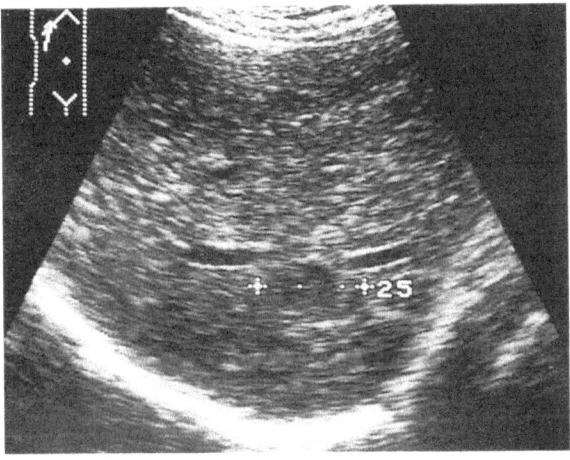

Fig. 2.10. Staging for carcinoma of the sigmoid colon. Prelaparoscopic sonography, longitudinal scan in left decubitus. At the deep portion of segment V a hypoisogenic nodule (diameter 2.5 cm) can be seen with signs of vascular compression. Echo-guided fine-needle biopsy revealed nonneoplastic tissue

and can be reached for biopsy. At laparoscopy the macroscopic findings were not clear but the biopsy showed a nodular focal hyperplasia, thus establishing a diagnosis. There are also cases in which laparoscopy is indicated, but where sonography demonstrates that the position of the lesion to be diagnosed will hinder endoscopic visualization. The patient shown in Fig. 2.10 had a carcinoma of

the sigmoid colon, and sonography demonstrated a round hypoechogenic area which appeared to be a nodule attached to a portal vein. Under guided biopsy using a fine needle a nonneoplastic material was obtained. As the diagnosis was uncertain, laparoscopy was indicated, if necessary, with a biopsy using a cutting needle. This was not performed, however, because as the lesion was found to be deeply seated, it would have been impossible to obtain a satisfactory laparoscopic finding.

Specific sonography is thus of great value, for it provides information for the *laparoscopic technique* itself and indicates the most suitable *method* to follow in each individual case. If the exmination is to be successful, it is very important to choose the best point to introduce the trocar and, of course, the laparoscope. This choice depends upon safety factors and technical criteria. The following must be avoided:

1. Areas of the abdominal wall that correspond to the liver, the spleen, the round ligament of the liver, and the epigastric arteries
2. Areas that correspond to any palpable masses
3. Surgical scars which may correspond to internal adhesions that could hinder the examination

Of course, the particular point for introduction of the laparoscope varies from patient to patient, depending also on the shape of the abdomen in relation to the organ or area to be explored. The points of introduction generally preferred are along the pararectal median line, to the left if above the umbilicus and to the right if below. The criteria now governing the choice of the point for introducing the trocar are much more precise and rational, thanks to sonographic findings.

Preliminary sonography allows us to establish the margins of the organs and to detect any masses more reliably. Above all, it tells us when organs are in an atypical position, a task that is otherwise impossible. It also indicates whether any hollow pathological formations (e.g., cysts, abscesses, and dilated vessels) are present in the abdominal walls or immediately under them, at the usual points for trocar or pneumoperitoneum needle introduction.

The most common finding is umbilical or periumbilical vein dilation due to portal hypertension; these can be damaged by trocar introduction, with serious consequences. These veins can be identified and localized very well using sonography. In Fig. 2.11 an example is shown of a superficial umbilical vein situated at one of the traditional

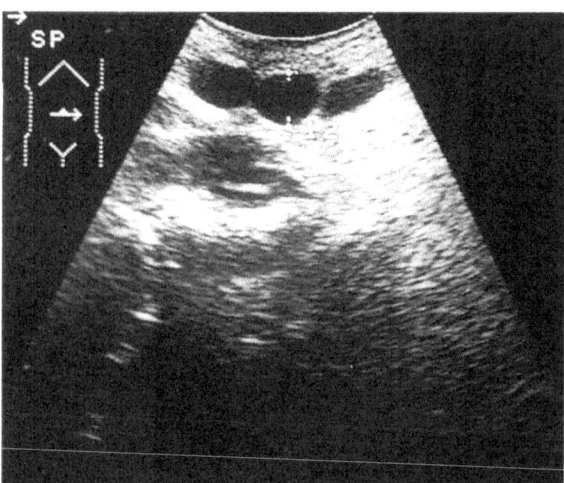

Fig. 2.11. A round anechogenic area attributable to a dilated umbilical vein at the abdominal wall

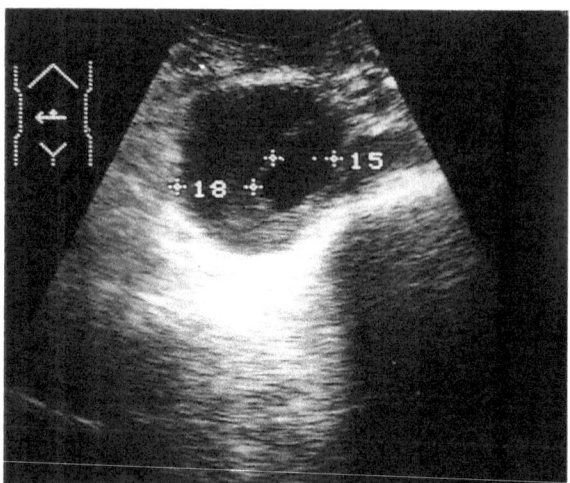

Fig. 2.13. Sonography for laparoscopy. Transverse subumbilical scan shows an extensive round anechogenic area attributable to an aortic aneurysm

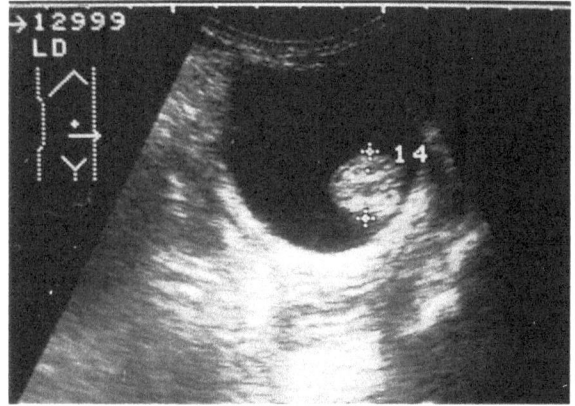

Fig. 2.12. An anechogenic area reaching the lower left abdominal quadrant contains round hyperechogenic formations due to an enormous hydropic gallbladder containing an adenomatous formation

points for trocar introduction. In this case, of course, the trocar must be inserted at another point.

The risk of a hydropic gallbladder being damaged by the trocar is fairly high; this organ is sometimes so enlarged and dilated that it reaches the lower quadrant of the left abdomen, as can be seen in Fig 2.12. If there is no echographic sign of this condition, there is a risk that the gallbladder wall will be perforated by the peritoneum needle, which is traditionally introduced at this part of the abdomen. The serious risks due to any aortic aneurysm can now be avoided if prelaparoscopic

findings are obtained, as shown in Fig. 2.13. Apart from reducing the risks, preliminary sonography enhances the diagnostic efficacy of laparoscopy, and the sonographic findings also indicate the more suitable laparoscopic method to follow in each individual case. If lesions are localized echographically in a particular area, then the endoscopic examination can focus upon that particular area; the patient can be placed in the most suitable position, and the appropriate endoscopic maneuvers can be made to expose the organ or part of the organ where any biopsies are to be taken.

In our experience, by following the trace indicated by the sonographic findings when performing laparoscopy, it has been possible to reach and diagnose lesions that would otherwise have escaped detection. Moreover, by integrating and comparing sonographic pictures we facilitate an interpretation of a particular condition and improve upon the precision and the reliability of the diagnosis.

2.2.2 Sonography After Pneumoperitoneum

In certain cases a sonographic examination can also be performed after pneumoperitoneum, as proposed by us in 1986. This may seem contradictory, because it is well known that gas is an obstacle to the transmission of echoes and therefore hinders diagnostic sonography. However, the gas in the peritoneum acts as a contrast medium, allowing the detection of abdominal adhesions [9, 10] which, secondary to peritonitis and to previous surgery, make laparoscopy difficult. They can, in fact, be so diffuse that they preclude any satisfactory pneumoperitoneum, thus making it impossible to perform laparoscopy. In other cases, the gas chamber may allow trocar introduction, but the adhesions may be so extensive and thick that exploration is limited or impossible.

Finally, adhesions considerably increase the risk of serious accidents such as hemorrhage or loop perforation which may occur where the trocar is introduced. The localization of abdominal adhesions is therefore an important preliminary step that allows us to reliably establish whether laparoscopy is technically feasible, whether it will yield useful findings, and whether it involves a high risk. In the past, in patients with possible adhesions, this evaluation was made through percussion and auscultation in order to ascertain the progressive diffusion of gas in the abdomen while initiating the pneumoperitoneum and then by checking whether there was a pocket of gas at the point chosen for trocar introduction. Any gas was then aspirated with the needle and syringe used for the anesthesia. Some information on the distribution of the gas could also be obtained by radiography after the pneumoperitoneum had been performed. But these methods were not accurate and only large adhesions were detected. Sonography performed after pneumoperitoneum, on the other hand, enables us to detect small adhesions and localize them in a reliable way.

At our center we considered the interpretation of images of abdominal conditions. Figure 2.14 is a typical echographic image of an abdominal cavity without adhesions and in which gas introduced for pneumoperitoneum is distributed evenly. It is characterized by a large cone-shaped shadow, in the central part of which can be seen some hyperechogenic streaks that probably represent echoes of the wall layers. This finding demonstrates that the cavity is free, and that laparoscopy can be performed and good results expected. If there are adhesions, the picture is irregular because of the presence of echoes like those shown in Fig. 2.15. The cone-shaped shadow is interrupted and limited by a large hyperechogenic area due to the presence of an adhesion that is clearly diffuse and remarkably thick. Around these hyperechogenic areas some intestinal loops can be seen grouped

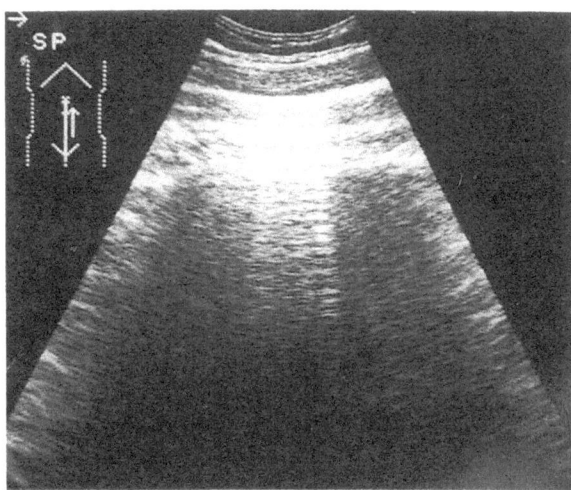

Fig. 2.14. Sonography for laparoscopy after pneumoperitoneum. Picture normal. A conical shadow can be seen under the wall with parallel transverse hyperechogenic streaks

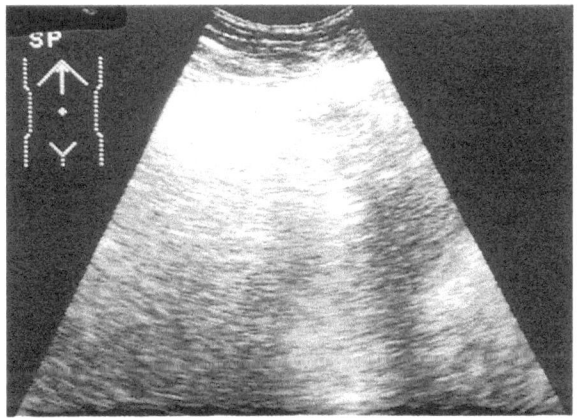

Fig. 2.15. Echography for laparoscopy after pneumoperitoneum. The conical shadow from pneumoperitoneum is interrupted by an extensive hyperechogenic band due to the presence of large adhesions

together. The typical loop structure is easily seen and the peristaltic movements of the intestine can be identified with the real-time apparatus (Fig. 2.16). If the entire surface and the different planes are carefully explored even the adhesions can be detected, and a clear map of the areas with adhesions and the free areas with gas in them can also be obtained. The only cause for error, and this is not frequent, may be an accidental insufflation of some gas from the abdominal wall or omental fat. The emphysema thus formed can alter the sonographic image of the peritoneum

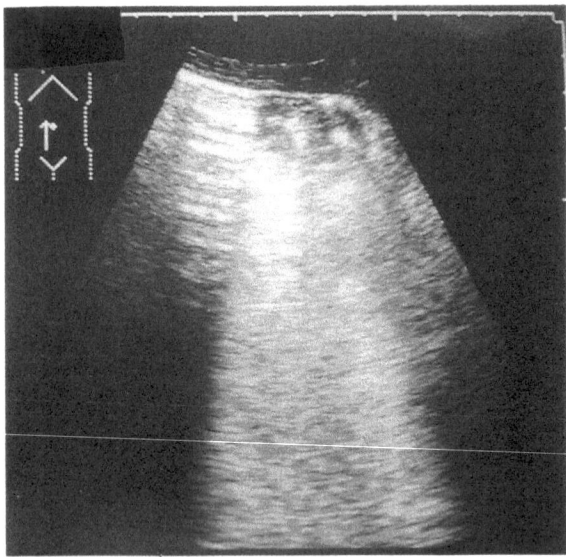

Fig. 2.16. Echography for laparoscopy after pneumoperitoneum. Underneath the wall can be seen an oval area corresponding to an intestine loop within adhesional tissue. Bilaterally, the conical shadow due to pneumoperitoneum is quite evident

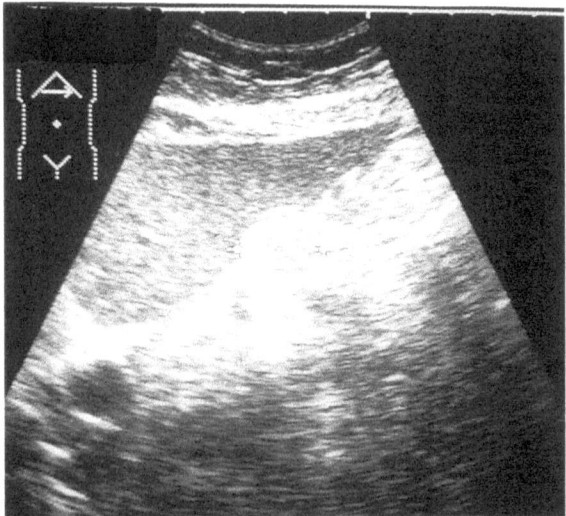

Fig. 2.17. Follow-up for carcinoma of the ovary. Echography for laparoscopy, longitudinal epigastric scan. Left lobe of liver is normal; the lower margin contains a nodule of the hepatogastric ligament tissue. This is fairly hyperechogenic, with a diameter of 2.1 cm and a hazy border. Metastasis to the small omentum suspected

even where adhesions are absent, thus giving rise to false negatives.

Sonography repeated after the pneumoperitoneum gives the important information necessary to reduce the risk and improve upon the efficacy of

the laparoscopy. It enables us to accurately study the diffusion of gas in the abdomen and to reliably ascertain whether there is a pocket of gas large enough to allow the laparoscopy to be performed. In addition, we can localize the chamber into which the trocar can be introduced without risking damage to the underlying formations adhering to the abdominal wall we can then choose the point for the introduction of the trocar, bearing in mind both the risk and the possibility of using the laparoscope to explore the parts of the abdomen that appear to be of particular diagnostic importance in each particular case. When the adhesions have resulted in the formation of multiple pockets of gas, the most suitable point for endoscopic observation is chosen on the basis of a sonographic map. In other words, the point for introduction and the course that the laparoscope can and must follow to reach its objective are decided upon on the basis of the sonographic findings.

Sonography after pneumoperitoneum helps us to ascertain, fairly reliably, a priori whether laparoscopy would be technically feasible but probably not useful. This is the case if the pocket of gas is large enough but closed by thick adhesions that greatly reduce the field for exploration. The decision whether to perform laparoscopy, and if so how, is thus guided rationally by preliminary sonography, and the chances of reaching a satisfactory diagnosis are thereby enhanced.

The following case is an example of laparoscopy guided by preliminary sonographic findings. A young woman was referred to our center for laparoscopy as a follow up for ovarian carcinoma while she was still under therapy. Along the right margin of the liver preliminary sonography demonstrated a round area that was slightly more hypoechogenic than the surrounding tissue (Fig. 2.17). It was necessary to ascertain whether this was a metastasis and, if so, whether it was a metastasis of the adipose tissue of the hepatogastric ligament (as it appeared to be), or of the liver, which was also possible. The outcome was important because in the case of the liver, the finding would mean that the disease stage was to be upgraded from III to IV. Laparoscopy was therefore definitely indicated, but the patient had already been operated on and had a puboumbilical scar. If she underwent surgery of the abdomen there would be adhesions that could prevent the trocar introduction and also hide the area to be explored. Echography after the pneumoperitoneum was therefore performed. It showed adhesions occupying the epigastric region

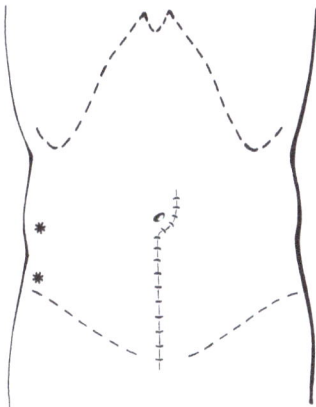

Fig. 2.18. Trocar insertion in an atypical site with a view to avoiding adhesions in the epigastric region

and the left hypochondrium: a pocket of gas to the far right, however, was found to be large enough to allow safe introduction of the trocar, and it appeared to give access to the site of the lesion. Laparoscopy was therefore considered possible. The trocar was introduced at an atypical point at the level of the umbilicus, to the right, outside the hemiclavicle or median pararectal line (Fig. 2.18) to avoid the median scar. Endoscopically, at the central part of the abdomen, up to the left hypochondrium, a thick adhesion was visualized attached to loops of the small intestine. At the left of the field a large opening was seen (Fig. 2.19), through which it was possible to reach a point from which the left lobe of the liver could be visualized. The margin was normal and only slightly raised by

the fat from the hepatogastric ligament, which appeared irregular (Fig. 2.20). This was due to neoplastic infiltration, as confirmed by biopsy.

Notwithstanding the considerable technical difficulties posed by this laparoscopy, it was possible to perform because of the sonographic information obtained, and the clinical doubts raised were completely resolved. A neoplastic spread of the ovarian carcinoma was demonstrated, but this was limited to the adipose tissue; the liver was intact.

2.2.3 Sonography After Laparoscopy

The integration of sonography and laparoscopy can be completed by postlaparoscopic sonographic control, which allows us to check the prelaparoscopic findings and to ascertain and reliability of the different images obtained, in light of the definite anatomopathological diagnosis made on the basis of the endoscopic examination. This check is made when the laparoscopic findings contradict those of the preliminary sonography. This occurs in many different conditions, but particularly in cases of abdominal tumors, above all those of the liver: lesions not detected by pre-

Fig. 2.19. Extensive adhesions containing an intestine loop are confirmed. Wide opening to the left

Fig. 2.20. The hepatogastric ligament is thickened and rigid and with heteroplastic tissue infiltrations. To the left can be seen the margin of the left lobe of the liver, which is normal

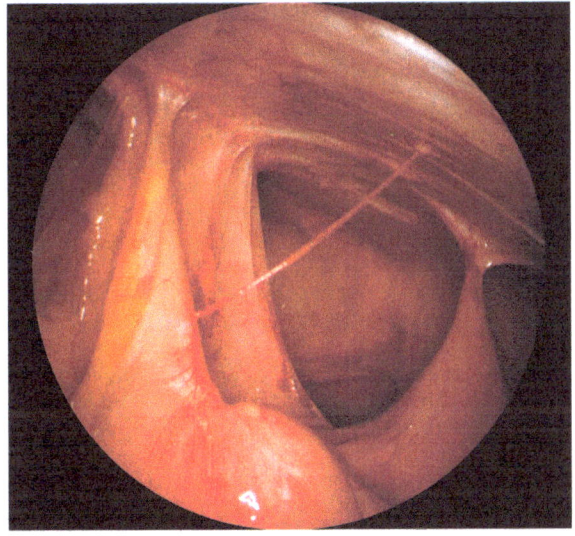

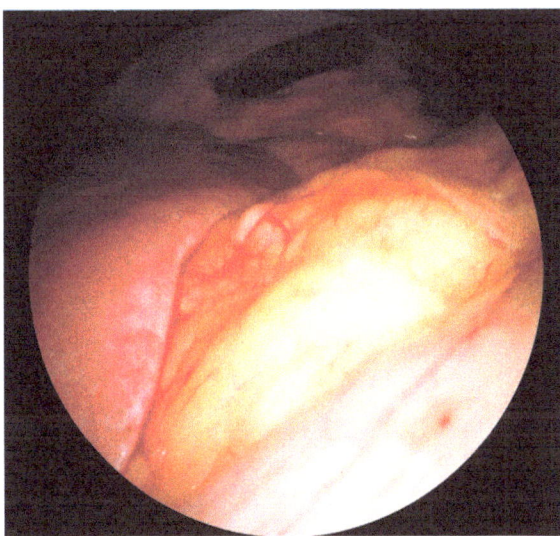

laparoscopic sonography are detected by laparoscopy, which is performed because a neoplasm was still suspected or considered possible. In such cases, a diagram is made to show the lesions observed laparoscopically (number, form, volume, distribution in the organs, etc.). On completion of the laparoscopy, the gas is completely expelled from the abdomen and sonography is repeated with a careful point-by-point exploration of all the areas in which the tumor has been demonstrated.

In our experience, about 25% of prelaparoscopic sonographic examinations give false negative findings that are often confirmed if the examination is repeated. The characteristics of certain lesions escape sonographic detection. In some cases, however, at the second sonographic examination a careful search at points indicated enables us to demonstrate a significant image, or at least an image that suggests the presence of a tumor. This confirms the crucial importance of expertise and patience in interpreting sonographic findings.

Finally, in areas in which laparoscopy demonstrates a malignant tumor, echography may show slight echostructural modifications or a diffuse reorganization that may appear due to a pathological process, but that according to traditional echographic diagnostics would not be interpreted as neoplastic.

Laparoscopy can be used to reveal incorrect interpretations of sonographic images. If, for example, an organ is misinterpreted, repeat sonography can show why an error was made and establish the value of particular signs that facilitate the correct interpretation of the given images. A similar check of the findings, made by comparing them with the anatomopathological diagnosis, also has an important role in improving upon sonographic diagnostics. In fact, as we shall see in Sect. 5.3, certain echographic signs that may not appear remarkable can, if interpreted properly, be of great diagnostic value.

2.2.4 Conclusions

1. Sonography for laparoscopy, performed as here proposed and described by us, acts as a further "filter" for patients, reducing to a minimum the number of unnecessary or useless laparoscopies through the rigorous control of indications that it provides and through its ability to reliably predict whether laparoscopy is technically feasible and, if so, whether it would give useful findings (localization and exploration of the organs and of any lesions to be examined, sonographic detection of adhesions after pneumoperitoneum, etc.).

2. Sonography improves upon the laparoscopy itself by indicating the most suitable method for the particular individual and by "guiding" endoscopic exploration in the most rational way possible.

3. It has drastically reduced the danger of accidents from trocar and needle introduction for pneumoperitoneum by detecting any risk situations (vessels, adhesions) and it improves upon echographic diagnostics because it allows us to check on findings where necessary by repeating sonography after laparoscopy.

References

1. Japan Society of Ultrasonics in Medicine (1966) Ultrasonics in medicine, principle, research and practice, 1st edn. Igaku-Shoin, Tokyo, p 311
2. Look D, Henning H, Yano N (1975) Direkte Ultraschallechographie der Gallenblase unter laparoskopische Sicht. In: Lindner R (ed) Fortschritte der Gastroenterologischen Endoskopie, vol 6. Witzsrock. Baden-Baden
3. Ohta Y, Fujiwara K, Sato Y, Niwa H, Oka H. (1983) New ultrasonic laparoscope for diagnosis of intra-abdominal diseases. Gastrointest Endosc 4: 289–294
4. Frank L, Bliesze H, Beck K, Hammes P, Linhart P (1983) Laparoskopische Sonographie. Dtsch Med Wochenschr 108:902–904
5. Bönhof JA, Linhart P, Battendorf U, Holper N (1984) Liver biopsy guided by laparoscopic sonography. A case report demonstrating a new technique. Endoscopy 16:237–239
6. Fukuda M, Mima S, Tanabe T, Haniu T, Suzuki Y, Hirata K, Terada S (1984) Endoscopic sonography of the liver – diagnostic application of the echolaparoscope to localize intrahepatic lesions. Scand J Gastroenterol 19 (Suppl 102):24–38
7. Marin G, Candiani F (1985) Ecografia laparoscopica. G Ital End Dig, 8:197–199
8. Dagnini G (1984) Il momento attuale della laparoscopia. Premesse per un bilancio. G Ital Endosc Dig 1:1–8
9. Marin G, Bergamo S, Miola E, Dagnini G (1986) L'ecografia prelaparoscopica nella prevenzione dei rischi della laparoscopia. G Ital Endosc Dig 9:189–193
10. Marin G, Bergamo S, Miola E, Dagnini G (1987) Prelaparoscopic echography used to detect abdominal adhesions. Endoscopy 19:147–149

3 Technical Innovations

3.1 Laparoscopic Exploration of the Pancreas

As the pancreas is located retroperitoneally, it is not usually visualized laparoscopically. However, with the improvements made in special techniques in recent years, laparoscopic exploration of the pancreas is no longer considered an impossible feat.

3.1.1 Technique

In 1972 a "supragastric" technique was first suggested to allow laparoscopic visualization of the pancreas through the transparent part of the lesser omentum [1, 2]. With the patient in lateral right decubitus while in an anti-Trendelenburg position, the laparoscope is used to raise the left lobe of the liver and push it back to expose the lesser omentum, which presents a transparent area. If the patient is not obese, the body of the pancreas is visible underneath.

This supragastric pancreatoscopy is relatively simple to perform and does not require special equipment, but in about one third of cases it fails to allow visualization of the body of the pancreas, either because excess fatty tissue has thickened the lesser omentum or because there are adhesions.

Another technique, the so-called infragastric pancreatoscopy, was proposed to overcome the above mentioned shortcomings [3, 4]. With this technique, the laparoscope is introduced into the epiploon retrocavity by passing underneath the stomach through a hole made, using diathermocoagulation, into the adipose tissue of the gastrocolic ligament.

Some authors [3] suggest that some gas should be insufflated through the laparoscopic canal to distend the epiploon retrocavity to create an exploration cavity. This technique usually allows the visualization of a large part of the body and tail of the pancreas, but it is complicated to perform and not always satisfactory. With it, moreover, two pincers must be introduced through holes made in the abdominal wall to grasp the two sides of the epiploon and keep it taut so that the cut through which the laparoscope is passed can be made. This technique is not risk free because, particularly in patients with pancreas tumors, quite large vessels can be hidden in the body of the greater omentum.

More recently, some Japanese authors described a more simple and effective technique [5–7], which uses a supragastric route for access, by means of omentotomy. The lesser omentum is held with pincers introduced from outside and held in tension; a small hole is then made by cutting the thinnest part, and through it the laparoscope is guided into the epiploon retrocavity (Fig.

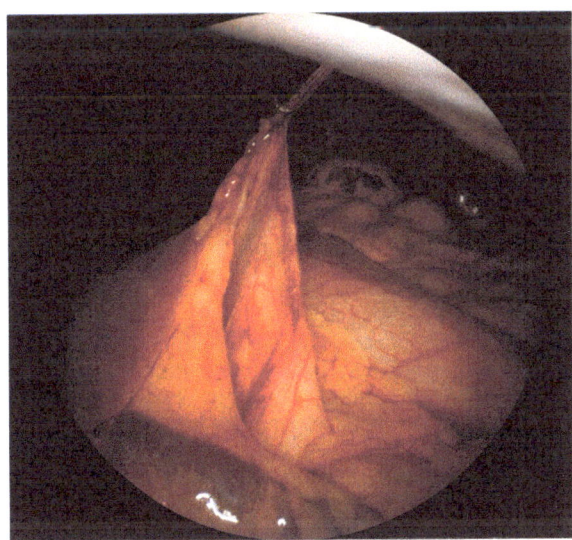

Fig. 3.1. The lesser omentum is grasped with the forceps and pulled upward. The hole for laparoscope insertion can be seen

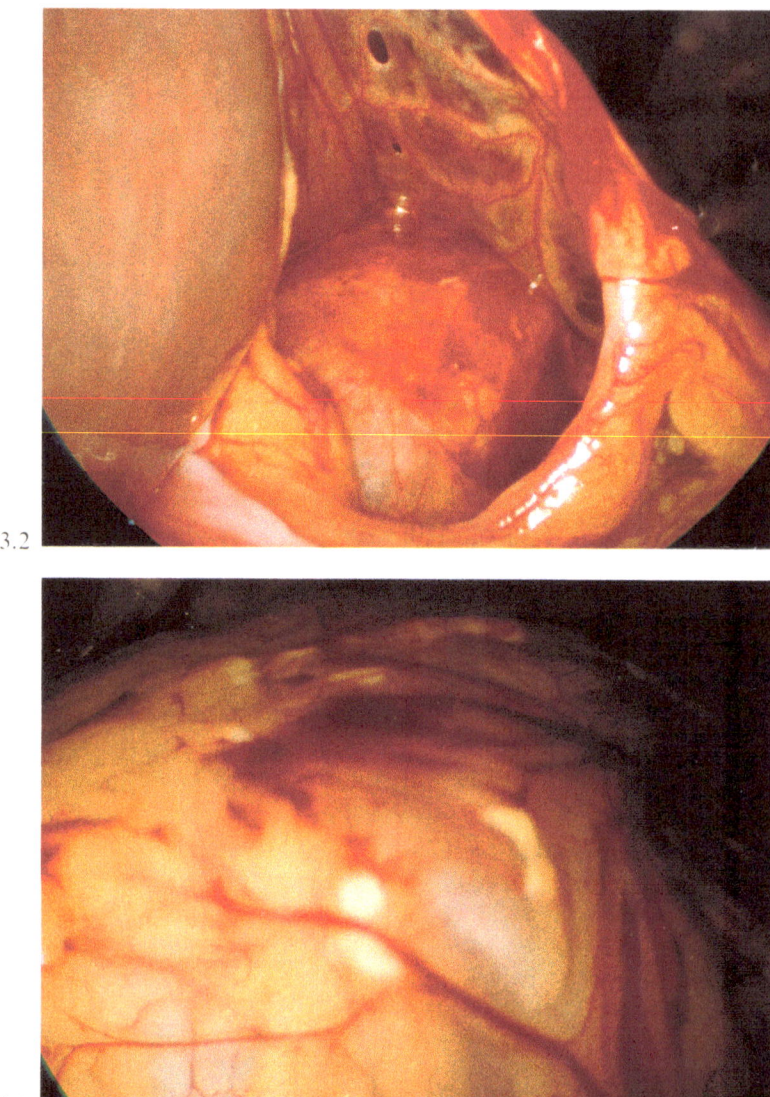

3.2

3.3

Fig. 3.2. *Acute edematous pancreatitis.* Through the large hole the pancreas can be seen; it appears enlarged, pale and edematous. The blood-stained tissue is due to a small hemorrhage from the cut omental fat

Fig. 3.3. *Subacute pancreatitis.* Numerous whitish-yellow patches from cytosteatonecrosis on the adipose tissue of the omentum. Part of it appears raised and adherent to the upper abdominal wall. Along the adhesion line can be seen initial fibrin formation, and there is slight passive congestion

3.1). The surface of the pancreas can thus be observed directly (Fig. 3.2). Supragastric pancreatoscopy with omentotomy is the most satisfactory technique; we, too, have used it successfully.

3.1.2 Interpretation of Laparoscopic Findings

Traditional laparoscopy allows us to collect findings outside the pancreas, and these *indirect signs* are of diagnostic importance [3, 8, 9]:

1. Cytosteatonecrosis manifests as small whitish-yellow plaques on the peritoneum and omentum; roundish or oval, they are easily recognized macroscopically (Fig. 3.3). Fatty tissue necrosis can be histologically confirmed if a biopsy is made, and is a sure sign of acute pancreatitis.
2. Congestion and edema of the greater and particularly the lesser omentum suggest edematous pancreatitis.

3. Subserous petechiae of the greater or lesser omentum strongly suggest acute hemorrhagic pancreatitis.
4. Taut gallbladder with a slight increase in volume, an over-thick and edematous wall, and signs of active congestion is considered to be an indirect sign of possible acute pancreatitis, because acute concomitant colecystitis is present in about half the cases of pancreatitis.
5. Signs of sectorial portal hypertension from thrombosis of the splenic vein are relatively significant, because this type of lesion is often associated with pancreatitis.
6. Slight serous or hemorrhagic abdominal leakage of liquid containing a large proportion of amylase indicates, respectively, edematous or necrotic hemorrhagic pancreatitis.
7. Adhesions and thickening of the lesser omentum and small cytosteatonecrotic spots without active congestion phenomena can have a diagnostic value because they may be caused by chronic pancreatitis.

Observation of the pancreas using the above-described techniques contributes to the diagnosis by also providing *direct signs* that can be decisive:

1. Swollen pancreatic parenchyma, pale pink, with an unclear lobular border that is harder than the norm at palpation with the probe, indicates an acute edematous pancreatitis.
2. Massive hemorrhagic suffusions with necrotic areas that appear darker on the pancreas body are typical of acute necrohemorrhagic pancreatitis.
3. An irregular, whitish, hard pancreas surface with cystic formations suggests chronic pancreatitis.
4. Carcinoma is suspected or diagnosed if nodules, hard whitish swellings of different sizes, are found, but it is difficult to distinguish between it and chronic nodular circumscribed pancreatitis.

Supragastric pancreatoscopy allows the direct exploration of a large part of the pancreas body and tail, but not the head; this is a great shortcoming because tumors are frequent at this site [10]. A tumor of the pancreas head can be diagnosed laparoscopically only if the neoplastic mass is large or if there are indirect signs caused by compression to the choledochus, signs typical of mechanical jaundice. However, at this advanced stage the diagnosis is no longer useful.

Of course, by visualizing the pancreas we can take biopsies that once were considered practically impossible because of the technical difficulties involved and the risk of damaging a hidden organ. These issues are discussed in Sect. 3.4.3.

3.1.3 Present Value

One of the great shortcomings of laparoscopy earlier was that it did not allow any exploration of the pancreas. Technical innovations now allow this hidden organ to be visualized, and we can obtain important laparoscopic findings that allow us to make accurate and reliable diagnoses in at least 75% of the cases of acute and 70% of the cases of chronic pancreatitis [5, 7, 11]. Diagnoses for carcinoma of the head of the pancreas are fewer (about 30%), while those for carcinoma of the body and tail reach 85% [5–7].). These recently reported results are of value in theory, but they have only a limited practical value for several reasons.

The techniques used for exploration of the pancreas are complicated and difficult to perform; the excellent results reported can be obtained only by extraordinarily skilled and experienced operators.

Various maneuvers are required to expose the pancreas (extra holes in the abdominal wall for the introduction of instruments, traction and incisions on the greater and lesser omentum, palpation and shifting of the organs with the probe) and the duration of the laparoscopy itself is considerably prolonged, so the patient experiences greater discomfort. Hypotensive crises making it necessary to discontinue the examination have occurred [11]. No deaths have been reported, but of the 71 patients reported on by Ishida [7], seven (3.3%) had complications: acute pancreatitis, necrotic tissue spreading into the cavity, hemorrhage, and leakage of pancreatic juice.

While strenuous efforts were being made to obtain these laparoscopic results, the boom in imaging techniques occurred. The first reports on their use were most eloquent: in diseases of the pancreas the sensitivity and the specificity of ultrasonography are high, ranging from 80% to 90% [12]. In the diagnosis of carcinoma of the pancreas, authors have reported a sensitivity of 94% and a specificity of almost 100% [13, 14]. These results, integrated as we shall later see with those of echo-guided fine-needle biopsies, reflect the great steps forward made in the diagnosis, of diseases of the pancreas. These techniques, moreover, are far less invasive.

So the improvements made in the laparoscopic technique have lost their practical value, and in this field laparoscopy cannot compete with the imaging techniques. Besides, in the diagnosis of diseases of the pancreas, the indications for laparoscopy are now very limited.

However, we should never forget that the pancreas can be explored directly when necessary, and that certain indirect laparoscopic signs are still of importance [8, 9], for they allow us to differentiate between particular pancreatic diseases and other abdominal conditions simulating them. Here, Haubrich's observation is both appropriate and amusing:

My choice of approach in most cases of body and tail carcinomas will still be fine-needle aspiration under ultrasound or CT guidance.

So, what should we do? Should we all seek to gain facility with the technique so well described and illustrated by Ishida? I would not think this is necessary, but each laparoscopist will answer for himself or herself. Perhaps in large centers dealing with vast numbers of patients with perplexing pancreatic problems, it might be well for one laparoscopist to be prepared to undertake probing of the pancreas.

For myself, I feel no great urge or need to climb Mount Everest, but I find it worthwhile knowing that a successful ascent can be made [15].

3.1.4 Conclusions

1. The visualization of the pancreas, a retroperitoneal organ that was once inaccessible, must be considered an important improvement in laparoscopy.

2. The techniques that enable us to expose and explore the pancreas are very complicated, however, and require skilled experts.

3. The working out of a technique for the laparoscopic exploration of the pancreas coincided with the boom in imaging techniques, which now allow us in the majority of cases to make a diagnosis easily, without exposing the patient to any risk.

4. The laparoscopic exploration of the pancreas is therefore important in theory but not in practice.

5. The indications for laparoscopy in the diagnosis of a pancreas disease are now quite few and far between. The examination may be indicated in particular situations, however.

3.2 Operative Laparoscopy

Laparoscopy is essentially the exploration of the abdominal cavity. It is not limited to the observation of organs as they appear at first sight; several maneuvers are made, either with the laparoscope itself or with other appropriate instruments. In order to obtain as much information as possible, the different organs can be palpated, shifted, or lifted by means of the rigid probe, and obstacles, particularly omental fat covering or hiding the surface of the liver or the spleen, for example, can be removed. Moreover, during laparoscopy organ biopsies are usually taken: In a sense, these are operative maneuvers, but they should be considered an important part of the normal technique for explorative laparoscopy. Strictly speaking, "operative laparoscopy" means the performance under laparoscopy of small "special" operations.

Fiberendoscopy has made extraordinary progress. It is now possible to perform "operations" that replace surgery. These operations done under endoscopy give magnificent results and have several advantages over surgery. The most important recent advances are outlined here.

Esophagogastroduodenoscopy makes possible (a) removal of foreign bodies, (b) polypectomy, and (c) sclerotherapy for gastrointestinal varices. *Endoscopic retrograde cholangiopancreatography* (ERCP) allows endoscopic papillostomy for (a) acute obstructive cholangitis, (b) benign papillary stenosis, (c) neoplastic obstruction, (d) biliary pancreatitis, (e) choledochal lithiasis, and (f) removal of foreign bodies. With *coloscopy* we can perform polypectomy and palliative resection of malignant tumors and we can remove foreign bodies. Thus, operative fiberendoscopy now has an important role in the field of therapy and in the prophylaxis of diseases of the digestive tract and of the hepato-biliary-pancreatic system.

Valid proposals and important achievements have been made in *gynecological laparoscopy*, or *celioscopy*. In fact, gynecologists now acknowledge the important diagnostic indications and have specified morbid conditions in which a small endoscopic operation could obviate surgery. Special techniques have been described and appropriate instruments devised, so that endoscopic operations now give results that are more than satisfactory.

The development of endoscopy in gynecology has depended greatly on the fact that it is performed in the operating room by surgeons who can pass rapidly from laparoscopy to surgery, if necessary. This is advantageous, and it guarantees that any accidents can be resolved in time. We have no experience of this and outline here only the main endoscopic operations being done at present [16, 17].

Multiple Biopsies of the Ovary: These are made only with forceps that allow a large fragment to be removed; they have satisfactorily replaced surgical resection in the treatment of anovularity, in particular of the Stein-Leventhal syndrome.

Salpingolysis: The resection of adhesions from previous inflammations involving the fallopian tubes, particularly at the fundus, and causing their stenosis is a delicate operation, but it has proved useful in cases of infertility due to tube closure.

Lysis of Peritoneal Adhesions: This is performed for diagnostic reasons to expose or free organs that are covered or hidden; it is also used for therapy when the adhesions cause pain.

Tubal Sterilization: This is the most frequent indication for gynecological laparoscopy in countries in which this procedure is allowed, above all in the United States [18] and Great Britain, where about 30000 sterilizations are performed a year [17]. This can be done by electrocoagulation and tube resection or by applying clips or rings to close the tubes.

Endoscopic Treatment of Tubal Pregnancies: This can be performed only when the fetus is localized in a less vascularized area of the tube and when the sac diameter measures up to 3 cm. If the sac measures less than 1.5 cm it can be removed by electrocoagulation alone, or with electrocoagulation followed by excision or aspiration. The results in such cases have been good and the risk entailed is low.

Therapy for Endometriosis: This can be achieved with electrocoagulation when the lesions are small and situated far from any parts that might be damaged by fulgurations. Carbon dioxide laser vaporization has also been successful.

Removal of Foreign Bodies: The most frequently found foreign bodies are intrauterine devices, such as coils, clips, or rings, that have perforated the wall and reached the small pelvis; they are often covered by the peritoneum or fixed by adhesions.

Treatment of Ovarian Cysts: These can be punctured and emptied both for diagnostic (complete examination of liquid) and for therapeutic reasons.

Retrieval of Oocytes: This is a procedure for in vitro fertilization. After the ovaries have been stimulated, four to six oocytes can be obtained.

Although, from a surgical standpoint, traditional gastroenterological laparoscopy has not made sensational progress, interesting innovations have been made in this field. Above all, the method used for diagnostic examination has gradually become more aggressive. For example, it is now considered safe to take biopsies from organs that were once considered "untouchable," such as the spleen, and under conditions of higher risk. Moreover, multiple biopsies are often taken. Even the technique described for pancreas exploration can be considered an operative procedure.

Finally, gastroenterological laparoscopy has been enhanced in recent years by some surgical procedures of great value. It is, however, necessary to accurately define the conditions in which it is both justified and convenient to perform a particular endoscopic procedure. Some [17] claim that operative laparoscopy should be performed: (a) in the operating room with the patient monitored intra- and postoperatively; (b) with the patient with general anesthesia, with endotracheal intubation and the use of muscle relaxants; and (c) using CO_2 for pneumoperitoneum if electrocoagulation is called for.

We are of the opinion, however, that laparoscopic intervention is justified in cases in which it (a) is simple to perform, (b) only slightly prolongs the operation, (c) can be performed with the patient under *local* anesthesia, and (d) does not involve maneuvers that are dangerous or poorly tolerated.

Traditional gastroenterological laparoscopy was introduced among internists and has always been considered mainly a diagnostic tool. Even surgeons who acknowledge the diagnostic value of laparoscopy tend a prefer major surgery to small endoscopic operations. If the endoscopy calls for general anesthesia and the complex equipment required for a true surgical operation, it is preferable to open the abdomen, for in such cases surgery is technically more simple and accurate;

the risk is minor, the patient's discomfort is the same, and the costs are no higher.

Operative gastroenterological laparoscopy is also performed for the following diagnostic and therapeutic purposes: (a) lysis of adhesions, (b) puncturing of cystic formations, and (c) puncturing of abscesses. Laparoscopic cholangiography, which some authors still consider one of the indications [17], should be discontinued because it is dangerous, and a perfect radiological picture of the biliary tree can be obtained with ERCP. This was our opinion years ago [19], and now echography, which allows a very accurate study of the gallbladder and the biliary tree, has made both laparoscopic cholangiography and laparoscopy itself useless in the majority of cases in which a differential diagnosis of icterus is required. The indications for operative gastroenterological laparoscopy are similar to those specified for operative gynecological laparoscopy. The main difference between the two is that with operative gastroenterological laparoscopy only local anesthesia is required, and the procedure lasts no longer than normal exploratory laparoscopy; discomfort to the patient is no greater and the costs are no higher.

3.2.1 Technique

The rules for gastroenterological laparoscopy are the same as those for normal laparoscopy. *Local anesthesia* (with the same exceptions as those made for classical laparoscopy) is preceded by routine premedication.

The *instruments* used are needles of different lengths and calibers, forceps, scissors, and small, very pointed and sharp drills; all can be connected to an electrocoagulator. When possible, the instruments are introduced through the operating canal, a second hole being made only when absolutely necessary.

For *pneumoperitoneum* we routinely use nitrous oxide, which causes no disturbances. Many are of the opinion that this gas is inflammable and that CO_2 should be used for electrocoagulation. However, CO_2 is not tolerated by the patient because it causes intense peritoneal irritation with serious disturbances. Where CO_2 is used, therefore, general anesthesia is necessary. Our experience has shown that NO_2 electrocoagulation entails no risks and that with it general anesthesia can be avoided.

After an endoscopic operation the patient has bed rest until the following day, just as do patients from whom one or more biopsies have been taken under laparoscopic guidance.

3.2.2 Lysis of Adhesions for Diagnostic Purposes

One of the most important and frequent causes of partial or total failure in laparoscopy is the finding of adhesions in the abdomen. The result of prior peritonitis and, more often, of surgery to the abdomen, if they are extensive they prevent a satisfactory endoscopic exploration.

The adhesions sometimes cover the organs entirely and adhere closely to their surface, or they may resemble "curtains" and fibrous or fibroadipose septums which hamper or even prevent, any exploration because they are stretched between the wall and the abdominal organs. In such cases the simpler maneuvers should be tried first. Using the probe or forceps, an attempt should be made to remove any obstacles, especially adipose tissue flaps covering the organs, and any natural opening in the adhesion walls through which the laparoscope can be passed should be searched for. Using very sharp drills or scissors, incisions can be made endoscopically in order to free the exploratory field as much as possible.

The most frequent and profitable operation is to open a gap through a taut adhesion in order to see beyond the obstacle. The *thinnest part* must be chosen, as this should be the easiest to cross; it should be *hypovascularized* and in an area that will provide a good view of the organ to be explored. The experience of the operator and his ability to make a quick appraisal are of vital importance. However, for extensive adhesions, the sonographic examination made after pneumoperitoneum (see Sect. 2.2.2) shows the topography of the abdomen with its air and the septa that delimit it, and thus establishes the course to follow in order to reach the organ to be examined; it allows us to choose the most suitable point at which to make an artificial space for laparoscope introduction.

It can be very difficult, sometimes impossible, to open the hole if there are numerous adhesion bands; this frequently is the case with adhesions of the mesentery or omentum. Then it is necesssary to take great care when making the cut, because the adherent tissue may be highly vascularized,

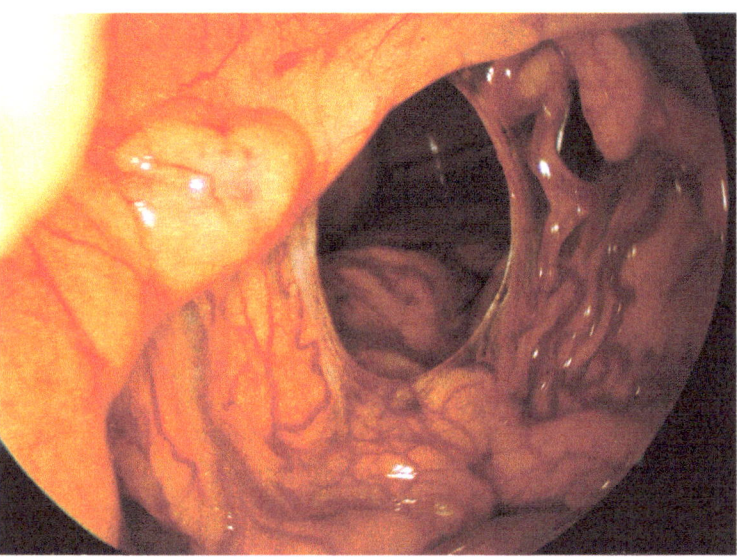

Fig. 3.4. Large space in adhesion, artificially opened, through which the laparoscope can pass for exploration of the right hypochondrium

the vessels being large but not always visible, as in portal hypertension, for example.

Electrocoagulation is always a good safeguard. Sometimes an intestinal loop may be hidden in the adhesion and, if lax, it may escape detection at both the direct endoscopic and the preliminary sonographic examination. However, if the necessary precautions are taken, the endoscopic operation is usually fairly simple and does not entail untoward risks. The results depend on the individual situation: if the curtain has a "simple" structure, forming a single barrier, then the laparoscope can freely explore the cavity behind it after being introduced. In the case shown in Fig. 3.4 a large opening was made, and this enabled us to see a large space beyond it, up to the diaphragm wall. It was thus possible to explore the left hypochondrial interior.

In some cases the results are not wonderful. The adhesion may in fact be "composite," that is, the curtain may be made up of more than one layer. As Fig. 3.5 shows, once the first layer has been cut, other adhesions may appear that prevent introduction of the laparoscope. In such cases new incisions should be made. Even if a space can be made to introduce the instrument, the field for frontal exploration may be small; here a laparoscope with a mobile head is very

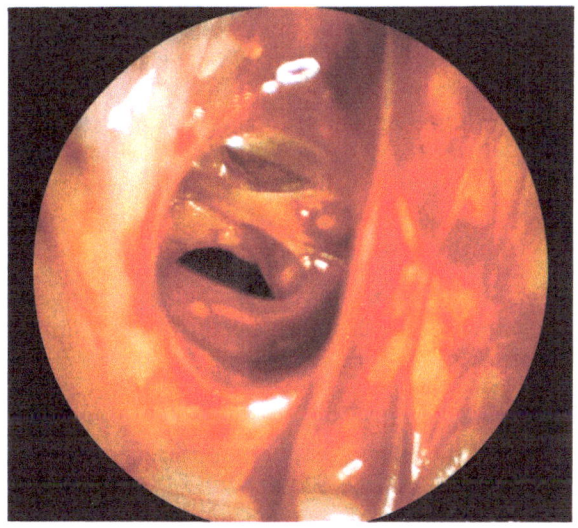

Fig. 3.5. Several layers of adhesions that prevent insertion; exploration impossible

useful for, by shifting it, a view can be had in all directions (see Sect. 1.2.2).

3.2.3 Lysis of Algogenic Adhesions

Abdominal pain is often attributed to "adhesions" following surgery, even if this is difficult to demonstrate. The results of a special laparoscopic study [20, 21] also negated this hypothesis.

Our experience, like that of other authors [17, 22], suggests that the phenomenon of pain from adhesions is quite probable, although it is not particularly frequent when we consider the enormous number of surgical operations performed on the abdomen. For example, it has been established that adhesions form in 0.2% of cases following a straightforward appendectomy and in over 10% of complicated cases, but only rarely do such adhesions cause complaints [21].

Laparoscopy enables us to make or confirm a difficult diagnosis of algogenic adhesions, and often it allows us to resolve any therapeutic problems by means of endoscopic resection. The indications for laparoscopy for resection in patients with abdominal pain must be controlled by highly selective criteria:

1. The patient should have had previous surgery to the abdomen or a clinical history of peritoneal inflammation several years before.
2. Other organic abdominal diseases should be ruled out after a complete clinical and instrumental study.
3. Pain that appears or diminishes with particular movements or in a particular position should be localized in a fixed point of the abdomen.
4. Pain should not be connected with mealtimes or with the digestion in general.

Thanks to sonography after pneumoperitoneum, any preliminary diagnosis can be confirmed on the basis of more concrete evidence. It is possible to use the difference between the cone-shaped shadow corresponding to the pneumoperitoneal gas and the echogenicity of the tissue corresponding to the adhesion itself to localize the lacinia between the peritoneal wall and the organ. Pain is most frequently caused by such adhesions because of the traction that they exert on the parietal peritoneum, which is highly innervated and therefore very sensitive.

The laparoscopic examination must demonstrate the presence of adhesions that can cause pain. During pneumoperitoneum, they resemble cords or curtains stretched between the organ and the abdominal wall (Fig. 3.6). Fairly reliable evidence that these formations are the true cause of pain can be obtained by grasping the adhesion with a forceps and tugging and pulling it downward. If this maneuver either causes pain or increases it, and the pain experienced has the same characteristics as that already mentioned by the patient, a diagnosis of algogenic adhesions is probable [23].

The resection can then be performed at the point where the adhesion is thinner and less vascularized. If a simple cord is found, a clean cut can be made with a scissors (Fig. 3.7). If, on the other hand, the adhesion is a large, thick curtain clinging fast to the wall along an irregular line, the operation is more difficult: small careful incisions must be made with coagulating scissors (Fig. 3.8). It is advisable to make the resection near to the peritoneal wall. As this is highly innervated, however, the heat from the fulguration, the scissor cuts, and the repeated traction can cause the patient great discomfort, particularly when the operation lasts several minutes. It is therefore useful to apply Novocain along the entire line of adhesion attachment, using a thin needle inserted through the laparoscope. If performed this way, the resection is tolerated well by the patient.

This operation has now been thoroughly tested in large series [17, 22, 24, 25] and no complications have been reported in the literature. The results obtained are highly satisfactory: rapid disappearance of, or a marked reduction in, pain in all operated patients. [22, 24–26]. The procedure has been successful in over 60% of cases [17].

Our series (29 cases in 1986) has now increased to 38 cases, with about 90% successful [27]. The long-term results are of great importance. In only one case did pain recur after a few months. In another the pain reappeared a year after resection; the patient asked us to repeat the operation and he then had total, permanent resolution of pain. New adhesions form only rarely following endoscopic resection; this is not the case when surgical resection is performed. The definitive resolution to painful symptoms with laparoscopic resection is yet another of the advantages of laparoscopy, and this simple procedure should be used more often.

→

Fig. 3.6. Algogenic adhesion: cord taut between the abdominal wall and the organs of the lower right quadrant from previous appendectomy

Fig. 3.7. Resection with electrocoagulation; pain arrested immediately

Fig. 3.8. Algogenic adhesion. Upper abdominal wall after resection of a thick extensive adhesion. Anesthesia was administered locally via endoscopy along the entire line of insertion

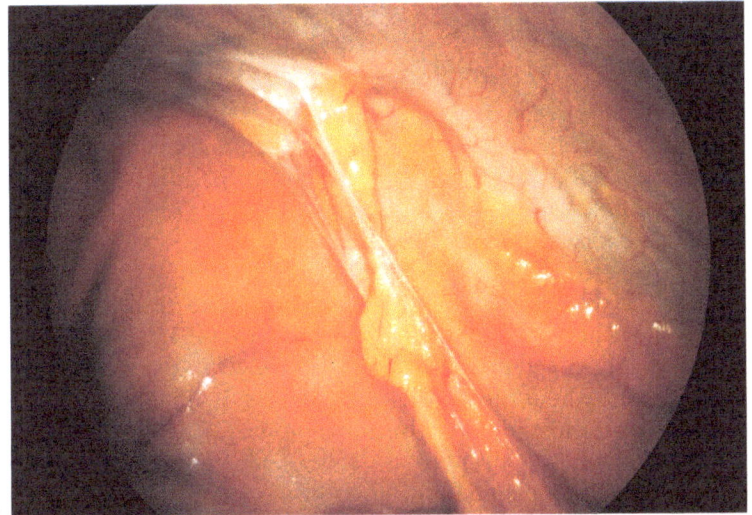

3.6

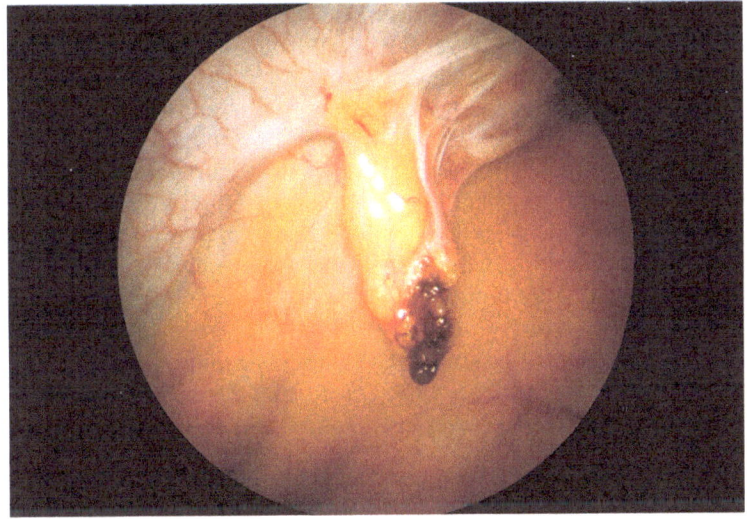

3.7

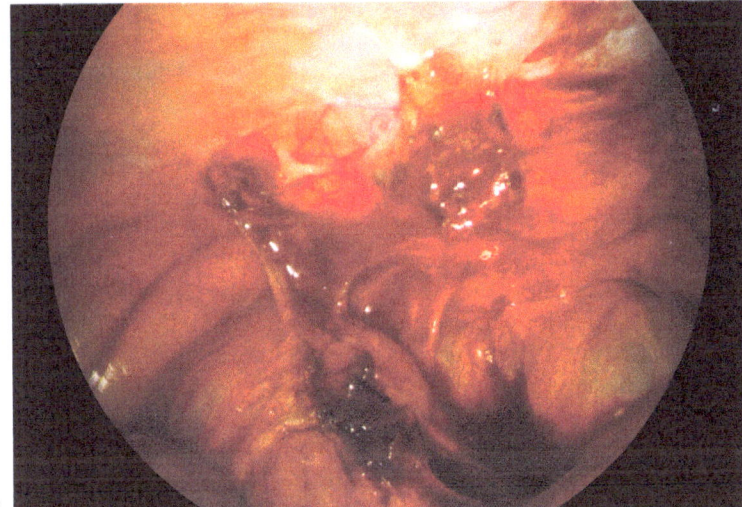

3.8

3.2.4 Puncturing and Drainage
of Cystic Formations

Cystic or pseudocystic formations can be punctured during laparoscopy for diagnostic or therapeutic purposes: a sample of liquid can be taken
for examination, or all the liquid can be drawn in
order to achieve a permanent cure. As already
mentioned, these endoscopic procedures are used
mainly in gynecological laparoscopy, and purely
gastroenterological indications are quite rare. Unexpected cystic formations are sometimes found,
however, and the laparoscopist who is not a gyne-
cologist must know how to deal with a cyst and be
able to correctly perform any minor operations.

Among the gynecological forms are epidermoid
cysts localized in various abdominal sites; they
usually require surgical removal. For the rare
forms of symptomatic nonparasitic cysts of the
spleen, which usually call for total or partial splenectomy, laparoscopic emptying has been proposed; it provides a definitive cure [28].

It is still controversial whether puncturing is
appropriate for patients with gynecological cysts.
Some are of the opinion that this technique is
always contraindicated for *ovarian cysts* because
if the cysts are malignant there may be liquid leakage to the peritoneum, with the spread of neoplastic cells. Others suggest that puncturing should be
performed only when the formation appears to be
benign, i.e., if (a) it has a thin wall with no
external papillary projections, (b) the diameter of
the cyst measures less than 5 cm, (c) it is entirely
mobile, and (d) it appears benign [16]. If a fine
(22-gauge) needle is used, the risk of leakage is
slight; a complete cytological, biochemical, and
bacteriological examination is made of the aspirated
liquid.

At endoscopic inspection totally benign *para-
ovarian cysts* appear to be separate from the
ovary. If large, they may require surgical removal,
but they can also be treated with aspiration under
endoscopy. *Benign cystic teratomas*, a frequent
finding, are easily recognized because the ovary
appears smooth and a yellowish color can be seen
through its capsule. Puncturing is not usually
opportune in such cases because any leakage
causes peritoneal irritation.

Cysts can easily be detected sonographically.
With the improvements in and the more widespread use of surgical sonography, echo-guided
transcutaneous puncturing has largely replaced
the indications for laparoscopy. This is understandable because not only is sonography noninvasive, but it also enables us to identify and
therefore puncture even deep sited formations that
are not visualized with endoscopic exploration. For
example, sonographically guided puncturing of
pancreatic pseudocysts, which is practically impossible under laparoscopy, has become a routine
procedure for both diagnostic and therapeutic
purposes.

Echo-guided transcutaneous puncturing is uti-
lized in treating rare symptomatic cases of *congenital hepatic cysts*. Either simple aspiration of
the liquid is done, with an improvement in the
symptoms [29] which, however, is not long-lasting
[30] or alcohol is instilled with favorable results,
even in cysts with a diameter of up to 20 cm [31].
Recently, because no complications occurred following accidental puncturing of hydatid hepatic
cysts, echo-guided puncturing with drainage has
also been attempted for parasitic cysts [32, 33].
The technique consists of puncturing with echo-
guided placement of a permanent drain and subsequent alcohol introduction. Long-term results
appear highly satisfactory, both at the clinical
and echographic follow-up, with a hyperechogenic image corresponding to scar tissue [34]. No
laparoscopic experience has been accumulated in
this field.

In gynecology, thin-needle echo-guided puncture and furnish material that is highly suitable
for a reliable diagnosis, but it is not widely used
for this purpose, mainly because of the risk that
the disease will spread. Unlike a diagnosis based
on a morphological macroscopic finding under
laparoscopy, a diagnosis based on an echographic
image does not allow us to reliably establish
whether the condition is benign or malignant
[34], and this explains the difficulty involved in
deciding whether it is opportune to puncture or
not.

We may therefore conclude that, in benign
cystic or psuedocystic formations on abdominal
organs, echo-guided transcutaneous puncturing
is very convenient for a variety of reasons. For
ovarian cysts, however, it is still preferable to
puncture during laparoscopy.

3.2.5 Puncturing and Drainage of Abscesses

Laparoscopic puncture has been practiced spo-
radically in the past, but it has never been employed systematically either to diagnose or to treat

abdominal abscesses. This technique now deserves consideration because some interesting observations have recently been made, favorable to laparoscopic puncture for abscesses of the liver. Experience gained with 108 cases shows that with this method a particularly accurate diagnosis and typing of a liver abscess can be obtained; moreover, with direct vision we can choose the most suitable point for needle insertion and for aspiration of material for examination [35]. Puncturing and drainage under laparoscopy have also been used successfully in the treatment of amebic or pyogenic cysts of the liver [36, 37].

The data from laparoscopic puncturing of abscesses are certainly of interest. But echo-guided transcutaneous puncturing, with drainage, where necessary, is widely used and has the edge over laparoscopic puncturing. In fact, it has enormous advantages over any other technique and can be used to resolve very serious pathological conditions without surgery being necessary. It has even been said that percutaneous drainage is one of the most important developments made in the past 10 years [38]. The numerous articles that have appeared in recent years are testimony to the progress made [39–50].

This technique can be used for all abdominal collections, mainly those of the liver, of the subphrenic space, and of the pancreas, *infected* (with positive or negative culture) and *noninfected* (hematomas, pseudocysts, etc.). Positioning of the catheter in the cavity for draining is achieved under sonographic or CT guidance. The therapeutic results – surgery being avoided – are brilliant. In 83.6% of 250 cases collected by Van Sonnenberg et al. [50] from three important US centers, the results were successful. Failures, which are few and far between, are due to such well-established factors as complicated abscesses or phlegmons, the presence of fistulas, or colliquative tumors simulating abscesses. Recurrences are not frequent. Echo-guided puncture is now the treatment of choice for all abdominal abscesses [51].

Recently, this technique has been proposed for *splenic collections*. Echo-guided puncture is done when the sonographic examination indicates the presence of a splenic collection: a complete examination of the aspirated material enables us to clarify the diagnosis and identify the microorganisms responsible for the process. Therapy involves apsiration of the contents and simultaneous lavage. If the collection is voluminous, a catheter can be introduced for drainage and left in situ for a few days to allows repeated lavage. Therapy is completely successful in approximately 80% of cases [52]. The results echo-guided puncturing in the diagnosis of, and therapy for, liquid collections localized in the abdomen have been so positive that there are now almost no indications for laparoscopy.

3.2.6 Endoscopic Operations for Laparoscopic Accidents

We have already discussed the various maneuvers for stopping a hemorrhage and cholorrhea following biopsy taking. We consider the above-described procedures an integral part of the usual laparoscopic technique, but it is important to stress that we can also intervene during laparoscopy to resolve some accidents. As far as frequency and seriousness are concerned, such accidents are just as important as those following biopsy: hemorrhage of the abdominal wall caused by laceration of the veins or arteries by the pneumoperitoneum needle or the trocar. If we respect all the rules for choosing the point for instrument introduction, if a fine needle is used for the pneumoperitoneum (see Sect. 1.1), and if, finally, a preliminary echographic exploration of the area is made (see Sect. 2.2), the larger vessels can be avoided. But we are just as likely to encounter a small artery or an anomalous course or a thick network of vessels that are turgid because the patient has portal hypertension.

As such a hemorrhage hardly ever stops spontaneously, it is necessary to resort to surgery when it occurs. But we should attempt to counteract such accidents endoscopically to obviate surgery where possible. Therefore, we usually perform electrocoagulation on any bleeding vessel that is located.

In order to reduce the chances of damaging a blood vessel, it is preferable to introduce the needle for pneumoperitoneum at the point where the trocar will be introduced, to ensure that there will be only one site of bleeding. In some cases, however, introduction of the instruments at two different points is more convenient, or unavoidable. It is therefore necessary to consider separately hemorrhages of the wall caused by the pneumoperitoneum needle and hemorrhages due to the trocar.

3.2.6.1 Hemorrhages Caused
by the Pneumoperitoneum Needle

The likelihood of bleeding from vessels damaged by the pneumoperitoneum needle must always be considered beforehand. Once the point for trocar introduction has been decided upon, it is advisable to introduce the needle at a point where the internal wall will be visible with and accessible to the laparoscope. The first step of the endoscopic examination is to control the needle protuding within the abdomen. Where a vessel is lacerated, bleeding can be evident immediately (Fig. 3.9); more often, however, as the needle works like a tampon, the bleeding is visible, or increases, only when the instrument is moved. If blood escapes from the hole in the wall when the needle is removed at the end of the examination, the wall must be pinched together with the thumb and forefinger to establish whether the hemorrhage is due to laceration of a superficial vessel. If this maneuver fails to arrest the bleeding, the telescope should be moved internally for a closer observation of the hole from which the blood escapes, and then a two-valved forceps or a probe should be introduced, connected to the electrocoagulator. Depending on the particular case, the abdominal wall can be pinched together at the appropriate point or the tip of the probe can be introduced into the hole and then the charge passed along it. Sometimes the maneuver must be made two or three times, but in the end a definitive coagulation is achieved (Fig. 3.10). Before the fine needle was available we successfully used endoscopic electrocoagulation in four patients with hemorrhaging from the Veress needle. We therefore suggest that this measure always be used in an attempt to stop bleeding before resorting to surgery.

3.2.6.2 Hemorrhage Caused by the Trocar

Hemorrhage from a lesion caused by the trocar can be very serious: when a large artery is damaged surgery is inevitable, and it is almost always emergency surgery. On other occasions, however, especially if we are dealing with hemorrhages of the veins and of the smaller arteries, the situation is less serious and it is therefore advisable to attempt to resolve the accident endoscopically. To arrest a hemorrhage of the abdominal wall, we advocate laparoscopy with electrocoagulation. This technique, which gave us excellent results in two cases, consists of the following steps.

1. Detecting the Hemorrhage. This might seem obvious, but hemorrhage from the wall can easily escape detection and thus become extremely serious. Laceration of a vessel may not cause bleeding while the trocar is in place, and the hemorrhage may start only after the instrument has been withdrawn. The trocar must therefore be withdrawn very slowly and the wall checked to rule out any

Fig. 3.9. Bleeding from puncture with Veress needle for pneumoperitoneum

Fig. 3.10. Same case as in Fig. 3.9; electrocoagulation

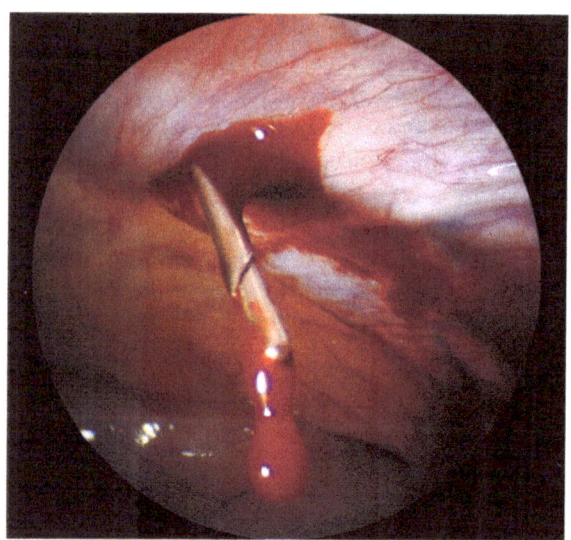

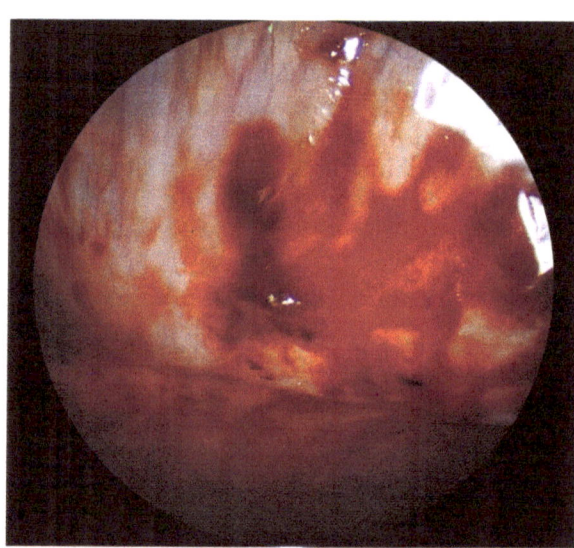

3.9   3.10

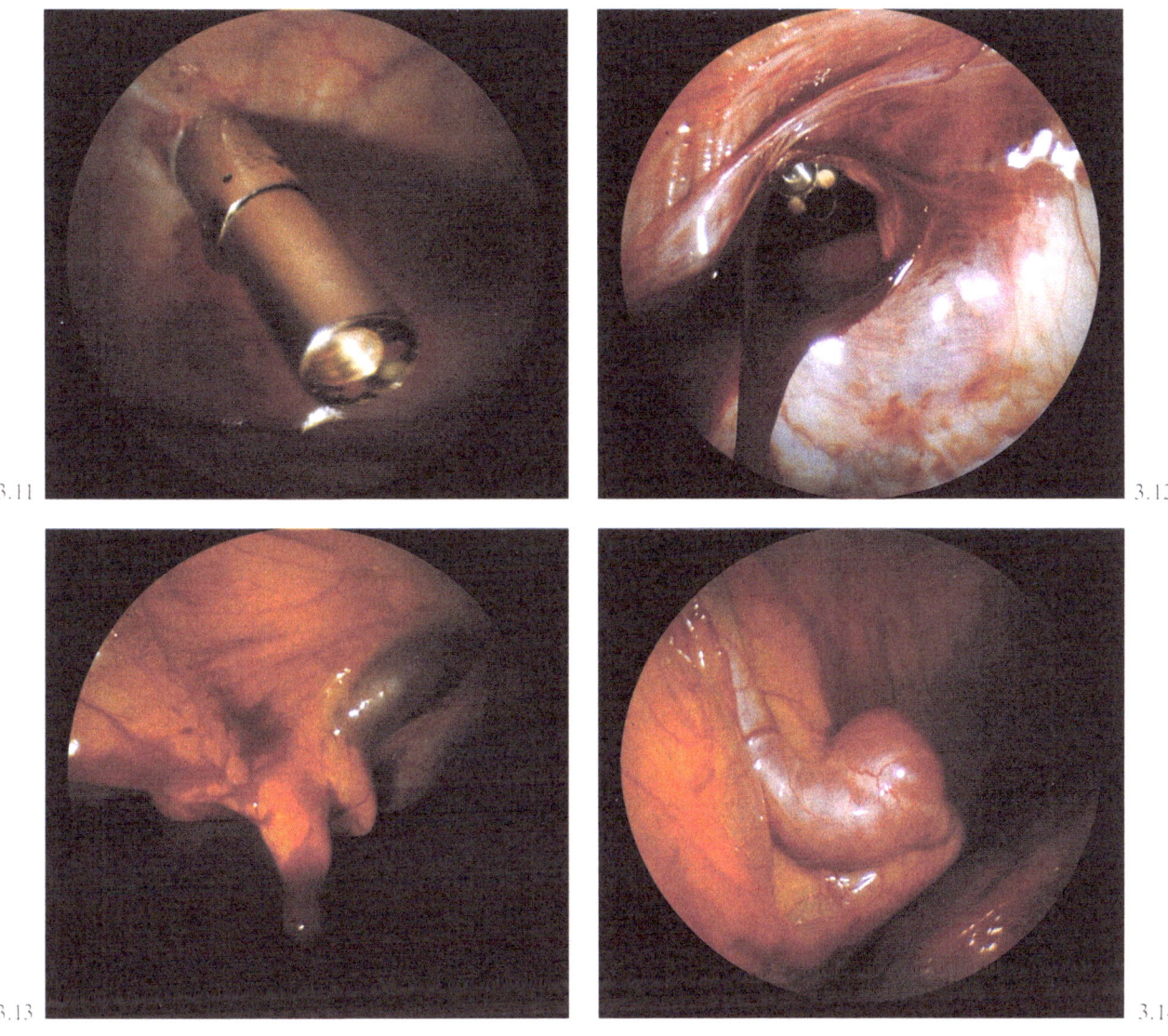

3.11

3.12

3.13

3.14

bleeding sites. This stage is so tricky that Menghini tried to facilitate inspection of the wall layers by inventing a special trocar with side windows [53]. In cases of hemorrhage the trocar and laparoscope must be resunk immediately, as this will temporarily plug the opening.

2. Exploration of the Interior of the Hemorrhage Site. In order to explore the hemorrhage site a second laparoscope must be introduced to determine how the accident happened and to establish whether electrocoagulation can be attempted and, if so, how to go about it. The second laparoscope can also be used to introduce the electrocoagulator (Fig. 3.11). The factors causing the accident can vary greatly, as demonstrated by the two cases

Fig. 3.11. Hemorrhage from trocar introduction. A second laparoscope is introduced

Fig. 3.12. On withdrawal of the laparoscope there is copious bleeding; hemorrhage due to laceration of a small artery of the wall

Fig. 3.13. A drop of blood shows that there is probably a lesion to a vein that is partly hidden by the upper wall fat

Fig. 3.14. Same case as in Fig. 3.13. The lacerated vein is the distal extremity of the recanalized umbilical vein due to portal hypertension. A large syphon can be seen at the base, and the vein is thinner at the upper part

observed by us: in one patient, the laparoscope in situ completely blocked the bleeding, which resumed if the instrument was withdrawn a few millimeters (Fig. 3.12); this indicated that the lesion lay immediately under the parietal serosa. In the other patient the hemorrhage evidently came from a terminal branch of an umbilical vein (Fig. 3.13) that was recanalized because of portal hypertension (Fig. 3.14).

3. Electrocoagulation. The forceps is connected to the electrocoagulator and introduced through the canal of the second laparoscope: the technical modalities used depend upon the particular findings. In the first of our two cases hemostasis was obtained by pressing the margins of the hole together point by point between the forceps and by applying the electric current at each step (Fig. 3.15). In the second case, once the vein had been detected, it was pinched together at several points with the forceps, the current being released until complete hemostasis was achieved (Fig. 3.16).

4. Checking the Results. After the hemorrhage is arrested, the interior must be examined in order to make sure the bleeding has permanently stopped before removing the instrument that caused the lesion. The instrument is then slowly and carefully withdrawn, the entire maneuver being checked with the second laparoscope.

In our view, these operative interventions should at least be attempted in cases of hemorrhage at the abdominal wall. The technique is simple; it can be performed by any laparoscopist with a fair amount of experience and often allows us to avoid surgery.

However, if endoscopic electrocoagulation is not clearly indicated, then no time should be lost in making attempts and no good outcome should be expected. It is highly unlikely that such hemorrhages will stop spontaneously, and the case should be considered an emergency and referred to the surgeon.

3.2.7 Conclusions

1. Gastroenterological laparoscopy has not made any sensational progress in the operative field, but interesting steps forward have been made because of small operations that are well tolerated by the patient under local anesthesia and that take no longer than a normal laparoscopy.

2. Lysis of adhesions due to prior surgery is simple but has been proven useful both for diagnostic purposes – because the field of vision is enlarged by moving partitions and opening spaces so that the laparoscope can be passed through – and for therapeutic reasons if the adhesions are causing pain.

Fig. 3.15. Same case as in Fig. 3.12. Electrocoagulation at the site of bleeding

Fig. 3.16. Same case as in Figs. 3.13 and 3.14. Electrocoagulation

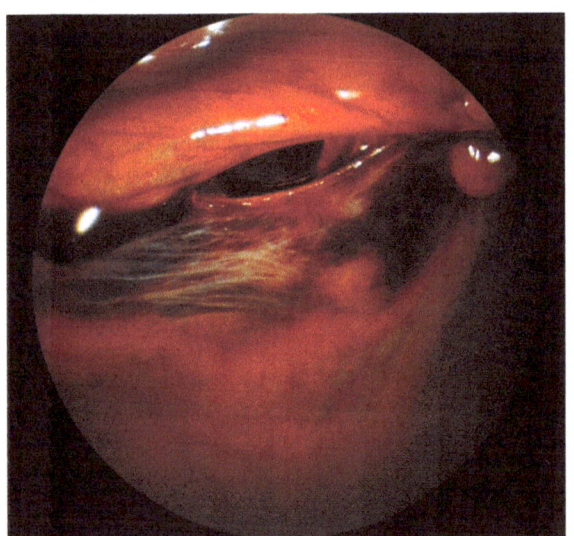

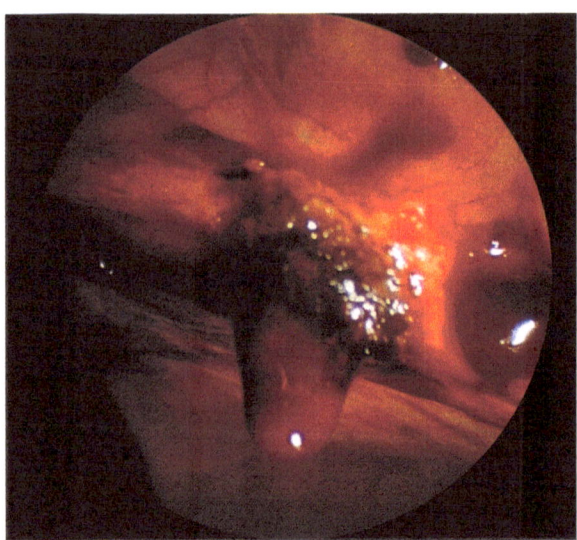

3.15

3.16

3. The laparoscopic puncturing of cystic formations is advisable mainly when they involve the ovaries. For other types of cysts echo-guided transcutaneous puncturing is now preferred.

4. The puncturing of abscess collections during laparoscopy gave highly satisfactory results, but it cannot compete today with echo-guided puncture, which is safer and simpler.

5. Finally, some surgical endoscopic procedures are of interest in accidents such as hemorrhaging from vessel lesions caused by the pneumoperitoneum needle or by the trocar. Endoscopic electrocoagulation can often resolve the accident and should always be attempted before surgery is resorted to.

3.3 Laparoscopy in Patients with Possible Endoabdominal Adhesions

Prior abdominal surgery and a history of inflammation of the peritoneum, gallbladder, stomach, uterus, or adnexa once constituted a contraindication for laparoscopy because of the risk of adhesions. Now, however, the problem is of practical importance because a large number of laparoscopies are performed in patients with a history of one or more surgical operations.

From 1980 to 1983, among a total of 2938 laparoscopies performed at our center, 693 (23.58%) were done in previously operated patients. This high number understandably gave rise to concern because it is well known that endoabdominal adhesions compromise laparoscopy. They can increase any risk and cause the patient greater discomfort and hinder or prevent the examination itself. In recent years, however, the situation has changed, and although the above conditions can still create technical difficulties, they no longer constitute a contraindication to laparoscopy, which can almost always be attempted, provided that certain precautions are taken.

3.3.1 Risks

The risks most feared are those of encountering with the needle, and particularly with the trocar, underlying adhesions running from the wall to the viscera, of lacerating vessels in the adherent tissue with consequent hemorrhage, or of perforating any conglobate intestinal loops adhering to the wall (Fig. 3.17). To reduce these risks to a minimum, the technical rules for laparoscopy must be scrupulously followed, particularly when pneumoperitoneum is performed [54]. If there

Fig. 3.17. Small intestine loops, omental fat, and vessels adhering to the upper wall of the abdomen at the umbilical region. Risk of lesions on trocar insertion

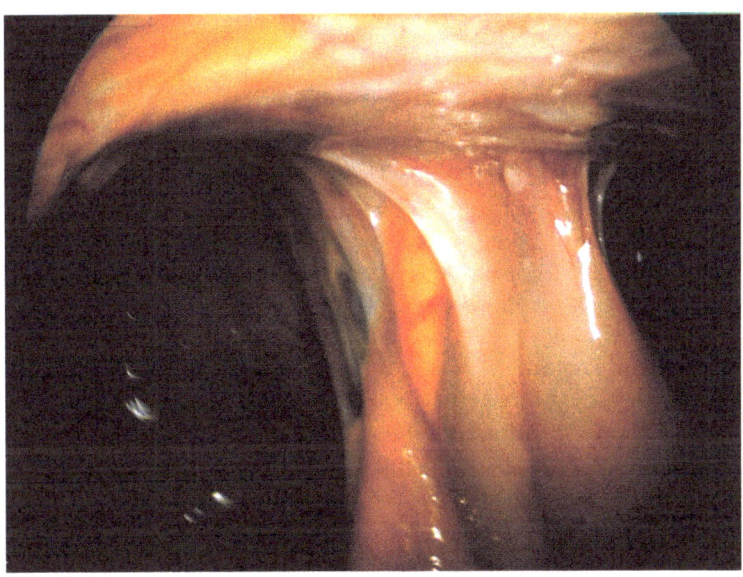

are abdominal scars, the needle for pneumoperitoneum should enter as near as possible to the traditional points but as far as possible from the scars; it should be kept in mind that, where necessary, altogether atypical sites can be chosen. It is also important to make sure that the needle tip is free within the cavity: this is achieved by using a syringe to inject 10–20 cc of gas. If the needle tip is free, the gas is injected without meeting any resistance because the pressure within the cavity is nil. It is difficult to inject gas when the needle tip is blocked and in such cases an attempt should be made to shift the needle; it this maneuver is not successful, a new point for introduction should be chosen.

The point chosen for trocar insertion is of great importance. There are some classical guidelines: the most suitable point is not necessarily the more commonly used one. In a previously operated patient, for example [55], the penetration should be made at least 5 cm from the edge or the extremity of each scar. The underlying peritoneal space must also be carefully explored, using a fine needle mounted on a syringe containing a physiological solution to ascertain whether, on aspirating gas, there is an adhesion-free chamber that is large and deep enough. Another precaution sometimes taken in the past was to make a roentgenogram after pneumoperitoneum to study the gas distribution in the abdomen. This technique can be useful, but the information it gives is not specific enough and is therefore unreliable. For cases in which adhesions are expected, a needle-shaped laparoscope with a diameter of 1.7 mm and frontal vision has also been proposed; it is introduced into the abdomen before hand to establish whether the laparoscopy itself will be successful. This technique has been advocated in gynecological laparoscopy with the patient under general anesthesia. A rapid inspection with this minilaparoscope allows tube sterilization to be performed even in patients for whom laparoscopy appears contraindicated because of previous surgery to the abdomen [56]. This technique is not popular and in any case appears inconvenient for gastroenterological laparoscopy.

The technical precautions mentioned are of vital importance for the safety of the examination. However, for trocar introduction, the most dangerous step, the problems entailed in choosing the point for introduction are practically overcome by our "echography after pneumoperitoneum" technique (see Sect. 2.2.2), which is always used

when it is presumed that there are postoperative adhesions and when adhesions from previous peritoneal inflammation are suspected. With this technique it is also possible to accurately establish whether there is a pocket of gas underneath the point chosen for trocar introduction and whether this chamber is large and deep, and free, so that we can continue with the procedure without incurring any risk. This is without doubt that safest and most rational system available, and the theoretical danger of accidents due to the presence of endoabdominal adhesions appears far greater than the effective risk.

In the more important series that have been reported over the past 10 years, the few accidents that have occurred have not been serious [54, 55, 57–59]. In their series of 836 laparoscopies performed in patients who had had one surgical operation or more, Marti-Vicente et al. reported no deaths, and only "minor" complications in 0.8% of cases; these resolved spontaneously. This percentage is no higher than that reported for laparoscopies performed under normal conditions [57]. From October 1980 to April 1983, i.e., before sonography after pneumoperitoneum was used systematically, we considered 693 laparoscopic examinations performed in 2938 patients who had already undergone abdominal surgery. In only two cases did important accidents requiring surgery occur: The first was perforation of a jejunal loop that adhered to the abdominal wall, and the second involved a copious hemorrhage due to detachment of adhesions from the wall, causing laceration of a vessel, the consequence of tension due to penumoperitoneum. With sonography after pneumoperitoneum the former accident could probably been avoided because the intestinal loop would have been detected. The second accident could not have been foreseen, however, and was therefore unavoidable. As this type of accident is rare, but not impossible, it is important not to interfere with the pneumoperitoneal tension.

It should be remembered that abdominal adhesions can also be found in nonoperated patients. In fact, "spontaneous" adhesions are quite frequent. Found in 7% of 1658 laparoscopies in the series reported by Pleissner et al. [58], these adhesions are particularly, insidious because, as the patients have no scars, adhesions are not suspected. It is indispensable to make a complete study and to take a careful clinical history of each candidate for laparoscopy, for in this way useful information is obtained. If these rules are scrupulously followed, no fear of accidents can now constitute a contraindication to laparoscopy.

Adhesions have also been considered the cause of abdominal pain irradiating to the shoulder during the examination, or in the hours following distension of the abdomen by pneumoperitoneum and consequent to traction on the adhesions themselves. We do not believe that there is a connection between the presence of adhesions in the abdomen and any discomfort to the patient, in particular, any pain. An interesting prospective study of laparoscopies performed in two groups of patients, one with and the other without adhesions, has provided significant findings: Pneumoperitoneum was performed in each patient in exactly the same way – with a gas flow of 500 ml/min and a mean insufflator pressure of 15 mm Hg. No statistically significant differences were found between the groups regarding tolerability [59], which was ascertained on the basis of the responses of the patients in both groups. Overall, therefore, adhesions do not appear to increase disturbances due to laparoscopy.

3.3.2 Results

Adhesions certainly cause technical difficulties and can prevent laparoscopy, or partially limit the field of exploration. So where adhesions are expected, it is important to decide whether or not the examination can be performed and, if so, whether it will be useful. This evaluation is difficult to make a priori, but the results of laparoscopy performed on operated patients over the past 10 years have been encouraging.

If we consider the larger series, which best guarantee experienced operators, in only a few cases was it impossible to introduce the trocar into the abdomen. Marti-Vicente et al. [55, 57] report that in 0.25% of their patients laparoscopy was "impossible" to perform; in one series of

ours laparoscopy was impossible or unsuccessful in 1.88% of previously operated patients.

Sometimes pneumoperitoneum and instrument introduction are achieved but the adhesions are so thick and diffuse that they preclude any useful finding; this happened in 1.17% of our cases. The percentage of total failures is negligible, however. The results of endoscopic exploration appear to depend on the extent of the adhesions and, in the operated patient, on the number, sites, and types of surgical operations already undergone. Not only can "unexpected" adhesions be found in patients who have never been operated on; quite a few operated patients have no adhesions whatsoever. In 167 of our 607 laparoscopies (27.5%) no adhesions were found, and in 144 (23.7%) the adhesions found were so minor that they did not influence the examination at all; thus, laparoscopy was performed without any hindrance in over half of our patients.

The results reported in the recent literature are promising [54, 55, 57–59]. Only De Groen and co-workers found that adhesions from surgery to the abdomen hindered the examination in two thirds of their patients [60]. Visualization of the liver was optimal in patients with subumbilical scars but more limited when surgery had been performed on the upper part of the abdomen, particularly in patients operated on more than once; in only 21% of the latter was it possible to visualize the entire liver [55] (Table 3.1). There is a correlation between the visualization of organs and the type of operation previously performed, as shown in Table 3.2, which reports Pleissner's experience with 467 cases [58].

Our experience was also encouraging, demonstrating that laparoscopy has a high diagnostic efficacy. When we evaluated our results, we took into account the capacity of laparoscopy to answer specific diagnostic questions in a *satisfactory, partially satisfactory,* or *unsatisfactory* way, rather than the explorability of each particular organ. Table 3.3 shows that when the exploration was

Table 3.1. Endoscopic visibility of the liver according to the site of previous laparotomy scars [55]

	No. of patients	Visibility of the liver			Laparoscopy not possible n (%)
		Total n (%)	Partial n (%)	None n (%)	
Supraumbilical scars	314	65 (21)	224 (71.5)	23 (7.5)	2 (0.5)
Infraumbilical scars	522	506 (97)	11 (2.1)	5 (0.9)	0

Table 3.2. Visibility after preceding laparotomy [58]

Kind of operation	Visibility of				
	R. liver (%)	L. liver (%)	Gall-bladder (%)	Stomach (%)	Spleen (%)
Good visibility after:					
Cholecystectomy	33	87	–	85	19
Operation of the stomach	76	59	42	–	24
Operation of the intestine	81	84	38	72	22
Partly visible after:					
Cholecystectomy	10	4	–	–	1
Operation of the stomach	4	3	1	–	–
Operation of the intestine	–	3	13	–	–
Not visible after:					
Cholecystectomy	57	9	–	11	80
Operation of the stomach	20	38	45	–	76
Operation of the intestine	19	13	47	22	78

Table 3.3. Results of laparoscopy in 607 patients with previous abdominal surgery

	Number	Percent
Exploration		
Complete	311	51
Incomplete	296	49
Adhesions		
None	167	27
Unimportant	144	24
Findings with regard to diagnostic question where exploration incomplete		
Satisfactory	187	31
Partially satisfactory	104	17.13
Unsatisfactory	5	1

incomplete, a satisfactory result was nevertheless had in 31% of cases, and in only 1% did we fail to obtain any useful information. As shown in Tables 3.4 and 3.5, the results vary considerably depending on the type of previous operation and the particular diagnostic goal.

As can be seen, although abdominal exploration was incomplete, the highest percentage of successful findings were in cases of diffuse liver disease. In such cases, it may be sufficient to visualize only a part of the liver and to take good biopsies to obtain an accurate diagnosis. On the other hand, laparoscopy was less satisfactory when tumors were searched for because here a reliable diagnosis can be made only if the ex-

Table 3.4. Answer to diagnostic question via laparoscopy in gallbladder-operated patients

Question	No. of cases	Satisfactory n (%)	Partly satisfactory n (%)	Unsatisfactory n (%)
Diffuse hepatopathies	61	50 (82)	10 (16)	1 (2)
Tumor diagnosis and staging	28	15 (53)	12 (43)	1 (4)
Other	11	10 (91)	1 (9)	0 (–)

Table 3.5. Answer to diagnostic question via laparoscopy in stomach-operated patients

Question	No. of cases	Satisfactory n (%)	Partly satisfactory n (%)	Unsatisfactory n (%)
Diffuse hepatopathies	46	36 (78)	6 (13)	4 (9)
Tumor diagnosis and staging	28	1 (39)	15 (54)	2 (7)
Other	10	8 (80)	1 (10)	1 (10)

Table 3.6. Results of laparoscopy lysis of adhesions that hindered exploration (65 cases)

	Number	Percent
Exploration		
Complete	23	35
Incomplete	42	65
Laparoscopic results with regard to diagnostic question where exploration was incomplete		
Satisfactory	19	45.2
Partially satisfactory	9	21.4
Unsatisfactory	14	33.3

ploration is complete, especially in patients with "negative" findings.

If the endoscopic maneuver described in Sect. 3.2 is used, the exploratory conditions are improved: any adhesions covering the surface of an organ can be resected and removed, or gaps between adhesions can be made for laparoscope introduction. We attempted endoscopic resection in 65 cases in which adhesions precluded any useful endoscopic finding. Lysis was technically successful in 83% of cases; in the remaining 17% the characteristics of the adhesions (thickness, extent, vascularization, multiple concamerations) prevented even a partial resection. These maneuvers enabled us to make a complete laparoscopic exploration in 35% of the cases. In 65% the exploration was only partial; in 30% of these cases, however, macroscopic findings were collected and biopsies taken, so a diagnosis was obtained (Table 3.6).

Is it important to stress the advantages of the systematic use of echography for laparoscopy, especially the greater diagnostic efficacy. Moreover, (see Sect. 2.2) with a preliminary echographic study after pneumoperitoneum we can fairly accurately predict whether or not the organs to be examined will in fact be visualized. This enables us to avoid performing useless laparoscopies. By studying the abdominal chart, the most suitable point for trocar introduction can be chosen, and in some cases we can decide a priori upon the route to follow in order to make the most profitable exploration.

3.3.3 Conclusions

1. Although abdominal adhesions are an obstacle to laparoscopy, they do not necessarily constitute a contraindication.

2. If the necessary measures are taken, the risk and the discomfort to the patient are no higher than those incurred in a "normal" examination.

3. Although the efficacy of the examination is reduced by adhesions, in only a small proportion of patients is it useless or impossible to perform a laparoscopic examination; a diagnosis can be made in a high percentage of patients, using special operative maneuvers and a laparoscope with a mobile head.

4. These results are important, because almost a quarter of the candidates for laparoscopy have had previous abdominal surgery, once or more than once.

3.4 Laparoscopic Biopsy

Organ biopsy is an integral part of laparoscopy. As is well known, liver biopsy is usually performed through blind, transcutaneous puncturing, and now thanks above all to Menghini's needle, this technique has become more widespread. Laparoscopy is certainly more of an undertaking but endoscopically guided biopsies are more satisfactory than blind biopsies. There are several advantages.

First, percutaneous biopsies can be taken only from certain parts of the liver, whereas with laparoscopy bioptic samples can be taken from the liver and from the *peritoneum*, the *omentum*, the *mesentery*, and the *ovaries*, as well as from *pathological abdominal masses*. Even splenic biopsies can be taken with laparoscopy. In theory they can also be obtained through a blind transcutaneous puncture, but this is not done because the procedure is too difficult and incurs too high a risk.

Second, laparoscopic biopsy is more fruitful. Samples taken under direct vision provide the most suitable material for examination, thereby reducing to a minimum the number of unsuitable samples and the percentage of false negatives.

Moreover, the histological diagnosis complements the macroscopic finding; in the majority of cases, this is decisive.

Third, laparoscopic biopsy is less dangerous. When the organ or tissue from which the biopsy must be taken can be visualized, there is no risk of inadvertently puncturing an intestinal loop, the gallbladder, a liquid collection, a cyst, or an angioma, and it is possible to avoid puncturing organs or tissues that are highly vascularized, edematous, or that present macroscopic evidence of a risk. For the liver in particular, biopsy can be extremely dangerous if there are signs of cholestasis. Direct vision also allows us to avoid taking a biopsy from an organ covered by adhesions that may hide any risk conditions.

When laparoscopy is performed, a thorough inspection can be made, and the probe can be used to palpate the tissue from which the biopsy must be taken to ascertain its consistency in order to choose the more compact parts. A preliminary "test puncture" can be made with a fine needle to rule out any doubts.

If an accident does occur during laparoscopy itself, we can immediately detect it and control it by following its course step by step; we can use the endoscope to resolve the accident – hemorrhages, for example, can be stopped by applying pressure from the probe below the biopsy hole thereby slowing down the blood flow and enhancing coagulation, and coagulants or electro-coagulation can be applied; or we can refer the patient for surgery as soon as we are sure that the accident cannot be resolved under laparoscopy.

Laparoscopic biopsy can be performed by introducing the various instruments either through the *operating laparoscopic channel* or through a *second hole*, passing the needle and forceps through the lumen of a small trocar. However, we feel it advisable to take a biopsy via the first channel for the following reasons:

1. A second puncture is not necessary and the operation is shorter and therefore better tolerated by the patient.
2. With the correct laparoscopic maneuvers, it is easy to take biopsies from several points on the same organ or from several organs.
3. As the operating laparoscope is under forward vision, it is easy to place the bioptic instrument right on the lesion.
4. Direct placement makes it easier to control any accidents and to take the steps required to resolve the situation.

We usually introduce the bioptic instruments through the operating laparoscope channel and use a second hole only in exceptional circumstances: when the lesion is too distant to be reached or when it is lateral to the laparoscope.

Several innovations have been made in the bioptic field: some of the changes concerning laparoscopic biopsy itself are certainly of interest, but we stress here the importance of the advent and subsequent widespread use of transcutaneous biopsies performed under sonographic and CT-scan guidance. This has radically changed the entire approach to biopsies of the abdomen, and a critical reappraisal of the topic is required to establish which of the traditional indications for laparoscopic biopsy are still valid.

Bioptic puncture is now a routine step in an echographic examination, just as organ biopsies are routinely taken to complete any laparoscopic exploration. The biopsies are taken by inserting a long fine needle through the abdominal wall into the abdomen and then guiding the needle along a sonographically indicated line up to the area indicated by the echographic examination.

Small tissue samples are then aspirated for cytological and histological study. This type of biopsy is often used for the liver, the lymph nodes, pathological abdominal masses, and also for the spleen. The indications for the biopsy and the results it gives vary depending on the organ or tissue to be studied and the diagnostic objective in each individual case, but overall, these biopsies enable us to accurately and reliably diagnose many different diseases in a high percentage of cases.

Any trauma from the maneuver is only slight and it is easily tolerated by the patient; local anesthesia is not required. The risk is minimal [61]: the percentage of deaths (almost always due to hemorrhage) in two large series ranges from 0.006 among 15000 punctures [63] to 0.008 in 11700 [62]. Moreover, in only a small number of cases have serious accidents requiring surgery occurred.

Fine-needle percutaneous biopsy can also be done under the guidance of *computerized tomography*. Real-time sonography calls for specific experience and great expertise, but it does appear to improve the results of abdominal organ biopsies. The equipment is convenient and economical, the spatial resolution is important in the parenchymatous tissues, and the image, which is three-dimensional, can be obtained on an infinite number of planes [64, 65]. It is thus evident why fine-needle transcutaneous guided biopsies have become very important in the diagnosis of abdominal diseases.

Once there was some discussion about whether it was more suitable to make blind percutaneous biopsies or laparoscopically guided biopsies. Now, however, the main and the most up-to-date alternative to laparoscopic biopsy is echo-guided fine-needle biopsy. It is therefore important to carefully consider when it is advantageous to use laparoscopic biopsy and when to perform echo-guided fine-needle biopsy.

We therefore report on innovations made in laparoscopic biopsies of various organs and tissues, but we also compare the two techniques and attempt to establish the indications valid for laparoscopic biopsy and those valid for echo-guided fine-needle biopsy.

3.4.1 Biopsy of Peritoneum, Mesentery, and Omentum

No important technical innovations have been made in this field. A two-valve forceps is still used: when the instrument is placed on the organ or tissue from which the biopsy is to be taken, the valves are kept open; when they are then closed, a tissue fragment is caught in the instrument and then detached through the pulling action made when the forceps is withdrawn.

An important methodological innovation has been made, however, in the use of multiple biopsies. The main use has been the staging of ovarian carcinomas. Often, small formations are found on the peritoneum (nodules, plaques, areas of thickening, or apparent fibrosis of the serosa). These signs may be due to small granulomas or indicate previous inflammation; they may be of no clinical importance, or they may be pathological processes of great importance. These suspect formatons, the macroscopic diagnosis of which is dubious, call for multiple biopsies. Some biopsies may in fact be positive for neoplasms while others may give findings that are not significant. This approach has enabled us to markedly reduce the percentage of false negatives made with single biopsies.

3.4.1.1 Comparison of Indications

Peritoneal diseases for which biopsy may be indicated are mainly neoplastic – primary and metastatic, or chronic inflammatory – in particular, granulomatous. These processes are often characterized by a few, fairly thick, small lesions localized on the abdominal wall or on the serosa of organs. The size and the position of the lesions, however, make it almost impossible for them to be detected sonographically, so there are no indications for biopsy because the US examination is negative and no target is found.

If there are clinical indications for performing a biopsy, laparoscopy is the only nonsurgical way of obtaining a tissue sample suitable for making an anatomohistological diagnosis. Laparoscopic biopsy is therefore still as valuable as it ever was in the majority of cases of peritoneal disease.

Guided fine-needle biopsy, on the other hand, can be performed only on larger, sonographically detected targets – in other words, where lesions of the peritoneum have the characteristics of a mass, as with neoplastic infiltration of the mesentery or the omentum or when a retroperitoneal mass invades the abdominal cavity. As the sonographic finding is clear, the needle can be guided correctly and enough material aspirated for the diagnosis. To obtain optimal results, several samples are taken from different points, particularly if the echographic structure of the mass is in homogeneous, with solid areas and areas of necrosis or of liquefaction.

The results reported in the literature are highly satisfactory: in the larger series an accurate diagnosis was made in an average of 94% of cases; the sensitivity is 91% and the specificity 98% [66].

The risks incurred with this maneuver are minimal: the needle is so fine that there is almost no risk of hemorrhaging; overlying structures, such as the stomach or intestine, can be crossed without causing any damage. In these cases it is therefore preferable to puncture with a fine needle, and laparoscopic biopsy is of little or no use.

Moreover, fine-needle biopsy is quite useful when there is sonographic evidence of a small abdominal fluid collection, because it is the only way of extracting enough material to make a diagnosis. The liquid can be studied in culture and a chemical and cytological examination made to clarify the nature of the process that may, for example, be a mesenteric cyst, a dried phlogistic collection, or a colliquative tumor.

Peritoneal pseudomyxoma, for example, is a lesion that gives different findings and that is indicated by sonography without its real entity being diagnosed. The sonographic finding may be aspecific abdominal masses, multiple liquid sac collections or, finally, ascites without masses [67]. A fine-needle biopsy with samples taken from different points in the solid areas as well as from the liquid collections enables us to make a diagnosis that would otherwise be extremely difficult. In all such cases we can avoid performing laparoscopy, which is useless if the collections are deep-seated or hidden.

3.4.1.2 Conclusions

1. No great innovations have been made in laparoscopic biopsy of the peritoneum, but the technique is still of value as far as traditional indications are concerned.

2. When solid masses or liquid collections are detected sonographically, however, echoguided fine-needle biopsy is of great diagnostic value and carries no risk; it should therefore be considered the technique of choice.

3.4.2 Liver Biopsy

Liver biopsy is the first type of closed-organ biopsy to be employed. It gives exceptionally valuable diagnostic and anatomohistological information on some liver diseases and on their evolution. Moreover, with the use of Menghini's needle blind transcutaneous biopsy is a valuable procedure that is also simple to perform and carries a relatively small risk.

The number of liver biopsies performed at the Royal Free Hospital of London [68] steadily increased from 1960, when about 300 were performed, until 1980, when over 1400 were performed. Only recently has the number dropped, and the reasons for this will be discussed later. Diffuse liver disease, in particular chronic hepatitis and cirrhosis, is the most prevalent indication for liver biopsy. These data, however, are from Britain, where laparoscopy is not widely used. They therefore pertain to transcutaneous biopsy.

Laparoscopic biopsy is particularly useful where *focal lesions* of the liver are suspected. The biopsy can be guided under direct laparoscopic vision, the sample thus being taken from a pre-established point, whereas with blind biopsy the sample can be taken only haphazardly from a diseased tissue, with a consequently high risk of false negatives being obtained. Another important indication for liver biopsy is suspected *diffuse liver disease*, and almost all authors [69–77] are of the opinion that laparoscopically guided biopsy gives far better results than blind biopsy.

The tendency to use laparoscopically guided biopsy in patients with diffuse liver disease has therefore increased considerably, as is borne out by the data reported by the two institutes of general medicine at Padua, specializing in liver diseases [78]. In 1974 the two divisions sent 130 and 120 blind biopsies respectively to the Institute of Pathology for a diagnosis of chronic hepatitis and cirrhosis. Only 14 and 53 laparoscopic biopsies respectively were taken. In 1983 the number of percutaneous biopsies taken fell to 48 and 17 respectively, while the number of larparoscopic biopsies rose to 101 and 67. The total number of blind biopsies received by the Institute of Pathology dropped from 322 in 1974 to 158 in 1983.

In recent years important advances have been made: technical innovations have enhanced the efficacy and reduced the risks of the procedure, and the advent of fine-needle biopsy, i.e., guided using noninvasive techniques, has greatly modified the indications for laparoscopic liver biopsy.

3.4.2.1 Technical Advances

The way in which a laparoscopic biopsy is taken has not changed. As a rule, we prefer to take a tissue sample by passing the instrument through the operating laparoscopic channel and make a "second hole" only in exceptional circumstances. This also applies to the liver, for which multiple biopsies are often required – from the right and the left lobe. The real modifications made have been in the instruments now used: cutting needles and the Bio-Plug.

Cutting Needles
The most widespread and traditional technique for transcutaneous and laparoscopic liver biopsy employs Menghini's needle and aspiration biopsy. Menghini's needle of course has several advantages over the other types of needles. But it also has a disadvantage, especially if the tissue is hard and friable: with puncture and aspiration we may obtain a small, fragmented sample that makes the

diagnosis difficult, sometimes even impossible. This shortcoming is widely acknowledged, even by those who continue to use the technique for various reasons [68] (it is safer, easier to use, and cheaper than other techniques). More satisfactory tissue fragments can be obtained with instruments that cut rather than tear the tissue because they reduce fragmentation and cellular trauma to a minimum. The first of these instruments, Vim-Silverman's needle, was made available in 1938 and is therefore certainly no novelty. The main part of the instrument consists of a slotted cannula with two cutting valves that slice off the fragment of liver tissue required.

Vim-Silverman's needle and others like it have been used successfully in many centers and are still in use at some [72, 77, 79]. They are more difficult to use than Menghini's needle, however, and because of this the biopsy obtained is not always satisfactory. They are also more dangerous than aspiration biopsy needles. We do not recommend Vim-Silverman's needle, and have always preferred a 1.9-gauge Menghini's needle, which has given good results.

Worthy of mention are Palmer's pincers and similar models, which consist of a pointed valve with a small chamber that can be closed in order to section and trap the tissue fragment in the chamber. Ideally, the pincers should be used to take biopsies of masses, but they have also proved satisfactory for liver biopsies, although they are now no longer used for this purpose.

A quite different model with a cutting needle has enabled us to obtain liver biopsies of far better quality and it has several advantages for the diagnosis. For several years now, the larger centers have preferred the *Bio-cut* or the *Tru-cut*, which are quite similar to each other because they are quite simple to use for laparoscopic liver biopsies and they provide good-quality fragments. We have routinely used the Bio-cut since 1978.

This needle, which has a stainless-steel 2-mm diameter cannula, is 15 cm long for introduction through a second hold and 47 cm long for introduction through the operating laparoscopic channel. Through the cannula runs a full cylindrical stylet, the distal end of which tapers for about 2 cm, ending in a flat blade with a very fine point (Fig. 3.18). The instrument is easy to use: its tip is made to touch the liver surface at a pre-established point. Using the left hand, pressure is exerted on the appropriate handle, and the stylet is moved forward alone until it penetrates 2–3 cm into the

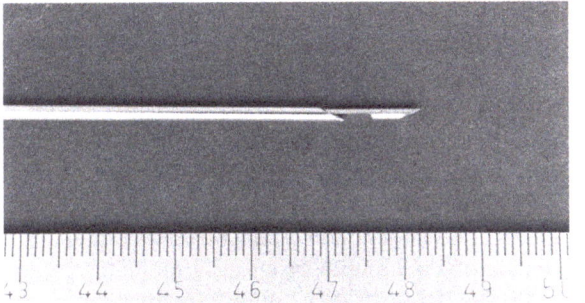

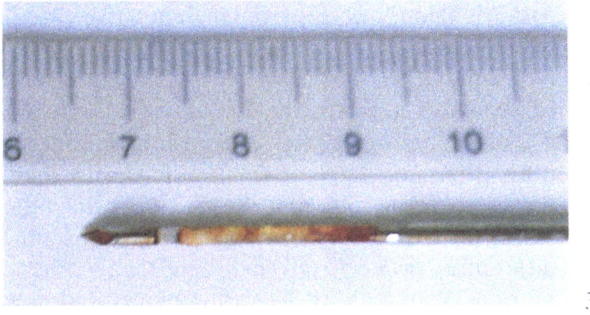

Fig. 3.18. Bio-cut, distal tip

Fig. 3.19. Bio-cut with cylindrical liver tissue fragment

parenchyma; then, using the right hand, the sheath is pushed forward so that a small cylinder of tissue is cut and trapped in the space formed by the sheath at the flat part of the stylet. The instrument is then quickly withdrawn. The entire maneuver is performed as quickly as aspiration needle biopsy. As every step is done under direct laparoscopic visual control, the Bio-cut needle guarantees the best yield with minimum risk. The Bio-cut can also be used for transcutaneous blind biopsy. As it cuts rather than tears, the sample obtained is an even cylinder (about 2 cm long) that is neither deformed nor coarctate; above all, it rarely fragments (Fig. 3.19).

The value of this type of cutting needle is particularly evident in cases of *diffuse liver disease*, especially where a differential diagnosis is to be made between chronic hepatitis and cirrhosis. With a hard liver, tissue fragmentation is more likely to occur. In such cases the size of the fragment is of vital importance to the pathologist because the diagnosis is based upon the tissue structure, so the larger the sample the more reliable the diagnosis. Orlandi and co-workers have demonstrated that there is a 59.6% agreement between macroscopic and histological findings in alcoholic liver disease when the bioptic fragment is under 8 mm, but when the sample measures over 9 mm the agreement rises to 79.7% [80].

Data from large series have been collected to compared the results of laparoscopic biopsies obtained with Menghini's needle and with Bio-cut. Sessa found that a diagnosis was made with 84.2% of aspiration biopsies obtained with Menghini's needle whereas a diagnosis was made with 98.5% of 1509 biopsies that were made afterwards with the Bio-cut [81]. In our center, an initial batch of 224 laparoscopic biopsies were taken with Menghini's needle from patients with chronic liver diseases; 14% of these tissue samples were not suitable for diagnosis [70]. In a later series of 306 cases in which the Bio-cut was used, only 4% of the tissue samples were unsuitable for diagnosis; the percentage of definite diagnoses therefore rose from 75% to 85% [75]. On the other hand, for focal lesions of the liver no substantial differences were found between the results of biopsies obtained with aspiration biopsy and those obtained with the cutting needles.

Bio-Plug
Although the Bio-Plug is discussed is length in Sect. 1.3, we consider it opportune to deal with it briefly here because it is not simply a technical innovation. It has also greatly modified traditional concepts regarding the risks, the consequences, and the limitations of laparoscopic liver biopsy [68]. It has, in fact, enabled us to use the laparoscopic channel to stop a severe hemorrhage or cholorrhea consequent to taking a biopsy, and we can therefore safely say that laparoscopic liver biopsy is now almost free of risk to the patient.

The importance of this claim is evident from all standpoints. Irrespective of any other considerations, laparoscopic liver biopsy should always be preferred to blind biopsy, for a considerable number of accidents have occurred with the latter, as is borne out by a recent report from the well-known and reputable Royal Free Hospital of London: among 6379 blind aspiration biopsies performed in the past 10 years, there have been "only two deaths" and 40 intraperitoneal hemorrhages that called for transfusions [68].

But not only has the Bio-Plug made the procedure almost risk free, it has also made biopsies easier to perform, and therefore more widespread, with a consequent increase in the diagnostic potential of the entire laparoscopic examination.

The fear of accidents, which is understandable, can condition the operator, who tends to rigor-ously respect all the contraindications (coagulatory defects, passive liver congestion, biliary stasis, etc.), and thus not to punctured if conditions are not ideal. He therefore tends to limit the number of biopsies taken with a view to reducing the risk of unpredictable accidents, such as laceration of an intrahepatic blood vessel or bile duct. However, it is well known that there is not always a correlation between postbiopsy hemorrhage and the coagulation index [82].

It is thus evident that if we do not perform a biopsy that could allow us to make an otherwise impossible diagnosis the problem remains unsolved, and that if we take a single biopsy when multiple biopsies are indicated we risk making an unreliable or incorrect diagnosis. Thanks to the Bio-Plug, the contraindications to liver biopsy are few and far between. So where it is indicated the biopsy can be safely taken, even in patients with coagulatory defects or with blood congestion or biliary stasis, thus allowing a diagnosis to be made in conditions that until recently were considered preclusive (Figs. 1.8–1.10). Moreover, up to four biopsies can be taken with complete safety from different points of the organ, thus increasing the probability of obtaining significant liver tissue. The diagnostic value of laparoscopic biopsy of the liver is thus far greater than it once was.

3.4.2.2 Echo-guided Fine-needle and Laparoscopic Biopsy

The advent of ultrasound-guided liver biopsy [83, 84] and its increasingly widespread use has brought about a radical change in the diagnostic approach to liver diseases. This technique is also a valid alternative to laparoscopic biopsy. In a large number of cases of liver disease it is now considered the method of choice, thanks to improvements made in the tissue sampling technique and in the preparation of materials, as well as to the ever increasing experience accumulated by pathologists.

We recognize that this technique is invaluable, but we also believe it inadvisable to be categorical, and a careful appraisal should be made to establish whether echo-guided liver biopsy should altogether replace laparoscopic biopsy or whether there are still valid indications for the latter. Different considerations should be made for the diagnosis of *diffuse disease* and *focal lesions of the liver*.

Diffuse Liver Disease

Sonography neither facilitates biopsy taking nor improves upon its diagnostic efficacy in diffuse liver disease. In cases of diffuse disease, the concept of a "guide" is considered untenable because the site for the biopsy is not indicated echographically. Yet among cases of diffuse liver disease there are those in which it is important to take a biopsy from one point rather than from another. During the direct laparoscopic examination the organ often reveals aspects that vary from site to site, with some areas apparently normal while others are fibrous or present scar retractions, areas of congestion, or isolated nodules from regeneration. These different characteristics reflect equally different situations and a target biopsy under direct visualization may enable us to make a more reliable and accurate diagnosis. Echography can demonstrate only diffuse alterations that are not particularly significant and usually fails to indicate the points where biopsies should be taken (Fig. 3.20).

So in cases of diffuse liver disease laparoscopy is the only available means to guide biopsy taking. Of course, echography is very useful because it enables us to avoid puncturing cysts, angiomas, and abscesses that may be deeply embedded and therefore overlooked at laparoscopy.

In diffuse liver disease, therefore, laparoscopic biopsy is still of diagnostic value and echo-guided

biopsy cannot be suggested as an alternative to it. The latter does not even seem to have any advantages over blind biopsy.

Focal Liver Lesions

Where lesions are focal, sonography is of fundamental importance as a guide for bioptic puncture. Echography provides clear findings and an accurate target for biopsy taking, and any point of the organ can easily be reached.

It is important to bear in mind that for lesions localized in the right lobe, and for subdiaphragmatic masses in particular (7th and 8th segments), the needle is introduced through the intercostal spaces, while for lesions of the right (5th and 6th segments) and the left lobes the subcostal route is used [85].

Biopsy is a necessary complement to the echographic examination: it either confirms or negates the sonographic finding and allows us first to establish whether the disease is benign or malignant, and then to specify the tumor type.

Sonographically guided biopsy for focal lesions of the liver can be made with different types of needles: large and fine, noncutting and cutting needles being used. *Large needles* have a caliber of over 1 mm. The most common are the Menghini cutting needles (18 gauge), although they are now used less than before because, as they are more traumatic than other types of needle, the patient must be hospitalized [86, 87], and improvements in preparation techniques for aspirated material and the experience gained by pathologists in reading the preparations has meant that highly satisfactory results are also obtained with *fine needles*.

Noncutting needles (Chiba's needle, 7 mm in diameter, 22 gauge; the spinal 21–25 gauge needle; etc.) have a point with a fluted lip that makes deep penetration as atraumatic as possible. With aspiration a collection of cells with only a little stroma is obtained.

The *cutting* needle may be either shaped like a drill bit (Otto, Franseen) or blunted circularly at a different angulation (Histocut, Surecut); it can section a small piece of tissue that is then aspirated. These needles enable us to take samples from more compact tissues and to obtain fragments that are larger and therefore more suitable for microhistological examination.

The material aspirated with fine needles is prepared following the cytological technique used for the smear test or with inclusion.

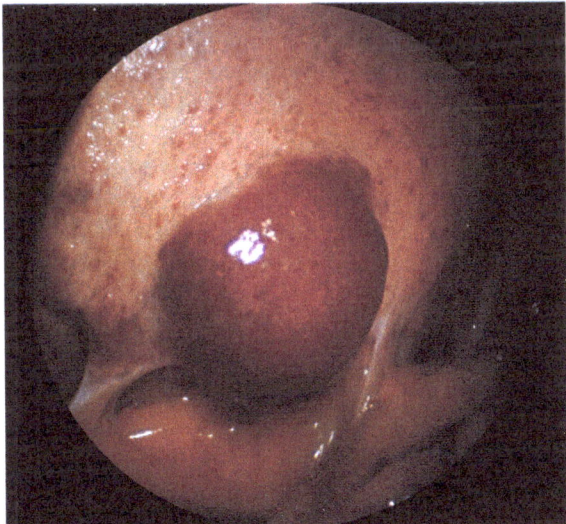

Fig. 3.20. Micronodular liver cirrhosis with a large regenerative nodule. Depending on the point from which the biopsy is taken, the biopsy finding may be cirrhosis or almost normal liver tissue

With smear cytology the cells are preserved very well; this means that an accurate study can be made and a detailed picture obtained. As it is rapidly performed, the quality of the biopsy can be immediately evaluated, and if the material is unsuitable, further samples can be taken.

Apart from cellular studies, microhistological examinations are made to evaluate the structure of the tissue. This increases our capacity to type and reduces the incidence of false negatives, above all in cases of well-differentiated neoplasias. The results of cytology for the inclusion of materials aspirated with fine noncutting needles appear superior to those of smear cytology [87–89].

The results of echo-guided transcutaneous biopsy are good and allow the diagnosis to be made in a high percentage of cases. The topic has been dealt with exhaustively by different authors, but we feel it opportune to stress the following point: Large needles appear to be more satisfactory. The initial comparative studies revealed that a malignant form was diagnosed in 92% [90] and 98% [91] of cases when an 18-gauge needle was used but in only 78% [90] and 84% [91] when 22-gauge needles were used. The information obtained with large needles is more complete, and there is a marked improvement in the diagnosis of the benign forms. However, now that results obtained with fine needles have been improved upon, the larger-gauge needles are being used less frequently. In fact, the diagnosis of focal lesions made with fine-needle biopsies is now optimal [87, 92–98], with a diagnostic accuracy of 94–95%, a sensitivity of 90%–94%, and a specificity of 100%.

It has been demonstrated that with a single "passage" using a fine needle, the diagnostic accuracy is limited to about 70%, while with multiple passages the accuracy increases to 80%–94% [83, 91, 92, 99, 100]. With multiple passages some authors have obtained adequate samples in 100% of cases using a fine needle, but in only 88% of cases when using a large needle [86]. Worthy of note is the important difference found in efficacy between the first and the second passage. In a series of 374 biopsies there was an overall sensitivity of 91.3%, a specificity of 100%, and a diagnostic accuracy of 94.6%. After the first passage the accuracy wasd 72.5% and after the second it rose to 90.2%. When a third passage was made, the accuracy rose to 94.6% [101]. In each individual case these authors evaluated the need for any further passages making use of rapid staining which, in only a few seconds, allows us to make a

decision on the basis of the results from the preceding biopsies. The results obtained from cytology associated with microhistology were more satisfactory than those obtained with smear or inclusion cytology alone [96, 102].

Tissue fragments for inclusion can be obtained with fine cutting needles, but in a large number of cases they are also obtained with noncutting needles, although special technical precautions such as gentle aspiration and needle and syringe heparinization must be taken [96, 103].

Echo-guided liver biopsy is therefore a highly effective method for the diagnosis of focal lesions of the liver and should be considered the technique of choice in this field. The highly satisfactory results obtained suggest that fine cutting or noncutting needles should be used in the first instance; the large needles should be used only when inclusion or smear cytology and microhistology fail to furnish a definite diagnosis [86, 87, 95, 104].

In view of the extremely high percentage of diagnoses obtained and the low risk incurred with transcutaneous echo-guided biopsies, it might be concluded that laparoscopic biopsy is no longer necessary. In most of the studies dealing with this topic, the bulk of which are from institutes of radiology, laparoscopy is not even mentioned, and some authors [104] are of the opinion that echo-guided fine-needle biopsy can replace laparoscopic biopsy in the diagnosis of focal lesions of the liver, because it (a) requires neither premedication nor local anesthesia, (b) carries none of the risks of laparoscopy, (c) is tolerated well by the patient, and (d) is more economical.

However, it must be borne in mind that the statistics reported in the literature on the sensitivity, specificity, and diagnostic accuracy of fine-needle biopsy are often from highly selected series and therefore cannot be considered absolutely reliable. In series consisting of patients with unknown tumors the percentages of diagnoses are lower [105].

Considerable difficulties are involved in diagnosing benign lesions [106], with the risk of obtaining false cytological negatives, and highly differentiated malignant forms, because their neoplastic cells are similar to those of normal hepatocytes [103, 104, 106].

Diagnostic failure can occur for the following reasons:

1. If the lesions are small and deep it may be difficult to guide the long, thin needle and the

biopsy may not be obtained from the diseased tissue.

2. The aspirated material may be necrotic and insufficient for a reliable reading.

3. As echo-guided biopsy and cytological and microhistological studies call for technical skill and considerable experience, technical errors and incorrect readings are more likely.

Finally, although the risk is low, there is a risk. Deaths have occurred [107], as have hemorrhages requiring surgery [92] or transfusions; some hemorrhages have resolved spontaneously [83, 87, 99, 104, 108]. Nor should we ignore the less serious accidents that have also been reported [91, 96, 102, 105].

It is thus evident that the indications for laparoscopic biopsy in the diagnosis of focal diseases of the liver have now been considerably reduced, especially where metastases are concerned. Echo-guided fine-needle biopsy is not without a doubt the approach of choice. However, laparoscopic biopsy is still indicated in the following circumstances [109, 110]:

1. When fine-needle biopsy is either impossible or unsatisfactory

2. When it is difficult to make a differential diagnosis between a benign or a malignant tumor

3. When the characteristics of the cells preclude an adequate diagnostic accuracy (distinction between primary or secondary neoplasia, typing of the tumor, etc.)

4. When the cytological and microhistological findings are negative but a malignant liver tumor is considered possible or is suspected on the basis of biohumoral or clinical findings. This aspect is dealt with in Sect. 5.3.

3.4.2.3 Conclusions

1. Laparoscopic liver biopsy is still a valid means for diagnosing liver diseases.

2. Two important technical innovations are the cutting needles now employed (e.g. Biocut) and the Bio-plug, both of which have markedly reduced the risks of this maneuver.

3. Laparoscopic biopsy is far superior to blind transcutaneous biopsy.

4. Echo-guided biopsy using a fine needle is the most important advance that has been made

in this field: it has literally revolutionized the diagnostic approach to diseases of the liver.

5. In diffuse liver diseases echo-guided biopsy is useless, so here laparoscopic biopsy is still the most effective available biopsy technique.

6. In focal lesions, on the other hand, the results obtained through the cytological and microhistological study of the material collected by means of echographically guided puncture are excellent. This highly effective and almost totally noninvasive technique has therefore become, in a short period of time, the diagnostic approach of choice in this particular field.

7. Until recently, laparoscopically guided liver biopsy was the best available means for making an accurate and reliable diagnosis of liver diseases.

8. This technique has lost many of its indications, but all.

9. The cytological and microhistological findings with echo-guided puncture may be uncertain or negative because the sample material is insufficient or inadequate. In 10%–25% of cases, in fact, a false negative is suspected, and in these cases laparoscopy with a biopsy taken under direct visualization is still indicated, as it can satisfactorily resolve the diagnostic problem.

3.4.3 Pancreas Biopsy

Until recently any exploration of the pancreas under laparoscopy was impossible because of the organ's retroperitoneal position; nor was it possible to obtain a biopsy of the pancreas: it was considered too difficult and risky to make a puncture in a deep, hidden area. In fact biopsy taking is not very effective and is risky when we cannot (a) take the biopsy from the most significant part of the organ, (b) avoid the risky areas (large vessels, cysts or pseudocysts, collections, etc.), (c) immediately detect any accidents caused by the biopsy taking, and (d) promptly take the measures necessary to deal with the accident. Thus, except for the odd attempt, biopsies of the pancreas were made only when it became possible to visualize the pancreas laparoscopically. Pancreatic biopsy should therefore be considered an innovation of theoretical importance.

Laparoscopically guided biopsy of the pancreas can be done directly with fine (diameter 0.6–0.8 mm) needles introduced transcutaneously or with Menghini's or Tru-cut needles; Robber's pincers can be used, but in this case the instruments must be introduced through a second hole [111, 112]. We have always used the Bio-cut, which is introduced through the operating laparoscope channel.

Even though the experience gained in this field is limited, we may safely say that with laparoscopic biopsy of the pancreas the risks are minimal. No deaths have been reported. Among the 215 biopsies performed by Ishida [112], important accidents occurred in seven cases (3.3%): pancreatic juice leakage, spread of necrotic tissue to the peritoneal cavity, and acute pancreatitis. These complications were all satisfactorily resolved with conservative therapy.

After performing biopsy it is advisable to press the sites of bleeding for a few minutes with the probe and to make sure that a clot has formed. Where necessary, the Bio-Plug can also be used to plug the biopsy hole.

3.4.3.1 Results

The series of Ishida [112], which consisted of 124 patients studied laparoscopically, gives a reliable picture of the results. In cases of acute pancreatitis a biopsy was not always necessary for a diagnosis; a sample taken from the cytosteatonecrosis plaques sometimes solved the problem. In half the cases, the diagnosis was made on the basis of findings from biopsies taken from true pancreatic tissue. In chronic forms of the disease biopsy is often indispensable because it is difficult to make a differential diagnosis macroscopically between circumscribed chronic pancreatitis and a tumor; in 70% of these cases it was possible to make a histological diagnosis. A histological diagnosis was made of 50% of carcinomas of the head and of 84% of those of the body and the tail. If the cytological examination (sample taken with a fine needle) and the histological results are combined results improve, reaching 74% and 88.7% for carcinomas of the head and of the body and tail respectively.

So important progress has been made in the diagnosis of diseases of an organ that, until recently, was almost impossible to study. However, in order to evaluate the practical importance of these results, they should be compared with those obtained with biopsies made under the guidance of the various imaging techniques available.

3.4.3.2 Echo-guided Fine-needle Biopsy

Sonography is an exceptionally important means for diagnosing diseases of the pancreas, but, although images indicating the presence of diffuse or circumscribed pancreas alterations are usually quite informative, often they do not enable us to specify the nature of the particular disease. Here, echo-guided fine-needle biopsies using the techniques described have proved invaluable, for they provide the material for accurate and reliable cytological and histological diagnoses.

Echo-guided biopsies are indicated in all patients with diseases of the pancreas that have not been sufficiently clarified, in particular for: (a) an early diagnosis of solid focal lesions; (b) a differential diagnosis between chronic forms of pancreatitis, particularly in the nodular circumscribed forms; and (c) the differentiation between benign or malignant cysts or pseudocysts.

The importance of the last-mentioned indication is stressed by Solmi and Bolondi for locular cysts with irregular walls. These may be benign cysts, but they may also be neoplastic processes, such as pancreatic cystadenocarcinoma [113]. An analysis of the results has demonstrated that echographically guided fine-needle biopsy has been highly effective ever since the first attempts were made, mainly concerning tumors: in 1975, Hancke et al. [114] obtained accurate diagnoses in 84% of their cases, false negatives being made in 16%; in 1976 Yamanaka et al. reported that correct diagnoses were made in 90% of their cases, with 10% false negatives [115]; and in 1980 Schwerk et al. [116] reported correct diagnoses in 87%, 10% false negatives, and 2% inconclusive. These data have been confirmed in the larger series that have been reported on since.

Minimum *sensitivity* is reported as 75% or 76% [117, 118] but more often it has a minimum of over 85% [119–121] and a maximum of over 90% [122, 123]. *Specificity* is generally 100%, and the *diagnostic accuracy* ranges from about 88% to 91%. With echo-guided fine-needle biopsy, however, slightly more malignant tumors of the liver than of the pancreas are diagnosed. The technique is valuable nevertheless in the diagnosis of solid pancreatic masses, even small ones, and it has been used more and more often in recent years.

As already mentioned, considerable technical difficulties are involved in the laparoscopic study of the pancreas. As it is essential to visualize the organ when obtaining a laparoscopic biopsy, laparoscopy can in no way compete with fine-needle biopsy, which is both fruitful and simple to perform. Overall, for the pancreas the results had with fine-needle biopsy appear to be better. The risk entailed is also minimal. In theory, the following complications can occur: hemorrhage, spread of infected material, acute hemorrhagic pancreatitis, and, where there are tumors, spread of neoplastic cells. In practice, however, accidents are negligible [114, 118, 120, 123–126]. Fine-needle biopsy should therefore be considered the technique of choice for the diagnosis of these diseases, particularly for pancreatic neoplasms; it is also probably the only valid means for reaching a diagnosis without performing surgery. It should always be kept in mind however, that a laparoscopic biopsy may be useful in particular situations.

3.4.3.3 Conclusions

1. Laparoscopic biopsy of the pancreas is an important novelty, but today it has only a theoretical value.

2. Echo-guided fine-needle biopsy is the technique of choice for a "pathological" diagnosis of a disease of the pancreas.

3. There may also be indications for laparoscopic biopsy, but these are few and far between. Nevertheless, it should be borne in mind that a biopsy can be taken under "direct" vision even from the pancreas.

3.4.4 Splenic Biopsy

Splenic biopsy is not a complete novelty. Yet its value in the diagnosis of diseases of the spleen has only recently been recognized, and as it is still considered a risky procedure it has not been developed as it should have. For these reasons it is dealt with in here.

Laparoscopic study of the spleen is based upon only macroscopic findings and has considerable limitations. Even with the patient in the appropriate position, it is not always possible to perform a satisfactory laparoscopic examination of the spleen because of its site. However, a sufficient part of it can almost always be visualized, above all if there is spleen enlargement. In addition, only the surface of the organ is visualized at laparoscopy: the fibrous capsule of the spleen is less transparent than that of the liver, and the underlying parenchyma is not easily seen; moreover, previous perisplenitis may have caused capsular thickening, and in these cases the splenic tissue is totally or partially hidden.

It is difficult to make a macroscopic diagnosis of splenopathy and to interpret the various findings. Although at laparoscopy a diseased spleen usually shows enlargement, it is important to bear in mind that some diseases of the spleen are not accompanied by enlargement of the organ. The spleen may also present surface alterations or have an apparently normal surface.

Changes visualized on the spleen surface may be flat, protruding, or excavated. *Flat lesions* may present as color alterations of uncertain origin with bluish or greenish patches or dark "tattoos". They may also be punctiform plaques or roundish or oval spots with irregular or clearly defined margins, whitish with a pink or yellow hue (Fig. 3.21). *Protruding lesions* may appear as small and miliary (Fig. 3.22) or larger nodules attaining the size of a walnut, and whitish with different densities, or they may be large, deeply embedded nodes covered by normal splenic tissue, resulting in irregular surface protuberances (Fig. 3.23). *Excavated lesions* are roundish, white, hard crater-like areas resembling scar tissue.

All of the above findings suggest that the spleen is diseased, but the lesions seldom have characteristics specific enough to reliably indicate a differential diagnosis. They enable us only to make quite different hypotheses concerning, for example, the nature and severity of the disease, the prognosis, and the therapy required. More reliable data are necessary for the diagnosis of a granuloma (tuberculosis, brucellosis, sarcoidosis, etc.), a malignant lymphoma, or a secondary neoplasm. A reliable diagnosis cannot be made on the basis of macroscopic data alone [127].

A diseased spleen does not necessarily present surface lesions. If splenomegaly is observed a disease can be suspected, but sometimes the size of the organ is normal and the spleen is considered normal on the basis of the laparoscopic examination. This can give rise to false negatives.

Other difficulties occur because nodular lesions are situated within the organ only and are not pres-

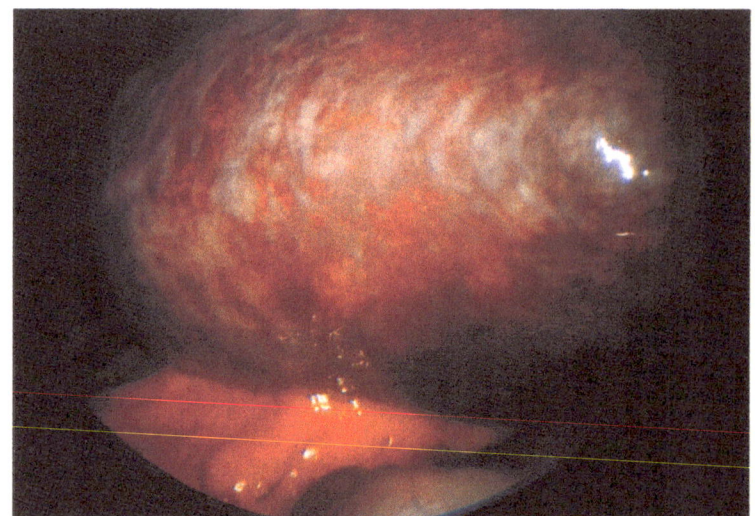

3.21

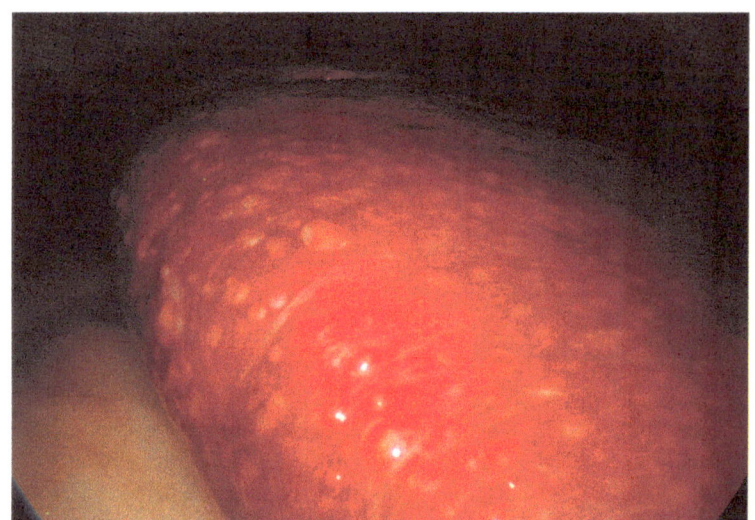

3.22

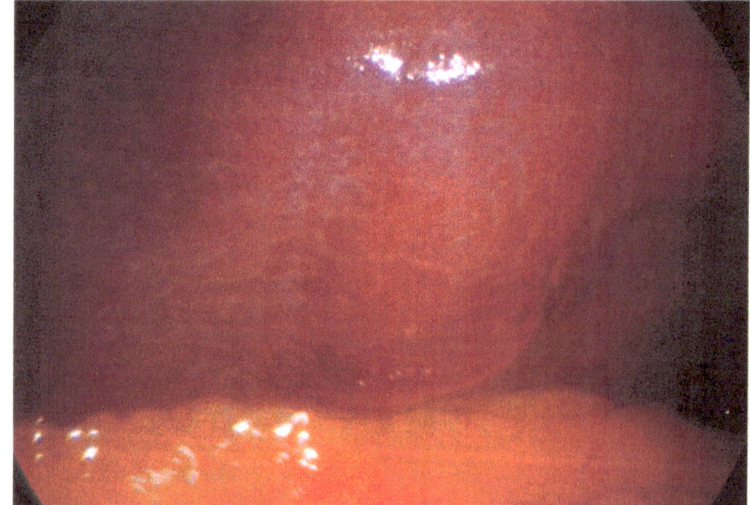

3.23

ent on the surface, or there may be a diffuse infiltration of the splenic parenchyma by a diseased tissue, but this spread may occur without giving rise to any macroscopically visible signs. In conclusion, if the spleen is studied laparoscopically and macroscopic findings alone are considered, there will be a high percentage of uncertain or mistaken diagnoses due to difficulty in interpreting visible lesions, as well as false negatives if the spleen is apparently normal.

3.4.4.1 Indications

It is essential to take a biopsy where diseases of the spleen are to be diagnosed, as is clearly demonstrated by the few examples cited here. Only by means of a histological examination is it possible to identify the nature of the different lesions and to establish whether or not:

1. Color variations are due to malignant lymphoma
2. Flat plaques are due to a Besnier-Boeck-Schaumann sarcoidosis
3. The numerous protuberant nodules (See Fig. 3.22) are due to diffusion in the spleen of non-Hodgkin's lymphoma
4. A tumefaction covered by normal tissue (See Fig. 3.23) is due to a nodular Hodgkin's lymphoma that does not reach the surface.

These are only a few of the many differential diagnoses that can be made on the basis of splenic biopsy findings. It is therefore evident that bioptic laparoscopy of the spleen is of great utility [128]. Yet it is only rarely performed and sometimes is

◄ ────────────────

Fig. 3.21. Splenomegaly of unknown nature: Infiltration from malignant lymphoma? Granuloma? Spleen has rounded medial margin. Under the capsule appear numerous whitish-rose pale areas of varying shape; they are either isolated or aggregated. Biopsy finding: *Besnier-Boeck-Schaumann sarcoidosis*

Fig. 3.22. Splenomegaly of unknown nature: Tuberculous granuloma? Malignant lymphoma? Surface of upper facies and the medial margin of the spleen with highly numerous protuberant yellowish nodules against a bright red background. Biopsy findings: *non-Hodgkin's lymphoma*

Fig. 3.23. Staging for a Hodgkin's lymphoma. Lower facies of the spleen: slightly protuberant tumefaction covered by apparently normal tissue. Pathological formations? Biopsy findings: *Hodgkin's lymphoma*

not even considered, as it is presumed to carry a high risk [129]. The spleen is, of course, a highly vascularized organ and there is a theoretical danger of severe hemorrhage. In practice, however, this risk is minimal.

Bioptic laparoscopy of the spleen is generally indicated where the clinical and instrumental studies have not led to a satisfactory diagnosis and where splenic involvement is considered likely or possible.

The main indications are:

1. The staging and follow-up of a Hodgkin's lymphoma
2. The staging and follow-up of a non-Hodgkin's lymphoma
3. Splenomegaly of uncertain nature
4. Suspicion of a splenic disease without evidence of splenomegaly

3.4.4.2 Technique

To visualize the spleen, the laparoscope should be introduced above the umbilicus, along the left supraumbilical line; from here the left hypochondrium can be well visualized, and the spleen is almost always found at a distance allowing the maneuvers necessary for taking the biopsy. In some cases, however, it may be necessary to introduce the laparoscope at a different point. With splenomegaly, it is opportune to introduce the laparoscope under the lower pole of the spleen in order to avoid damaging it. The point most appropriate for each individual patient is decided upon on the basis of a preliminary echographic exploration, however, (see Sect. 2.2.1); in this way risks are minimized and a more satisfactory examination can be performed.

The most appropriate *position for the patient* in splenic exploration is right, almost complete decubitus in an anti-Trendelenburg position. The Intestinal loops and the greater omentum are thus displaced downward and medially through the force of gravity and the organ is exposed. Even if the spleen is normal or reduced in size, most of its surface is visible. Of course, the inferior pole, the posterior surface, and the lateral border cannot be explored in this position.

In some cases, however, even when the most appropriate possible technique is used, the spleen either cannot be, or is only partially, visualized. The spleen may very small or deeply situated; it may be that the omental fat covering the organ cannot be removed using the probe either because it is too thick or because, consequent to a previous perisplenitis, it adheres to the organ; finally, adhesions closing the left hypochondrium and hiding the spleen may be found. In these cases however, if the adhesions are not too thick, a hole can be cut with small scissors introduced through the laparoscope, and through this hole the laparoscope can be passed in order to examine the organ. These three technical difficulties can complicate biopsy taking. Among our 2167 patients 2105 splenic biopsies were performed; in 62 cases biopsy was indicated but precluded by one or more of these factors.

3.4.4.3 Instruments

Needles of different types and sizes are used for laparoscopic biopsy of the spleen; in particular, Menghini's needle (diameters 1.2 and 1.4 mm) is used for aspiration biopsy.

We also used Menghini's needle for several years, performing 886 of our 2105 splenic biopsies with it. For the past 3 years, however, we have preferred to use a cutting needle (diameter 1.8 mm), with which we have performed 1184 biopsies. It is not more dangerous than Menghini's needle, and it allows us to obtain abundant and compact cylindrical (2 cm long) tissue samples. Splenic tissue is rather friable and not very compact and Menghini's needle almost always gives a fragmented, powdery material, resulting in a less accurate, unreliable, histological diagnosis. Palmer's forceps was once used in certain cases, mainly where there were large compact protruding nodules, but it is rarely used today.

When obtaining a biopsy we find it more convenient to introduce the needle through the laparoscope, without making a second hole. This gives an anterior view, allowing us to direct the instrument accurately. By moving the laparoscope in different directions, multiple biopsies can be taken at points in the organ that are quite distant from each other.

We make a further hole only when the biopsy must be taken from a point too distant to be reached from the laparoscope point or when the laparoscope cannot be directed perpendicular to the surface and the needle cannot be given the angulation necessary to penetrate the parenchyma.

Of course the biopsy is guided, for it is made under direct visualization from the point most appropriate for obtaining a satisfactory tissue sample. Where lesions are visible, the biopsy must be taken from the lesions themselves. If, on the other hand, lesions are not evident but splenic involvement is suspected, it is opportune to take random multiple biopsies at different points in the organ. The points should be far from each other so that as much material as possible can be obtained, with the greatest possible probability of including diseased tissue.

The tissue samples should be examined immediately under magnification; this allows us to decide whether or not the sample is satisfactory. If not, further biopsies can be taken.

As with the liver, bioptic puncture of the spleen is usually allowed by bleeding, which can be profuse. In most cases, however, the bleeding diminishes gradually until it stops with the formation of a clot. It is useful to exert continuous pressure under the hole with the probe to slow down the blood flow and facilitate coagulation. When the bleeding has stopped, the clot should be gently removed to uncover the hole and to check it for a few seconds to make sure hemostasis has been achieved.

In some cases bleeding is profuse and shows no sign of stopping even with pressure from the probe. If the bleeding continues after 5–6 min it is advisable to insert a Bio-Plug in the biopsy hole (see Sect. 1.3). This fibrin cartridge closes the hole perfectly and stops the hemorrhage immediately (Fig. 3.24). If the entire plug is inserted, it is always effective. We used to apply pressure with the laparoscope, inject coagulating substances into the hole, and apply, electrocoagulation, but results were often disappointing and we believe this approach should no longer be used. If a hemorrhage cannot be arrested, the patient must undergo emergency splenectomy.

3.4.4.4 Contraindications

There are general and local contraindications to splenic biopsy, the general contraindications being identical to those specified for liver biopsy. The main *local* contraindication is congestive splenomegaly, for in this case it is risky to perform biopsy, and the biopsy itself hardly ever yields useful results. Each individual case must be considered carefully and in the light of the laparoscopic findings, which indicate whether or not the biopsy can be performed.

Splenic biopsy is also in advisable when the surface of the organ is partly or entirely covered

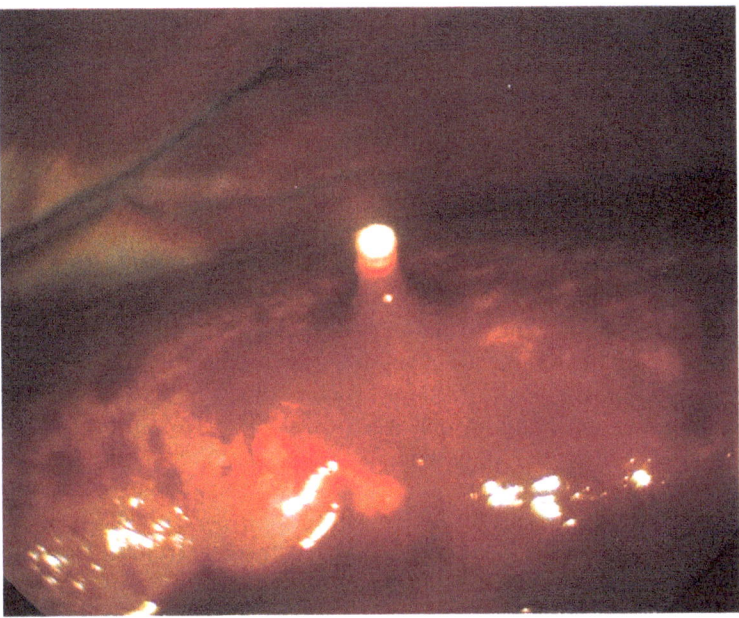

Fig. 3.24. Most of upper spleen surface covered with blood from severe hemorrhage after biopsy. At the center the Bio-Plug can be seen protruding; it immediately arrested bleeding

by fat and visualization of the biopsy hole is prevented, and when the spleen is rather inaccessible because it is small and mobile – in such cases it may be difficult to make the maneuvers necessary to stop bleeding. Liquid collections such as cysts and angiomas, which are not considered an indication for biopsy, are discussed elsewhere (see Sect. 3.2).

3.4.4.5 Accidents

As the spleen is highly vascularized, splenic biopsy is rarely performed for fear of hemorrhage. In our experience, however, the effective risk is far lower than the theoretical risk. In the literature few accidents due to splenic biopsy have been reported, but it should be borne in mind that the number of splenic biopsies performed is far smaller than the number of liver biopsies performed.

The data from our series are of value, however, for they are from 2105 splenic biopsies performed among a total of 13 520 laparoscopies. Only two of the patients (0.095%) had intractable hemorrhages – both patients underwent splenectomy and recovered; there were no deaths [128].

Moreover, both of these accidents occurred before August 1981. We then started using the Bio-Plug; since then, profuse hemorrhaging has always been resolved endoscopically, and emergency splenectomy is no longer necessary in such cases.

Whether blind or performed under laparoscopy, liver biopsy is now considered to carry little risk. Yet from a recent report on a large series of patients who underwent liver liopsy [130] it emerges that the proportion of serious accidents requiring surgery was greater than the proportion cited in cases of splenic biopsy; deaths have also been reported. Manenti and co-workers [131, 132] reported severe hemorrhage in 0.871% of cases and death in 0.261%.

Our series of hepatic biopsies [133] published in 1982 reports 0.058% severe hemorrhages and 0.022% deaths. If we add to these the patients with cholorrhea who underwent laparotomy (0.058% in our series and 0.348% in that of Manenti and co-workers) and deaths (0.011%). We must conclude that splenic biopsy is certainly no more risky than liver biopsy.

3.4.4.6 Echo-guided Fine-needle Biopsy

The improvements made in interventional echography and the excellent results obtained with fine-needle biopsies prompted the use of this technique in the study of diseases of the spleen.

Echography can, in fact, be used to detect focal lesions of the spleen and has been shown to be even more sensitive than CT. However, it does not, clearly define the type of disease process: it can only distinguish between liquid or solid lesions. So the picture it provides is not specific enough to enable us to diagnose the nature of the disease in question.

Moreover, lesions of the spleen are almost always very difficult to ascertain on the basis of the macroscopic anatomical finding made under laparoscopy. So it is almost impossible to diagnose the nature of a lesion on the basis of major or minor variations in its echogeneity, which is not specific. Biopsy is therefore the only basis for a satisfactory diagnosis.

Yet, although it is obviously important, fine-needle splenic biopsy has not often been used, due to the fear of accidents. We reported on the low risk from splenic biopsy when a 1.8-mm caliber Bio-Cut is used under laparoscopy. Also, experienced with echo-guided fine-needle biopsy confirms that any accidents from splenic puncture are negligible, even though this organ is highly vascularized [134–137].

Echo-guided splenic biopsy is performed using fine (outer diameter 0.7–0.8 mm) noncutting or cutting needles. The material aspirated is treated using the same methods as those described for the cytological and microhistological study. The puncture can be made intercostally or, in cases of splenomegaly, subcostally.

The indications for echo-guided diagnostic splenic fine-needle biopsy are the same as those for laparoscopic biopsy: (a) lymphoma staging, (b) splenomegaly of uncertain nature, and (c) suspected spleen disease without evidence of splenomegaly. Depending on the clinical situation, echography can show focalized single or multiple lesions, diffuse modifications in the echogenicity, or a normal picture. Where there are apparently solid focalized lesions a biopsy is of course taken, under echographical guidance, from the most significant point or points. The cytological and microhistological examinations may show a lymphoma or a metastasis from a malignant tumor, also revealing whether it is, for example, a tubercular process or an aspecific granuloma.

If the echographical examination reveals a formation with a liquid content and there is no doubt about the diagnosis – as is the case, for example, with simple congenital cysts and polycystic spleno-

pathy – biopsy is not required. But if the echographical finding is uncertain, as with so-called complex cysts, a puncture is indicated, because by studying the elements in the aspirated liquid a more accurate diagnosis can be made, and any dermoid, epidermoid, or false cysts (encapsulated post-traumatic hematomas, liquid collections consequent to an infarct, etc.) can be detected. It is advisable to avoid puncturing parasitic cysts, which have enough echographical characteristics to make them recognizable.

When the echography demonstrates an abscess, echo-guided puncture is useful for diagnostic purposes: an examination of the aspirated material enables us to identify the causal agent and to confirm the diagnosis, and then to choose the appropriate therapy.

If the echographical examination evidences a diffuse alteration of the splenic parenchyma, then fine-needle biopsy is indicated. In these cases there is no target, and echography is useful only because it enables us to direct the needle toward the spleen and to avoid damaging any large vessels near the hilus. In these cases we are more likely to obtain diseased tissue by making multiple biopsies, because echography fails to indicate any lesions.

Finally, if the spleen appears normal on echography but a disease is suspected on clinical or biochemical grounds, then fine-needle biopsy is indicated. Here, too, the likelihood of making a diagnosis is enhanced if multiple biopsies are taken from different points on the organ.

The results obtained with echo-guided splenic biopsy are satisfactory, both in diffuse infiltration [136] and in sonographically detected focal lesions [134, 137, 138], particularly in the diagnosis of non-Hodgkin's lymphomas. However, the results have not been adequately compared with those obtained through laparoscopic biopsy or splenectomy. It is therefore difficult to ascertain its diagnostic accuracy. As with the liver, fine-needle splenic biopsy may be the first invasive step in diagnosing diseases of the spleen because it can, if the result is satisfactory, resolve the problem.

Laparoscopic inspection through visually guided biopsy should be undertaken if the finding is uncertain or if findings are negative, even though a spleen disease is either suspected or considered possible.

Regarding splenic biopsy, however, the following points should be considered: First, as it is very difficult to make a histological diagnosis of splenopathy the number of dubious findings or false negatives is large, even when excellent tissue samples are obtained using the Bio-cut during laparoscopy. It should be borne in mind that a diagnosis based on single cells or small samples obtained using fine needles can give rise to even greater difficulties.

Second, echo-guided fine-needle puncturing of the spleen does not appear to incur excessive risks. In our experience, however, any danger of severe hemorrhage following laparoscopic biopsy of the spleen depends not on the size of the needle used, but on capsule laceration. This is more likely to occur when transcutaneous biopsy is performed, particularly if the intercostal route is used. As this technique does not allow us to immediately discover the accident, the necessary measures to resolve it are often taken too late. During laparoscopy, on the other hand, any bleeding can be controlled under direct vision until coagulation has taken place, and the hemorrhage can be stopped, if necessary, by inserting a fibrin plug through the biopsy hole.

It is therefore not yet possible to say whether echo-guided fine-needle biopsy is preferable to laparoscopic biopsy in the diagnosis of diseases of the spleen.

3.4.4.7 Conclusions

1. Laparoscopy performed alone is not useful in the diagnosis of a splenic disease; laparoscopic splenic biopsy is indispensable.

2. A combined macroscopic and histological study allows us to establish some important indications for laparoscopy in the diagnosis of diseases of the spleen.

3. The risk of accidents during splenic biopsy is small, and it is certainly no greater than that known, and considered acceptable, for biopsy of the liver.

4. The results of echo-guided fine-needle splenic biopsy in clinical practice have been promising; it may become the invasive technique of choice, also in the diagnosis of splenopathies. However, are of the opinion that in this field laparoscopic biopsy is still more reliable for the diagnosis and also perhaps carries less risk. Laparoscopy is always indicated where echo-guided fine-needle biopsy fails to provide satisfactory results.

3.5 Disinfection of Instruments

Infection following laparoscopy has never been an important problem. In the literature any cases of infection reported are negligible even though the laparoscope is an invasive instrument, for it directly enters a normally sterile part of the human body and should therefore in theory by "sterilized." As the instrument is routinely treated as "semi-invasive", it is only "disinfected" and in most centers kept in a closed container holding formalin gas for 18–24 h; the gas is produced by formaldehyde tablets. Formalin does not sterilize, for it cannot destroy all forms of life, but it does destroy pathogenic agents.

Our laparoscopes are disinfected using this simple method, and in our experience of over 16000 laparoscopies performed from 1966 to 1988, no cases of infection have come to our notice.

Today, however, viral agents for hepatitis, and especially AIDS, are more widespread and we must take steps to make sure that endoscopy never becomes a vehicle for the spread of these infections [139, 140]. We must ascertain therefore whether this examination entails a real risk of spreading infection and what preventive measures should be taken if any.

The risk of transmission of infection is difficult to determine because where laparoscopy is concerned, data are scarce. We observed no cases of laparoscopically transmitted infection, nor did Henning in his series, notwithstanding the "high" percentage of laparoscopies he performed on HBsAG- and HBeAg-positive patients [141].

Important information is available, however, regarding experience with digestive endoscopy. Although the data are not quite comparable because the techniques used are different, they do give us useful guidelines, especially if we bear in mind the fact that during most of these examinations invasive maneuvers are made, either for diagnostic biopsies or for therapeutic purposes (polypectomy, papillostomy, sclerosis of varices, etc.).

Data on the hepatitis viruses are consoling. The *hepatitis A* virus, an endovirus eliminated through the feces, has an elective oral transmission, although parenteral transmission cannot be ruled out. In theory, therefore, the risk of transmission of this disease through fiberendoscopic examinations would appear high. Yet no cases of infection transmitted through this examination have been reported, either from patient to examiner, from patient to patient, or from examiner to patient [142].

The *hepatitis B* virus (HBV) in particular has been studied from this standpoint. HBV is transmitted parenterally; a very small dose can cause infection. It is resistant even in an extra-human environment and it can be present in organic liquids. The chronic HBsAg carriers in Italy average 2.5%, ranging from 0.5% to 10% depending on the particular area and the category of patients considered. If we consider the invasive maneuvers made, the risk of the virus being transmitted through endoscopic examination is theoretically high. In practice, however, the risk is low. Infection from patient to examiner is negligible: in fact, the serological signs of a previous infection from HBV in endoscopists are no more frequent than those found in, for example, internists and gastroenterologists, who do not perform endoscopy. It is also important to bear in mind that the simple hygienic precautions taken in the past 10 years have drastically reduced the risk of infection from HBV in all hospital staff, to levels only slightly higher than those in the general population [143].

Data reported in the literature demonstrate that the risk of hepatitis B being transmitted from patient to patient following fiberendoscopic examinations is very low. Overall, therefore, the risk of transmission of the hepatitis virus through endoscopic instruments gives no cause for concern, and therefore no changes need be made in the procedures used in this field to date.

AIDS, on the other hand, poses a different problem: as yet there has been no evidence of transmission of the HLT VIII virus following endoscopic examinations [144], but this lack of evidence is not grounds for concluding that there is no such risk.

3.5.1 Current Precautions and Disinfection Procedures

It is necessary to answer the following questions [140]:

1. Should all patients about to be examined undergo systematic clinical and serological control?
2. If an infection is found, what measures should be taken to prevent any transmission?

Regarding question 1, it would probably be adequate to submit only those patients at risk to a rigorous control. Concerning question 2, the disinfection procedures for the environment, and for endoscopic instruments in particular, should be reviewed. Disinfection of the environment (room, furniture, operating table, etc.) is of minor importance. As these are "noninvasive," only cleaning with hot water or low-concentration disinfectants is required [144]. Invasive instruments should be washed with soap and water, as this measure is essential for good disinfection [144, 145]. Any residual organic material must be mechanically cleared by simple washing with soap and water: it has been demonstrated that the most thorough sterilization process, capable of killing bacterial spores, cannot destroy even vegetative bacteria if they are protected by dried blood or ascites, for example. As the number of germs is also markedly reduced by thorough washing, the efficacy of the disinfectant is enhanced. For more thorough and rapid washing, it is advisable to use a special apparatus [145].

For satisfactory disinfection of certain endoscopic instruments two substances are considered particularly suitable: glutaraldehyde and ethylene oxide. *Glutaraldehyde*, a saturated dialdehyde chemically linked to formaldehyde, acts on microorganisms through alkylation of the protein, amine, and sulfide groups and binding of the nitrogen atoms to the purine bases. In a 2% H_2O solution it is a powerful disinfectant and also provides sterilization if left for 3–10 h to act.

Ethylene oxide acts as a bactericide through alkylation of proteins. It is highly active but more difficult to use than other bactericides because it requires special equipment and sensitive controls.

At present, glutaraldehyde is the most widely used substance; it has given satisfactory results. We no longer use formalin gas, but prefer glutaraldehyde in a 2% solution to disinfect the laparoscope and the accessories that enter the abdomen or penetrate the parenchyma. "Sporicidine" is the most up-to-date glutaraldehyde preparation available. [145, 146]. It consists of a tampon of sodium phenolate and sodium tetraborate associated with an activator, glutaraldehyde, and is supplied as a ready-to-use solution containing only 0.13% glutaraldehyde stabilized to a basic pH of 7.9. The solution, which is stable for up to 30 days, destroys all microorganisms including HBV, herpes, and HIV [146]. As it destroys these viruses, we may assume that Sporicidine also destroys other, often associated, viruses such as the non-A and non-B virus or cytomegalovirus.

Sporicidine takes only 10 min to act completely, although an immersion period of 20 min is advisable. It also has the advantage of being well tolerated. Up to 37% of the staff using gluteraldehyde have had allergic skin reactions, while staff using Sporicidine have had no side effects, thanks to its low glutaraldehyde concentration. Sporicidine is as active as more concentrated solutions because its efficacy is guaranteed by the synergism of the phenolate tampon and the activator, gluteraldehyde.

Sporicidine therefore appears to be the most advantageous and reliable substance available for the sterilization of endoscopic instruments. Some believe that it is better to set aside instruments to be used exclusively for endoscopic examination of AIDS patients [147]. We are of the opinion that this precaution is unnecessary if the measures for disinfection are scrupulously followed.

3.5.2 Conclusions

1. In the past the risk of contracting an infectious disease through laparoscopic examination was considered negligible.

2. The high incidence of viral hepatitis and the problems due to AIDS, however, have led to a reappraisal of this aspect.

3. It can be concluded that it is advisable to disinfect laparoscopes with substances that are more effective than formaldehyde. Data are scarce, but we can assume that good washing of instruments followed by treatment with glutaraldehyde will provide adequate protection against transmission of either hepatitis or AIDS.

References

1. Meyer-Burg J (1972) The inspection, palpation and biopsy of the pancreas by peritoneoscopy. Endoscopy 4:99–101
2. Look D, Henning H, Lüders CJ (1972) Darstellung und Biopsie des Pankreaskopfes bei der Laparoskopie. Z Gastroenterol 10:209–214
3. Strauch M, Lux G, Ottenjan R (1973) Infragastric pancreoscopy. Endoscopy 5:30–32
4. Cuschieri A, Hall AW, Clark J (1978) Value of laparoscopy in the diagnosis and management of pancreatic carcinoma. Gut 19:672–677
5. Ishida H, Furukawa Y, Kuroda H, Kobayashi M, Tsuneoka K (1981) Laparoscopic observation and biopsy of the pancreas. Endoscopy 3:68–73
6. Komatsu K, Moriai N, Nishimura S, Stao W, Takahashi H (1982) Laparoscopic biopsy of the pancreas. In: Abstracts of the World Congress in Stockholm.
7. Ishida H (1983) Peritoneoscopy and pancreas biopsy in the diagnosis of pancreatic disease. Gastrointest Endosc 3:211–218
8. Dagnini G (1982) What can be expected of laparoscopy in the diagnosis of acute pancreatitis? In: Hollender LF (ed) Controversies in acute pancreatitis. Springer, Berlin Heidelberg New York
9. Dagnini G, Marin G (1988) Laparoskopie. In: Hollender LF, Peiper HJ (eds) Pankreas chirurgie. Springer, Berlin Heidelberg New York (Die Praxis der Chirurgie)
10. Vilardell F, Marti-Vicente A (1987) Laparoscopy of abdominal tumors. In: Sivak MV (ed) Gastroenterologic endoscopy. Saunders, Philadelphia
11. Arbeiter G, Marsch-Ziegler U, Leonhardt H, Schäfer JH (1981) Retrospektive Erhebungen zum Wert der Laparoskopie bei der Differenzierung von akuter ödematöser und akuter hämorrhagischnekrotisierender Pankreatitis in der Frühphase der Erkrankung. Z Gastroenterol 19:173–177
12. Lawson TL (1978) Sensitivity of pancreatic ultrasonography in the detection of pancreatic disease. Radiology 128:733–736
13. Taylor KJW, Buchin PJ, Viscomi GN, Rosenfield AT (1981) Ultrasonographic scanning of the pancreas. Prospective study of clinical results. Radiology 138:211–213
14. Pollock D, Taylor KJW (1981) Ultrasound scanning in patients with clinical suspicion of pancreatic cancer: a retrospective study. Radiology 47:1662–1665
15. Haubrich WS (1983) Probing the pancreas (editorial). Gastrointest Endosc 29(3):244–245
16. Yuzpe AA (1987) Gynecologic laparoscopy for the gastroenterologist. In: Sivak MV (ed) Gastroenterologic endoscopy. Saunders, Philadelphia
17. Berci G, Cushieri A (1986) Interventional laparoscopy. In: Practical laparoscopy. Bailliere Tindal, London, pp 95–121
18. Phillips JM, Mulka JF, Peterson N (1984) American Association of Gynecologic Laparoscopists 1982 membership survey. J Reprod Med 29:592–594
19. Dagnini G (1980) Jaundice. In: Dagnini G (ed) Clinical laparoscopy. Piccin Medical, Padua
20. Williams JA (1987) Le aderenze causano dolore? Br Med J (Ital edn) 7:5–6
21. Kresh AJ, Seifer DB, Sachs LB, Barrese I (1984) Laparoscopy in 100 women with chronic pelvic pain. Obstet Gynecol 23:191–200
22. Harndt HJ, Greutzfeldt W (1976) Abdominalschmerzen durch Adhäsionen und ihre laparo-

skopische Beseitigung. Dtsch Med Wochenschr 101:395–398

23. Nord NJ (1987) Technique of laparoscopy. In: Sivak MV (ed) Gastroenterologic endoscopy. Saunders, Philadelphia

24. Kleinhaus S (1984) Laparoscopic lysis of adhesions for postappendectomy pain. Gastrointest Endosc 5:304–305

25. Salky B, Bauer J, Gelernt I, Kreel I (1985) Laparoscopy for gastrointestinal diseases. M Sinai J Med 3:228–232

26. Kaplan LR (1981) Laparoscopy with adhesion lysis in chronic abdominal pain. Gastrointest Endosc 3:136

27. Marin G, Caldironi MW, Miola E, Dagnini G (1986) Resezione laparoscopica di aderenze algogene. G Ital End Dig 2:188

28. Salky B, Zimmerman M, Bauer J, Gelernt I, Kreel I (1985) Splenic cyst – definitive treatment by laparoscopy. Gastrointest Endosc 3:213–215

29. Roemer CE, Ferrucci JT, Mueller PR, Simeone JF, Van Sonnenberg E, Wittenberg J (1981) Hepatic cysts: diagnosis and therapy by sonographic needle aspiration. AJR 136:1065–1070

30. Saini S, Muller PR, Ferrucci JT, Simeone JF, Wittenberg J, Buch RJ (1983) Percutaneous aspiration of hepatic cysts does not provide definitive therapy. AJR 141:559–560

31. Bean WJ, Rodan BA (1985) Hepatic cysts: treatment with alcohol. AJR 144:237–241

32. Mueller PR, Dawson SL, Ferrucci JT, Nardi GL (1985) Hepatic echinococcal cyst: successful percutaneous drainage. Radiology 155:627–628

33. Ben Amor N, Gargouri M, Gharbi HA, Golvan YJ, Kchouk H (1986) Essai de traitement par ponction des cistes hydatiques abdominaux inoperables. Ann Parasitol Hum Comp 61:689–692

34. Dughetti S, Brunetti E, Pirola , Filice C (1988) Drenaggio percutaneo ecoguidato di cisti idatidee epatiche: risultati e follow-up. Atti V Corso di Ecografia operativa, Piacenza

35. Hitanant S, Tan-Ngarm Trong D, Damrongsak C, Chinapak O, Boonyapisit S, Plengvanit U, Viranuvatti V (1984) Peritoneoscopy in the diagnosis of liver abscess. Gastrointest Endosc 30(4): 234–236

36. Staples C, Dale A (1980) Peritoneoscopically guided needle aspiration of amebic liver abscess. Gastrointest Endosc 26(1):21–22

37. Salky B, Finkel S (1985) Laparoscopic drainage of amebic liver abscess. Gastrointest Endosc 31: 30–34

38. Welch CE, Malt RA (1983) Abdominal surgery. N Engl J Med 308:353–360

39. Gerzof SG, Robbins AH, Birkett DH, Jonson WC, Pugatch RD, Vincent ME (1979) Percutaneous catheter drainage of abdominal abscesses guided by ultrasound and computer tomography. AJR 133:1–18

40. Haaga JR, Weinstein AJ (1980) CT-guided percutaneous aspiration and drainage of abscesses. AJR 135:1187–1194

41. Gerzof SG, Robbins AH, Johnson WC, Birkett DH, Nabseth DC (1981) Percutaneous catheter drainage of abdominal abscesses. N Engl J Med 305:653–657

42. Johnson WC, Gerzof SG, Robbins AH, Nabseth DC (1981) Treatment of abdominal abscesses: comparative evaluation of operative drainage versus percutaneous catheter drainage guided by computed tomography or ultrasound. Ann Surg 194:510–520

43. Gronvall S, Gammelgaard J, Hubek A, Holm HH (1982) Drainage of abdominal abscesses guided by sonography. AJR 138:527–529

44. Kuligowska E, Connors SK, Shapiro JH (1982) Liver abscess: sonography in diagnosis and treatment. AJR 138:253–257

45. Martin EC, Karlson KB, Fankuchen EI, Cooperman A, Casarella WJ (1982) Percutaneous drainage of postoperative intraabdominal abscesses. AJR 138:13–15

46. Van Sonnenberg E, Ferrucci JT, Mueller PR, Wittemberg J, Simeone JF (1982) Percutaneous drainage of abscesses and fluid collections: technique, results and applications. Radiology 142:1–10

47. Herbert DA, Rothman J, Simmons F, Fogel DA, Wilson S, Ruskin J (1982) Pyogenic liver abscesses: successful non-surgical therapy. Lancet 16: 134–136

48. Berger A, Osborne DR (1982) Treatment of pyogenic liver abscesses by percutaneous needle aspiration. Lancet 16:132–134

49. Halasz NA, van Sonnenberg E (1983) Drainage of intra-abdominal abscess: tactics and choices. Am J Surg 146:112–115

50. Van Sonnenberg E, Muller PR, Ferrucci JT (1984) Percutaneous drainage of 250 abdominal abscesses and fluid collections. Radiology 151:337–341

51. Nielsen L (1988) US-guided percutaneous treatment of intraabdominal abscesses. Atti V Corso Ecografia operativa Piacenza

52. Bretagnolle M (1988) Interventions spléniques non vasculaires. Atti V Corso Ecografia operativa Piacenza

53. Menghini G, Miscusi GD (1983) The windowed trocar: a useful tool for a safer and efficient laparoscopy. Gastrointest Endosc 29:40–42

54. Ahn YW, Owens B (1979) Technique for laparoscopy on patients with previous abdominal surgery. Int J Fertil 24(4):264–266

55. Marti-Vicente A, Villalona-Rodriguez J, Martinez-Alcala F (1979) Peritoneoscopy examination following abdominal operations. Gastrointest Endosc 25(2):144–145

56. Cook WA (1977) Needle laparoscopy in patients with suspected bowel adhesions. Obstet Gynaecol 49:105–106

57. Marti-Vicente A, Villalona-Rodriguez J, Martinez-Alcala F(1980) La laparoscopia en pacientes con cirugia abdominal previa. Rev Esp Enferm Apar Dig 57(Suppl 3):85–91

58. Pleissner J, Berndt H, Gutz HI (1978) Laparoscopy following abdominal operations. Endoscopy 10:187–191

59. Terruzzi V, Introzzi G, Minoli G, Imperiali G, Rossini A (1981) Abdominal adhesions and laparoscopy in liver diseases. Acta Endosc 6:397–407
60. De Groen PC, Rakela J, Moore SC, Mc Gill DB, Burton DP, ott BJ, Zinmeister AR (1987) Diagnostic laparoscopy in gastroenterology – a 14-year experience. Dig Dis Sci 32:677–681
61. Livraghi T, Solbiati L (1986) Complicanze e controindicazioni. In: Livraghi T, Solbiati L (eds) Ecografia inteventistica. Masson, Milano
62. Livraghi T, Damascelli B, Lombardi C, Spagnoli I (1983) Risk in fine-needle abdominal biopsy. JCU 11:77–81
63. Smith EH (1984) The hazards of fine-needle aspiration biopsy. Ultrasound Med Biol 11:629–634
64. Bree RL (1985) Needle aspiration and biopsies; C.T. or ultrasound guidance? Appl Radiol 14:9–13
65. Damascelli B, Segre D (1986) Altre metodiche di guida. In: Livraghi T, Solbiati L (eds) Ecografia interventistica. Masson, Milano
66. Livraghi T (1986) Masse addominali di natura da determinare. In: Livraghi T, Solbiati L (eds) Ecografia interventistica. Masson, Milano
67. Yen HC, Shapir MK, Slaber G, Meyer RJ, Cohen BA, Geller SA (1984) Ultrasonography and computer tomography in pseudomyxoma peritonei. Radiology 153:507–510
68. Sherlock S, Dick R, Van Leeuwen DJ (1984) Liver biopsy today – the Royal Free Hospital experience. J Hepatol 1:75–84
69. Lindner H (1973) Why laparoscopy? Acta Gastroenterol Belg 36:595–602
70. Zotti S, Papaleo E, Marin G, Patella M, Bergamo S, Caldironi MW, Cecchetto A, Dagnini G (1981) Laparoscopy and liver biopsy in the morphological diagnosis of cirrhosis: concordance and diagnostic validity. Ital J Gastroenterol 13:14–17
71. Dagnini G (1984) Why laparoscopy? 1983. Cont Ed Gastroenterol 1:46–47
72. Pagliaro L, Rinaldi F, Craxì A, Di Piazza S, Filippazzo G, Gatto G, Genova G, Magin S, Maringhini A, Orsini s, Palazzo V, Spinello M, Vinci M (1983) Percutaneous blind biopsy versus laparoscopy with guided biopsy in diagnosis of cirrhosis. A prospective, randomized trial. Dig Dis Sci 1:39–43
73. Henning H, Look D (1985) Laparoskopishe Biopsie. In: Henning A, Look D (eds) Laparoskopie. Thieme, Stuttgart
74. Centeno F, Elizondo J, Robles-Diaz G, Wolpert E (1985) Liver biopsy (LB), blind percutaneous transhepatic (BPT) or by laparoscopy (L). An assessment of 1668 biopsies. Gastrointest Endosc 31:152
75. Dagnini G, Zotti S, Marin G, Caldironi MW, Patella M, Cecchetto A (1986) Laparoscopy and guided biopsy in the diagnosis of cirrhosis. Ital J Gastroenterol 18:93–96
76. Boyce HW (1987) Laparoscopy. In: Schiff L, Schiff R (eds) Diseases of the liver. Lippincott, Philadelphia
77. Brady P, Goldschmid S, Chappel G, Slone FL, Boyd P (1987) A comparison of biopsy techniques in suspected focal liver disease. Gastrointest Endosc 33:289–292
78. Piccigallo E, Battan R, Miola E, Cecchetto A, Parenti A (1985) Rilievi sull'impiego della biopsia epatica transcutanea e laparoscopica nel complesso universitario-ospedaliero di Padova. G Ital Endosc Dig 3:372
79. Nord HJ (1987) Technique of laparoscopy. In: Sivak M (ed) Gastroenterological endoscopy-Saunders, Philadelphia
80. Orlandi F, Study Group on Randomized Clinical Trials (1979) Observer error in morphological diagnosis of chronic active hepatitis and cirrhosis. Ital J Gastroenterol 11:5–8
81. Sessa R, De Nucci C, Forte G, Calise F, Mazzarelli R, Acconciagioco G (1982) Il bio-cut nella biopsia epatica laparoscopica. Minerva Dietol Gastroenterol, 28:227–236
82. Ewe K (1981) Bleeding after liver biopsy does not correlate with indices of peripheral coagulation. Dig Dis Sci 26:388–393
83. Haaga JF (1979) New techniques for CT-guided biopsies. AJR 133:633–641
84. Tao LC, Donat EE, Ho CS, MC, Loughlin MJ (1979) Percutaneous fine-needle aspiration biopsy of the liver. Cytodiagnostics of hepatic cancer. Acta Cytol (Baltimore) 23:287–291
85. Fornari F, Civardi G, Buscarini E (1986) Il fegato. In: Livraghi T, Solbiati L (eds) Ecografia interventistica. Masson, Milano
86. Jacobsen GK, Gammelgard J, Fuglo M (1983) Coarse-needle biopsy versus fine-needle aspiration biopsy in the diagnosis of focal lesions of the liver – ultrasonically guided needle biopsy in suspected hepatic malignancy. Acta Cytol (Baltimore) 2:152–156
87. Fornari F, Cavanna L, Civardi G, Foroni R, Tansini P, Distasi M, Buscarini E, Buscarini L (1985) Ultrasonically guided fine-needle aspiration biopsy: first-stage invasive procedure in the diagnosis of focal lesions of the liver. Ital J Gastroenterol 17:246–251
88. Livraghi T, Pilotti S, Ravetto C, Sangalli G, Solbiati L (1985) Inclusion cytology versus smear cytology in fine-needle abdominal biopsy. Eur J Radiol 5:111–114
89. Sangalli G, Livraghi T, Giordano F (1984) Smear and inclusion cytology in Chiba-needle aspiration biopsy of hepatic tumors. Appl Pathol 2:49–53
90. Haaga JR, Li Puma JP, Bryan PJ, Baesara KJ (1983) Clinical comparison of small- and large-caliber cutting needles for biopsy. Radiology 146:665–667
91. Pagani JJ (1983) Biopsy of focal hepatic lesions. Comparison of 18- and 22-gauge needles. Radiology 147:673–675
92. Nosher JL, Plafker J (1980) Fine-needle aspiration of the liver with ultrasound guidance. Radiology 136:177–180
93. Matter D, Spinelli G, Stoeckel E, Diebolt F, Warter P (1982) Guidage echoscopique des ponctions

biopsies transcutanées. J Radiol 63:667–672

94. Bret PM, Fond A, Bretagnolle M, Bret P (1982) Technique des ponctions biopsies percutanées sous guidage échoscopique avec appareil à balayage linéaire. Ann Radiol (Paris) 25:561–563

95. Montali G, Solbiati L, Croce F, Ierace T, Ravetto C (1982) Fine-needle aspiration biopsy of liver focal lesions ultrasonically guided with a real-time probe. Br J Radiol 55:717–723

96. Schwerk WB, Durr HK, Schmitz-Moormann P (1983) Ultrasound-guided fine-needle biopsies in pancreatic and hepatic neoplasms. Gastrointest Radiol 8:219–225

97. Ierace T, Solbiati L, De Pra L, Ravetto C (1983) Agoaspirazione sotto guida endoscopica nella patologia epatica, pancreatica e renale. Ultrasuonodiagnostica 4:15–23

98. Fornage B, Touche D, Lemaire A, Deshayes JL, Simatos A, Faroux MJ (1984) Apport en cancérologie de la ponction-aspiration à l'aiguille fine d'organes abdominaux sous controle échographique en temps réel. A propos de 265 observations. J Radiol 65:533–544

99. Martino CR, Haaga JR, Bryan PJ, Li Puma JP, El Yousef SJ, Alfidi RJ (1984) CT-guided liver biopsies: eight years' experience. Radiology 152:755–757

100. Ho CS, Mc Toughlin MJ, Tao LC, Blendis L, Evans WK (1981) Guided percutaneous fine-needle aspiration biopsy of the liver. Cancer 47:1781–1785

101. Civardi G, Fornari F, Cavanna L, di Stasi M, Sbolli G, Buscarini L (1988) Value of rapid staining and assessment of ultrasound-guided fine needle aspiration biopsies. Acta Cytol 32(4):552–554

102. Cornud E, Vissuzaine C, Sibert A, Oliver A, Lenoir S, Bocquet L, Benacerraf R (1985) Peut-on faire à l'aiguille fine le diagnostic histologique des métastases hépatiques? A propos de 70 ponctions hépatiques guidées par échographie. Ann Gastroenterol Hepatol (Paris) 21:23–25

103. Noguchi S, Yamamoto R, Tatsuta M, Kasugai H, Okuda S, Wada A, Tamura H (1986) Cell features and patterns in fine-needle aspirates of hepatocellular carcinoma. Cancer 58:321–328

104. LabadieM, Berger F, Liaras A, Bret Pa, Bretagnolle M, Fond A, Minaire Y (1985) Can cytological puncture-aspiration of hepatic lesions replace biopsy-aspiration? Acta Endoscop 4:281–286

105. Ranieri F, Basile PN, Bonneau HP, Cano N, Martin F, Di Costanzo J (1983) Diagnostic étiologique des masses hépatiques par la ponction percutanée guidée par les ultrasons. Etude réalisée chez des malades sans néoplasie connue. Presse Med 12:87–89

106. Wittenberg J, Mueller PR, Ferrucci JT, Simeone JF, Von Sonnenberg E, Neff CC, Palermo RA, Isler RJ (1982) Percutaneous core biopsy of abdominal tumors using 22-gauge needles: further observations. AJR 139:75–80

107. Smith EH (1984) The hazards of fine-needle aspiration biopsy. Ultrasound Med Biol 11:629–634

108. Damascelli B, Spagnoli I, Garbagnati F, Ceglia E, Milella M, Masciadri N (1983) Massive lymphorrhoea after fine-needle biopsy of the cystic haemangiolymphangioma of the liver. Eur J Radiol 4:107–109

109. Fedeli G, Rapaccini C, Rabitti C, Asunis A, De Vitis I, Marra G, D'Amato M (1985) La biopsia ecoguidata con ago sottile e la laparoscopia nella diagnosi di neoplasia epatica: studio prospettico. G Ital Endosc Dig 3:370

110. Buscarini L, Sbolli G, Civardi G, Di Stasi M, Fermi S, Buscarini E, Cavanna L, Fornari F (1987) La biopsie percutanée guidée sous écographie modifie-t-elle les indications de la laparoscopie en hépatologie? Acta Endosc 2:85–88

111. Ishida H, Furukawa Y, Kuroda H, Kobayashi M, Tsuneoka K (1981) Laparoscopic observation and biopsy of the pancreas. Endoscopy 3:68–73

112. Ishida H (1983) Peritoneoscopy and pancreas diseases. Gastrointest Endosc 3:211–218

113. Solmi L, Bolondi L (1986) Pancreas. In: Livraghi T, Solbiati L (eds) Ecografia interventistica. Masson, Milano

114. Hancke S, Holm HH, Koch F (1975) Ultrasonically guided percutaneous fine-needle biopsy of the pancreas. Surg Gynecol Obstet 140:361–364

115. Yamanaka T, Kimura K (1979) Differential diagnosis of pancreatic mass lesions with percutaneous fine-needle aspiration biopsy under ultrasonic guidance. Dig Dis Sci 24:694–699

116. Schwerk WB, Schmitz-Moorman P (1980) Sonographisch gezielte perkutane transperitoneale Aspirationsbiopsie raumfordernder Pankreasprozesse. Dtsch Med Wochenschr 105:1019–1023

117. Moreau J, Sabatier JC, Cassigneul J, Rozental G (1983) L'échographie interventionelle en pathologie pancréatique. JEMU 14:47–53

118. Hancke S, Holm HH, Koch F (1984) Ultrasonically guided puncture of solid pancreatic mass lesions. Ultrasound Med Biol 10:613–615

119. Mitty HA, Efremides SC, Yeh H (1981) Impact of fine-needle biopsy on the management of patients with carcinoma of the pancreas. AJR 137:1119–1121

120. Tatsuta M, Yamamoto R, Yamamura H, Okuda S, Tamura H (1983) Cytologic examination and CEA measurement in aspirated pancreatic material collected by percutaneous fine-needle aspiration biopsy under ultrasonic guidance for the diagnosis of pancreatic carcinoma. Cancer 52:693–698

121. Carrilho-Ribeiro JM, Moreira ML, Baptista A (1983) Ultrasonically guided percutaneous biopsies of abdominal masses: personal experience. Endoscopy 15:183–185

122. Jerace T, Solbiati L, De Pra L, Ravetto C (1983) Agoaspirazione sotto guida ecografica nella patologia epatica, pancreatica e renale. Ultrasuonodiagnostica 4:15–23

123. Buscarini L, Fornari F (1987) Application of interventional ultrasonography in gastroenterology.

Imaging and visual documentation in medicine. Elsevier Science, Amsterdam, pp 487–498

124. Lutz H (1983) Ultrasonically guided fine-needle puncture in gastroenterology. Endoscopy 15: 180–182

125. Otto R, Deville P, Pedio L (1983) Biopsia percutanea dei tumori del pancreas per aspirazione con ago sottile guidata ecograficamente sotto controllo visivo permanente. Minerva Dietol Gastroenterol 29:71–76

126. Grant EG, Richardson JD, Smirniotopoulos JG, Norman MJ (1983) Fine-needle biopsy directed by real-time sonography: technique and accuracy. AJR 141:29–32

127. Garcia Molinero MJ, Solis Herruzo JA, Munoz Yagüe MT (1981) La laparoscopia en el estudio de las esplenomegalias. Gastroenterol Hepato 4(10):515–519

128. Dagnini G, Caldironi MW, Marin G, Patella M (1984) Laparoscopic splenic biopsy. Endoscopy 2(16):55–58

129. Berci G, Cuschieri A (1986) Practical laparoscopy. Balliere Tindall, London, 91

130. Henning H, Look D (1985) Laparoskopie. Thieme, Stuttgart, p 42

131. Manenti A, Manenti F, Villa E, Ferrari A, Malagoli M, Cortesi M (1980) Complications de la laparoscopie: expérience sur 6563 observations. Acta Endosc 10:(5–6):373–379

132. Manenti A, Ferrari A, Gibertini G, Borruto A, Manenti F, Cortesi N (1983) Biopsie hépatique sous contrôle laparoscopique. Expérience de 3000 cas. Acta Endosc 13:21–27

133. Dagnini G, Bergamo S, Caldironi MW, Marin G, Papaleo E, Patella M (1980) Incidenti della laparoscopia: rapporto su 7870 casi. G Gastroenterol Endosc 3(3):9–13

134. Cavanna L, Fornari F, Buscarini E, Foroni R, Rossi S, Buscarini L (1985) Ultrasonically guided fine-needle aspiration biopsy of abdominal lesions in pathological staging of non-Hodgkin's Lymphomas. Haematologica (Pavia) 70:132–135

135. Cavanna L, Croce F, De Gasperin R (1986) Milza e linfonodi. In: Livraghi T, Solbiati L (eds) Ecografia interventistica. Masson, Milano

136. Jansson SE, Bondestam S, Heinonen E, Grohn P, Vuopio P (1983) Value of liver and spleen aspiration biopsy in malignant disease when these organs show no signs of involvement in sonography. Acta Med Scand 213:279–281

137. Solbiati L, Bossi MC, Bellotti E, Ravetto C, Montali C (1983) Focal lesions in the spleen: sonography patterns and guided biopsy. AJR 140:59–65

138. Suzuki T, Shibuya H, Yoshimatsu S, Suzuki S (1987) Ultrasonically guided staging splenic tissue core biopsy in patients with non-Hodgkin's lymphoma. Cancer 60:879–882

139. Galambos JT (1986) Transmission of hepatitis B from providers to patients: how big is the risk? Hepatology 6:320–325

140. Cheli R (1987) Infezioni ed endoscopia digestiva. G Ital Endosc Dig 10:95

141. Henning H, Look D (1985) Sterilität, Asepsis, Instrumentenpflege. In: Henning H, Look D (eds) Laparoskopie. Thieme, Stuttgart, pp 77–78

142. Chiaramonte M, Floreani A, Naccarato R (1987) Le epatiti virali. G Ital Endosc Dig 10:103–106

143. Osterholm MT, Garayalde SM (1985) Clinical viral hepatitis B among Minnesota hospital personnel. Results of a ten-year statewide survey. Jama, 254:3207

144. Bovero G (1987) Il problema della disinfezione strumentale ed ambientale in endoscopia digestiva. G Ital Endosc Dig 10:109–111

145. Rey JF, Davranche E, Kassentini P, Sempere Y, Greff M (1987) Désinfection des endoscopes par un complexe phénate-glutaraldéhyde (Sporicidine). Acta Endosc 1:47–49

146. Yoshii Y, Kasugat T, Nakamura T (1985) Disinfections effect of endoscopes using new washer model EW 10. Gastroenterol Endosc 27:361–365

147. Spire B, Nugeyre MT, Dormont D, Chermann JC, Barre-Sinoussi F (1985) Inactivation du "limphadenopathy AIDS virus" (LAV). Med Hyg 43:1614–1621

148. Martinelli G, De Mercato R (1987) Endoscopia e AIDS. G Ital Endosc Dig 10:97–99

II Present Uses of Laparoscopy

4 Traditional Indications for Laparoscopy

4.1 Ascites

Ascites has different causes, and the first step in making a diagnosis is to distinguish between *transudative* and *exudative* ascites, which are caused by completely different diseases, by examining the properties of the liquid, which can be withdrawn by means of exploratory abdominal puncture. In many cases ascites can be put into the context of a particular group of laboratory and instrumental symptoms and can therefore be satisfactorily interpreted. On other occasions, however, ascites is a single symptom or is associated with signs that are not particularly significant. So, where only clinical means are used, it is quite difficult to detect the disease causing the ascites, and laparoscopy has always been of value in its diagnosis.

The diagnostic hypothesis depends on whether or not the ascites is transudative, which is caused by only a few conditions. These diseases have transudative effusion as their dominant symptom, and they are therefore difficult to diagnose: (a) intrahepatic, metahepatic, or prehepatic *portal hypertension*, due to different types of processes that have few, or atypical, symptoms and cannot be detected clinically and (b) rare *gynecological diseases*.

Laparoscopy has a high diagnostic efficacy in such cases because it enables us to make a macroscopic and histological examination of the liver. In our series of 725 cases [1] of ascites that were clinically undiagnosable, 24 patients had transudative effusion. Laparoscopy revealed cirrhosis that had been overlooked at the clinical examination; in 14 of these cases there were endoscopic signs of portal hypertension, and in 2 there was liver carcinoma with cirrhosis. These findings allowed us accurately to interpret ascites as the consequence of intrahepatic portal hypertension. Since liver stasis was found, laparoscopy indicated that very probably (two cases in our series) effusion was caused by metahepatic portal hypertension as in the "genuine" (through occlusion or external pressure on the suprahepatic veins) or "pseudo" Budd-Chiari syndrome (from stasis of the blood flow into the right atrium in constrictive pericarditis).

Moreover, a laparoscopic picture consisting of the following was significant: (a) normal liver, (b) sectorial collateral venous circulation affecting only the vessels of the omentum, phrenocolic ligament, and abdominal wall at the left hypochondrium; and (c) any splenomegaly. In two of our cases the latter finding, compatible with prehepatic portal hypertension, gave a likely explanation for the ascites.

Laparoscopy also enables us to identify any diseases of the female genitalia, such as benign or malignant neoplastic ovarian or uterine cysts (two cases in our series). This finding allowed us to interpret ascites as a sign of Meigs's syndrome or pseudosyndrome. In our experience, in the presonographic age in cases of transudative ascites of uncertain origin, laparoscopy allowed a certain diagnosis to be made in 66% of cases, a probable diagnosis in 25%, while in 8% it failed to allow a diagnosis to be made at all.

Exudative or *hemorrhagic* abdominal effusion is almost always caused by *inflammatory* or *granulomatous* peritoneal diseases or by *primary* or *secondary* tumors.

With laparoscopy we can explore almost all the parietal, and a large part of the visceral, peritoneum, mainly by examining the patient in different decubitus positions and by shifting the organs with the probe. So any lesions are unlikely to be overlooked in a thorough examination. The proportion of laparoscopic diagnoses in these cases is notoriously high, above 90%. An exudative abdominal effusion left undiagnosed has always been considered a definite indication for laparoscopy.

4.1.1 Present Indications for Laparoscopy

The diagnostic approach to patients with ascites has also changed, thanks to the advent of imaging techniques. It is now easier to detect ascites, whether free or a sac collection, and this finding is made earlier because now even a small collection can be detected. Echography is the most sensitive available technique for detecting effusions of even 200–300 ml. Moreover, when the collection is small, we can use echography to guide an explorative puncture in order to obtain a sample of the fluid for examination. When considering the repercussions that noninvasive techniques have had on the indications for laparoscopy, we must make a clear distinction between *transudative* and *nontransudative* ascites.

4.1.1.1 Transudative Ascites

As is already known, the most frequent cause of undiagnosed transudative ascites is clinically undetected portal hypertension. With imaging techniques any portal hypertension causing ascites is unlikely to be overlooked. The sonographic symptomatology for portal hypertension is now both exhaustive and accurate, allowing a clear distinction to be made between intrahepatic and prehepatic or metahepatic portal hypertension. Prehepatic hypertension from portal thrombosis can be detected because the finding of a hyperechogenic area in a normally anechogenic area denotes the lumen of the vena porta with its main branches. Any splenic vein obstruction is also almost always detected, although this can be hindered by intestinal gas. Moreover, with sonography the Budd-Chiari syndrome can be diagnosed and the ascites accurately interpreted. In these cases the hepatic vein is either not visualized or it presents a reduced lumen, unlike cases of circulatory decompensation, where the hepatic vein appears dilated. Any failure to visualize the hepatic vein indicates a tumoral infiltration. Furthermore, with sonography we can detect practically any genital disease causing ascites in *Meigs's syndrome.*

Today, thanks to imaging techniques, there are very few cases of unsatisfactorily explained ascites. Consequently, laparoscopy is only indicated on rare occasions, depending on the evaluation of each particular case. For example, there have been reports of cases of clinically undiagnosed transudative ascites that at laparoscopy were found to be peritoneal tuberculosis, but these are exceptional [2, 3].

4.1.1.2 Nontransudative Ascites

Serous or serohemorrhagic nontransudative ascites is almost always due to a peritoneal disease and in these cases the diagnostic efficacy of the imaging techniques is poor; it can in fact only detect peritoneal and omental "masses," which generally present hypoechogenic images, appearing nodular, in the form of plaques (mantle or sheet-like), or irregularly shaped. But in the majority of cases the lesions are small, flat, or thin, and the sonographic finding, except for the finding of ascites, is negative.

It must also be added that even when sonography demonstrates serosa lesions, it does not provide reliable information on the nature of the process, and this can only be obtained if the masses are large enough targets for echo-guided fine-needle puncture. In such cases, the cytological or histological diagnosis is more reliable, but the disease is usually advanced, and the diagnosis late, so any chance of an effective cure is compromised. With imaging techniques, therefore, no great reduction in the number of clinically undiagnosed cases of non-transudative ascites has been achieved.

On the other hand, progress has been made in recent years in the study of the ascitic fluid. Cytological techniques have been refined and greater experience gained by the examiners, so now this technique contributes more to the diagnosis, mainly in cases of neoplastic ascites. However, peritoneal tuberculosis is more difficult to detect through examination of the liquid. The finding of manifest lymphocytosis is an indication, but it is not enough, and only in rare cases can we find mycobacterial tuberculosis of the ascitic fluid; it is isolated in culture in under 10% of cases [3–6]. Therefore laparoscopy is indicated when the cause of a nontransudative abdominal fluid collection must be discovered, and this aspect in the diagnosis of ascites is the same as it was in the past. Let us therefore stress only that:

An abdominal leakage with these features mainly occurs in organic diseases of the peritoneum. The most frequent forms are *tuberculosis* and *primary* and *secondary tumors*, which are more frequent.

Laparoscopy enables us to visualize directly the lesions on the parietal and visceral peritoneum in the great majority of cases. They cannot be diagnosed when the disease causing the exudation has a limited spread and is localized in inaccessible areas. In laparoscopy, peritoneal lesions can easily be recognized but it may be difficult to distinguish between the diseases causing ascites because the pictures may be polymorphic, resulting in poor specificity.

An intensely and diffusely congested peritoneum, damaged by numerous small slightly raised miliary-form nodules, gives a picture typical of miliary tuberculosis of the peritoneum (Fig. 4.1) and provides a sufficiently reliable diagnosis. The finding shown in Fig. 4.2 is quite similar: the parietal peritoneum is red and tumid, and has a clearly "inflammatory" aspect: it presents numerous tiny nodules, which are only slightly raised and of miliary-form. The macroscopic diagnosis of tuberculosis may therefore appear to be equally reliable. In the former case, biopsy confirms the tuberculosis, whereas in the latter it shows a metastatic carcinoma spread from the large intestine that had been overlooked.

The miliary-form spread itself therefore appears to be tubercular on the parietal peritoneum, and may lead us to suspect a noninflammatory process, because there is little or no congestion, as is found in cases of neoplastic spread (Fig. 4.3). In fact, the biopsy demonstrates carcinosis secondary to an overlooked ovarian carcinoma.

On other occasions the serosa is tumid with small, but not miliary-form, nodular lesions that are slightly raised and that have confused borders. There is no congestion and only small subserous hemorrhagic suffusions are observed. (Fig. 4.4). The picture is similar to that shown in Fig. 4.3. but the intestinal loops tend to adhere to each other and this suggests neoplasia. The histological examination, however, specifies tuberculosis. Yet it is known that tubercular lesions are polymorphic: fleshy nodular formations may be seen on the peritoneum with no sign of inflammation; they are described as "neoplastiform." A fairly specific feature of tuberculosis, even if it is not exclusive to this disease, is the presence of an important fibrinous exudative component. The fibrin may be suspended in the fluid or deposited between the intestinal loops, resulting in fusion, or it may form taut "curtains" between the wall and the organ.

Primary peritoneal tumors have no morphological features that facilitate their macroscopic detection, but lesions in the form of soft, raised, shiny plaques that are seen and then easily removed with the pincers lead us to suspect mesothelioma (Fig. 4.5).

It was long held that explorative laparotomy was required for the diagnosis of mesothelioma but it has been demonstrated that laparoscopy allows an equally reliable diagnosis to be made [4, 5], thanks to target biopsy. It should, however, be kept in mind that it is also difficult to make a histological diagnosis, and particularly exhaustive examinations must be made on several tissue samples, so multiple biopsies must be taken [6].

The examples here presented show the morphological features most frequently found in peritoneal diseases, stress the crucial importance of biopsy, and demonstrate that only through a direct examination, with the possibility of making an anatomo-histological evaluation, can a diagnosis be made. For these reasons the noninvasive imaging techniques provide decisive findings only in the occasional case. So even in the sonographic era laparoscopy with biopsy is still the technique of choice for the diagnosis of nontransudative ascites. This applies of course only after an exhaustive study has already failed to provide the diagnosis.

The more recent literature [7–10] confirms the above opinion. Laparoscopy with biopsy provides very good results, a reliable diagnosis being made in 100% of cases in which it is possible to find the peritoneal lesion from which the biopsy is to be taken. On the other hand, only a "probable" diagnosis is made in cases of serous or serofibrinous leakage with diffuse peritoneal congestion, which can be very copious, sometimes with numerous fixed adhesions. Since in these cases none of the lesions have specific features, target biopsy cannot be performed and any peritoneal fragment obtained fails to provide useful data. One can only make the following hypotheses: (a) aspecific exudative peritonitis, which is very rare; (b) spontaneous bacterial peritonitis (if there is associated cirrhosis); or (more probably) (c) tubercular peritonitis "without lesions."

Our series of 91 cases of serous effusion with exudative features is shown in Table 4.1: in 83.5% certain diagnoses were made, in 15.3% the diagnosis was probable, and in 1.09% diagnostic failures were recorded.

In serohematic effusions the process is almost exclusively tubercular or neoplastic and there are manifest lesions from which biopsies can always be taken; in 24 such cases we studied, a certain diagnosis was made in 100%. We therefore agree with Boyd [10], who in 1987 stated that in his

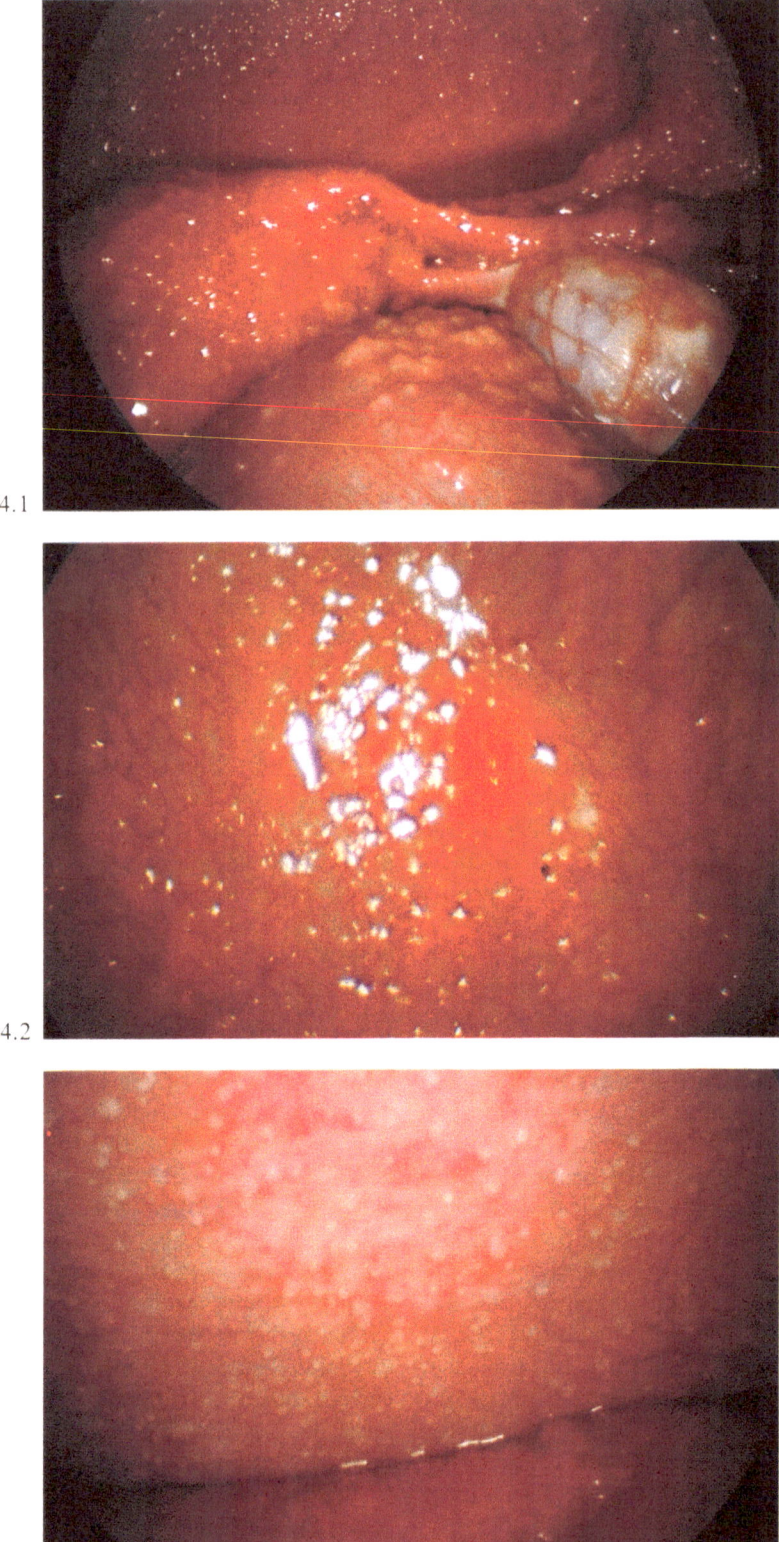

4.1

4.2

4.3

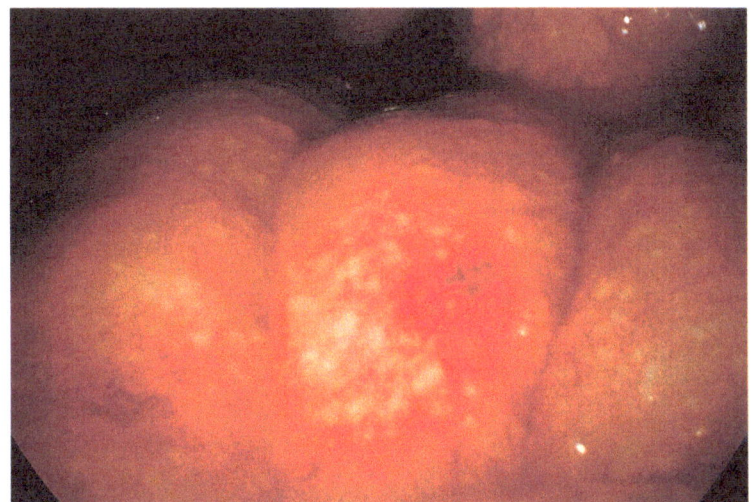

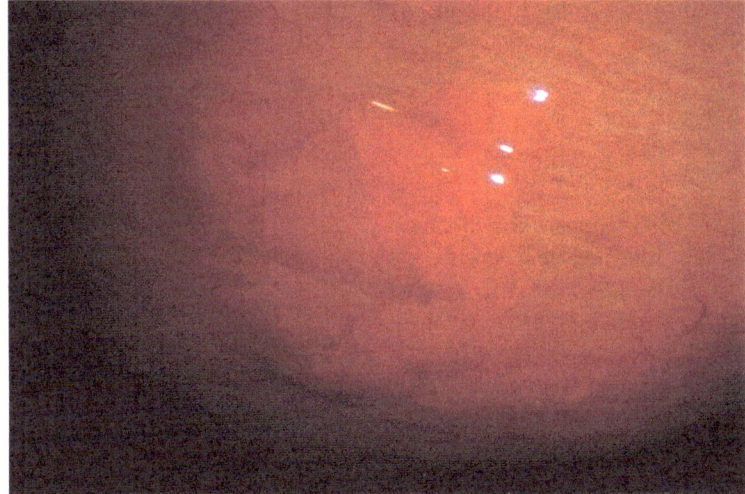

Fig. 4.1. Laparoscopic view of the pelvis: *to the left* can be seen the right half of the uterus, right adnexum, and ovary; *in the foreground*, an intestinal loop. The serosa is congested and has multiple whitish-pink nodular formations that are isolated or confluent. Also the parietal peritoneum, which can be seen in the background, appears highly congested and covered with miliary-form granules that are illuminated by the flash. *Peritoneal tuberculosis?* Histological confirmation

Fig. 4.2. Parietal peritoneum under high magnification. Active and passive congestion (small, turgid, distinct vessels). Numerous small nodules revealed. *Peritoneal tuberculosis?* Biopsy: *peritoneal diffusion from over-looked carcinoma of the intestine*

Fig. 4.3. Parietal peritoneum is not congested: dissemination of whitish nodules. *Peritoneal carcinosis? Tuberculosis?* Biopsy: *peritoneal diffusion of overlooked carcinoma of the ovary*

Fig. 4.4. Intestinal loops immersed in serohematic fluid tend to join together. Visceral peritoneum is not congested, but has subserous hemorrhagic spread with multiple whitish nodules with hazy borders. *Tuberculosis? Metastatic carcinoma?* Biopsy: *tuberculosis of the peritoneum*

Fig. 4.5. Parietal peritoneum of the abdominal arch that is slightly congested and scabrous. Fleshy, tumid deposit with an irregular shape. *Mesothelioma?* Biopsy: *mesothelioma of the peritoneum*

Table 4.1. Laparoscopic diagnosis in exudative ascites (91 cases)

	Diagnosis	
Certain diagnosis (76 cases)	Peritoneal tuberculosis	21
	Peritoneal mesothelioma	6
	Metastatic peritoneal tumor	49
Probable diagnosis (14 cases)	Tuberculosis peritonitis	6
	Secondary peritoneal tumor	2
	Liver cirrhosis	5
	Pancreatitis	1
Diagnostic error (1 case)	Cirrhosis (liver carcinoma)	1

experience "the importance of laparoscopy is underscored by the failure of CT to detect metastatic peritoneal lesions."

4.1.2 False Ascites

In 1980 I specified that before performing laparoscopy to diagnose ascites, the insidious nature of abdominal cysts, especially those of the ovary, should always be borne in mind [4]. When enormous, these formations can occupy a large part of the abdominal cavity and clinically simulate a free fluid ascites. I thus stressed the need for a particularly thorough clinical study in order to avoid mistakenly introducing the laparoscope in a large cyst: using a fine needle, fluid could be withdrawn from the cyst in an attempt to study its features. In doubtful cases some fluid should be withdrawn and some gas introduced and then a radiological study made of its distribution in the abdomen. If there are cysts, the gas forms a semicircle – its straight base is due to the fluid level and its convex border points upwards.

I believe that now, thanks to sonography, above all "sonography for laparoscopy," this danger is unlikely. However, some echographic and CT errors are still reported: among eight cases of enormous cysts (four ovarian and one pancreatic) echography and CT gave a diagnosis of free ascites in five [11].

4.1.3 Conclusions

1. Laparoscopy is a highly effective tool in the diagnosis of ascites.

2. In cases of transudative ascites, imaging techniques can now almost always explain the condition by demonstrating that there is clinically overlooked portal hypertension, the most frequent cause. Laparoscopy is therefore indicated only in exceptional cases.

3. In the large majority of cases, non-transudative ascites is caused by inflammatory or neoplastic peritoneal diseases with lesions that often are not detected or diagnosed with sonography and CT. So laparoscopy has kept almost all its traditional indications and is still the ideal diagnostic technique for exudative ascites.

4.2 Hepatomegaly

When hepatomegaly is the only or the main clinical symptom a number of different diseases should be considered: severe steatosis, sclerosis, hypertrophic "monosymptomatic" cirrhosis, abscess, parasitic and non-parasitic cysts, benign tumors, and malignant primary or secondary tumors. The diagnosis can pose problems that are extremely difficult, sometimes impossible, to resolve.

Of course, laparoscopy integrated with target biopsy does have limitations, but it can ensure a satisfactory diagnosis in a high percentage of cases. In the presonographic era, therefore, undiagnosed hepatomegaly was considered an absolute indication for laparoscopy [12–14].

The noninvasive imaging techniques have substantially modified the approach to these patients: hepatomegaly is an obvious indication for sonography, which enables us to recognize the features of certain processes, and establish whether the liver disease is due to a disease characterized by *diffuse* or *focal lesions*.

The improved diagnostic potential and the basic distinction now made between types of liver disease has radically changed the indications for laparoscopy because the diagnostic problems can often be overcome with sonography and CT. The indications for laparoscopy, in fact, do not depend upon the simple finding of liver enlargement.

Therefore *hepatomegaly of an uncertain nature* is no longer considered a "formal" indication for laparoscopy. However, any diagnostic problems not solved by imaging techniques must still be overcome. They are discussed in the chapters dealing with liver diseases.

4.2.1 False Hepatomegaly

When at palpation hepatomegaly is found we must always consider whether it might reflect *true* or *false* hepatomegaly. The clinical symptoms are not always reliable and a similar finding at the right hypochondrium or at the epigastrium, even if all the features of hepatomegaly are present, may not necessarily be due to liver enlargement. Some diseases can perfectly simulate hepatomegaly, for example: (a) gallbladder diseases (hydropic gallbladder covered by adherent omental fat, gallbladder with pericholecystitis, primary neoplasm involving the surrounding tissue, forming a compact mass that adheres to the liver and following its movements at inspiration and expiration, etc.); (b) neoplastic infiltration of the greater omentum that adheres to the liver, particularly to the left lobe; and (c) a large retroperitoneal tumor that raises and pushes the liver forwards and downwards.

In the above situations grossly mistaken interpretations can be made. Laparoscopy is performed to ascertain the nature of hepatomegaly. However, it also establishes whether or not the "hepatomegaly" itself is genuine. The laparoscopic finding of a normal-shaped and -sized liver dislocated by a mass which is sometimes directly visualized and sometimes hidden could presumably demonstrate false hepatomegaly; the real site of the lesion could be established and, in many cases, an exact diagnosis of its nature obtained. Nowadays the noninvasive techniques provide accurate insight and so any organ error is highly unlikely.

However, when there are no recognizable differences in the echogenicity of the organs and their contiguous structures, echography fails to establish reliably whether the finding of hepatomegaly at palpation really corresponds to a liver disease or not. In such cases laparoscopy is still definitely indicated as is borne out by the following example.

During a clinical examination a patient was being staged for cancer of the esophagus; questionable hepatomegaly was found and sonography demonstrated that the left lobe of the liver was raised and compressed by a formation, the nature of which

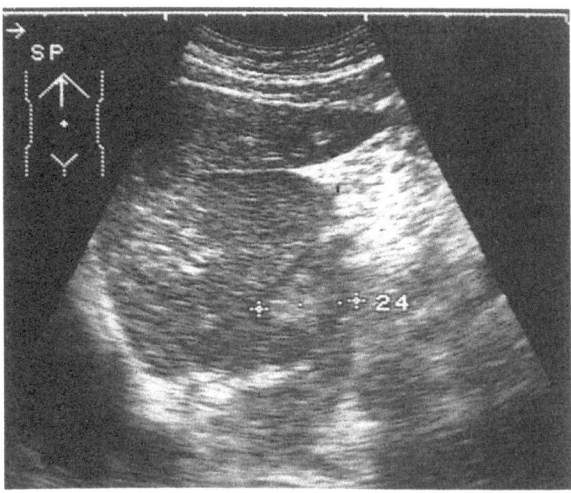

Fig. 4.6. Longitudinal echographic epigastric scan. The left lobe of the liver appears normal and is shifted and raised upwards by the caudate lobe, which is enlarged, has irregular margins, and has a dishomogeneous and hyperechogenic structure. *Neoplastic infiltration of the caudate lobe suspected*

was dubious (Fig. 4.6). This could have been an enlarged and infiltrated caudate lobe or a mass outside the liver. When staging, it is very important to establish reliably whether any tumor diffusion affects the liver or not because the stage specified also depends on this. In order to clarify the doubt a laparoscopy was performed. Endoscopically the liver appeared normal; the left lobe was shifted by a mass mainly covered by fat; its neoplastic nature was easily recognized – through the presence of an irregular nodule that appeared, in part, on the surface (Fig. 4.7). Biopsy confirmed metastasis from esophageal cancer, which, however, did not affect the liver.

4.2.2 Conclusions

1. Hepatomegaly of an uncertain nature was once a classical indication for laparoscopy, but is no longer considered so because ultrasound can demonstrate "localized lesions" irrespective of the presence of liver enlargement.

2. Laparoscopy may still be indicated when the echographic finding is doubtful, since it can establish whether the hepatomegaly is genuine or false.

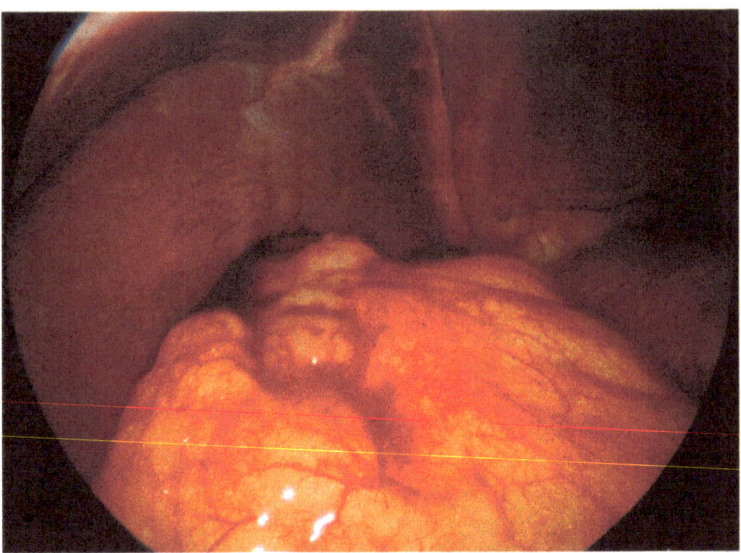

Fig. 4.7. Laparoscopy. Left lobe of the liver shifted upwards and medially by a large fat-covered mass at its tip, from which protrudes a fleshy nodule. *Metastasis of the omentum.* Biopsy: *metastasis from epidermoid carcinoma of the esophagus*

4.3 Splenomegaly

A clinical finding of splenomegaly can give rise to diagnostic problems that are difficult to resolve. This does not apply to splenomegaly when it is part of a complete and clear clinical picture and when it is a fundamental symptom of, for example, leukosis, hemolytic anemia, or polycytemia. In other instances, however, spleen enlargement may sometimes be an unexpected single finding or it may be the main symptom in a clinical picture that has no other significant elements. So here the diagnosis can be made only by studying the spleen, and in these particular cases laparoscopy proved it could resolve the diagnostic problem, either completely or partly.

As already stated (see Sect. 3.4.4) the spleen is a difficult organ to study laparoscopically and this is due to:

1. Technical reasons; in 10% of cases it is not easy to explore.
2. Difficulty in interpreting the different findings, which are often insignificant.
3. In many splenopathies the surface and macroscopic characteristics of the organ may appear normal.

Notwithstanding these difficulties, which are largely overcome if biopsy is used, the diagnosis of *clinically undiagnosed splenomegalies* has always been considered an important indication for laparoscopy.

4.3.1 Present Indications for Laparoscopy

Now with imaging techniques our diagnostic approach has changed and in certain types of splenomegaly a satisfactory diagnosis can be made. Obviously in these cases, any endoscopic examination would be superfluous, and the number of "clinically undiagnosed splenomegalies" has decreased. However, sonography cannot resolve the diagnostic problem in all cases of splenomegaly, so laparoscopy still has some valid indications.

4.3.1.1 False Splenomegalies

The semeiological distinction between *true* and *false splenomegaly* poses far greater problems than might at first be imagined; the finding at palpation can give rise to terrible mistakes. Because of its site, characteristics, and mobility a particular type of splenomegaly may simulate another abdominal condition, above all an enlarged left lobe of the liver; it may be mistaken for a tumor of the kidney or of the retroperitoneum, a neoplastic infiltration of the omentum, or a cyst. Several abdominal diseases, above all enlargement of the left hepatic lobe or a retroperitoneal tumor, can have the same site and can be mistaken for an enlarged spleen. With sonography many doubts are clarified and we can accurately establish whether or not there is true enlargement of the spleen. In some cases, however, the echographic finding is not clear, particularly in cases of infiltrating neoplasms that envelop the spleen, making it difficult echographically to distinguish between the infiltration tissue and the spleen. When the sonographic finding does not enable a diagnosis to be made, laparoscopy is indicated and it can be decisive. A false picture of splenomegaly may be due to a deep-seated mass that can shift or cause lateral or downward displacement of a normal spleen. In some cases direct vision of any such mass enables us to make an immediate diagnosis and with a target biopsy the nature of the process itself is easily established.

4.3.1.2 True Splenomegalies

Splenomegaly can be caused by *focal lesions* and by *diffuse alterations.*

1. Focal Lesions. Sonography can detect the presence of splenic focal lesions whether they have a *liquid* or *solid content.* Of course in the vast majority of *formations with a liquid content* sonography allows us to make an accurate diagnosis of *simple and complex, parasitic, epidermoid cysts or cystic lymphangioma,* etc. Intrasplenic *hematomas* are fairly easy to recognize: such diagnoses can moreover be confirmed and made even more accurate with fine-needle target biopsy.

The sonographic diagnosis of angioma, however, may pose problems. The difficulties encountered may be due to the fact that the picture is not always significant and in such cases biopsy is risky and, moreover, usually fails to provide enough data. Clearly when sonography shows a lesion with a liquid content the indications for laparoscopy are now few and far between, being limited to the cases (hemangiomas with an uncertain diagnosis, abscesses, or colliquated tumors, etc.) in which the echographic finding and fine-needle biopsy give rise to doubts.

In patients with *solid focal lesions,* sonography usually evidences diseased tissue even when the structural modifications are slight with respect to the parenchyma. And with sonography it is almost impossible to diagnose the nature (inflammatory, granulomatose, neoplastic, etc.), but with fine-needle biopsy it can be clarified.

The latter has proved promising, but its findings are still not comparable with those provided by laparoscopy and direct biopsy. Therefore where there is sonographic detection of solid focal lesions of the spleen, there are still several indications for laparoscopy.

2. Diffuse Alterations. In a considerable number of splenomegalies sonography can only confirm that the organ is enlarged but it does not allow a diagnosis to be made. There may in fact be diffuse alterations in the echogenicity with no particular characteristics being revealed, or the picture may even appear quite normal. The patient may have splenomegaly from *diffuse disease* or from *focal lesions* that, however, cannot be detected sonographically because they are too small or because there is little echogenic difference between them and their surrounding parenchyma. The diagnosis may then be made by using fine-needle transcutaneous biopsy, but the results are not always satisfactory. So in splenomegaly with an uncertain or negative sonographic finding, laparoscopy still offers the best chances of making a reliable and accurate diagnosis.

It is necessary here to refer to diagnostic "probability" because, as we shall see, neither laparoscopy nor multiple biopsies can always guarantee that the diagnostic difficulties will be overcome. A very large number of splenomegalies are never diagnosed or are insufficiently clarified because in many cases neither the macroscopic nor the histological finding can be correlated to a well-defined disease.

4.3.2 Main Laparoscopic Findings

In patients with splenomegaly laparoscopy can show: (a) focal lesions on the surface of the organ, (b) diffuse alterations of an uncertain nature, and (c) an apparently normal macroscopic picture.

1. Focal Lesions. If there are visible focal lesions with the characteristics described (see Sect. 3.4.4), it is difficult to make a decision on the basis of the macroscopic picture, but with target biopsy a diagnosis can be made in the great majority of cases. However, in only a small number of cases of splenomegaly is a similar finding made. Among our series of 221 patients with splenomegaly of an uncertain nature, only 31 (13%) had surface alterations that were probably pathological (Fig. 4.8);

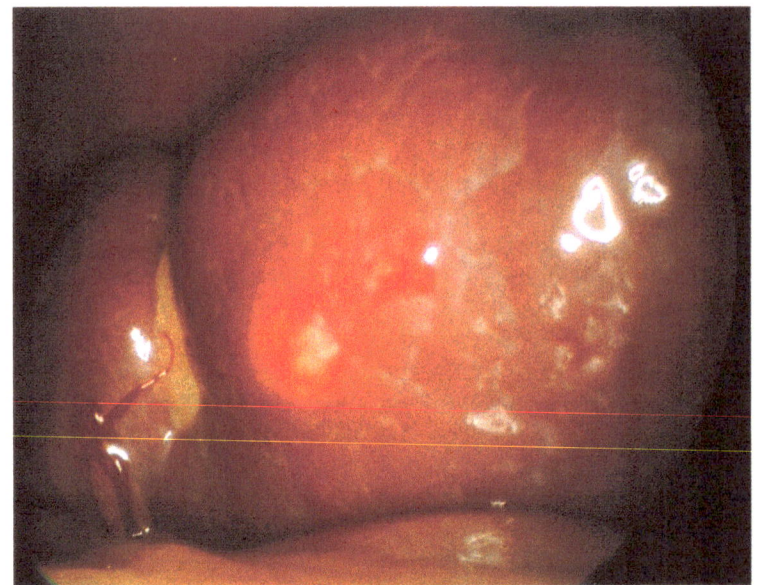

4.8

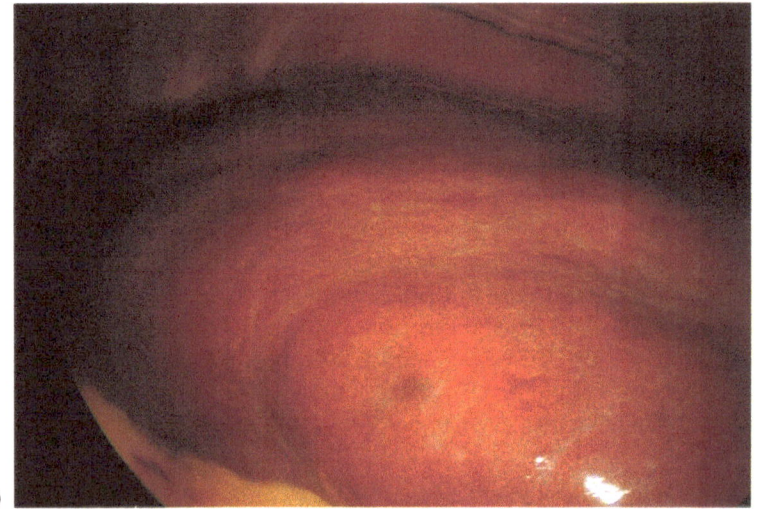

4.9

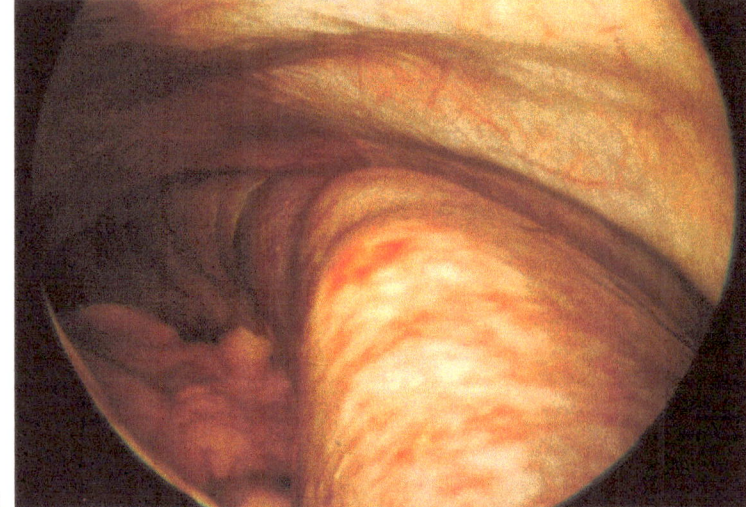

4.10

with one target biopsy, or more, a preliminary diagnosis of its nature was made in 23 cases [11 Hodgkin's disease (HD) lymphomas, 8 non-Hodgkin's disease (NHD) lymphomas, 2 sarcoidoses, 2 tuberculoses] while in the other 8 the finding was negative or uncertain [15].

2. Splenomegaly Without Visible Lesions. If at laparoscopy an enlarged spleen is found but no modifications in its shape and no significant alterations in its surface are observed, then the diagnosis is complex because the evidence needed to make it is missing. Unlike the liver, the spleen has a highly uncertain laparoscopic semeiology and in very few cases do variations in color or appearance have significant characteristics. In 80.8% of the 99 cases of splenomegaly examined by Garcia Molinero et al., no significant alterations were observed in the macroscopic picture; the spleen was enlarged and reddish or reddish-gray but no anomalies that indicated the diagnosis were found [16]. Where there is an isolated splenomegaly of this type the only hypotheses that can be put forward are: (a) splenomegaly due to a graunlomatous or neoplastic productive process localized within the organ, but hidden; and (b) a so-called "fibrous splenomegaly" or "fibrocongestive" splenomegaly or in any case a "primary splenomegaly," accepting all the etio-pathogenetic gaps and the nosographic uncertainties in this field.

We must, however, bear in mind that sometimes fibrocongestive splenomegalies have characteritics that are fairly distinct. The spleen may appear both enlarged and swollen, and its consistency may be increased; it may be congested, with small hemorrhagic subserous suffusions and it may have a slightly *rough* surface (Fig. 4.9). Otherwise, if there is prevalent fibrosis, the organ appears

---

Fig. 4.8. Splenomegaly. On the organ surface can be seen a small, slightly raised, roundish, yellowy-white small plaque. *Malignant lymphoma?* Biopsy: *Hodgkin's disease lymphoma*

Fig. 4.9. Splenomegaly. Marked enlargement of organ with an irregular surface that has small subcapsular hemorrhagic suffusions. *Congestive splenomegaly probable*

Fig. 4.10. Advanced splenomegaly: medial margin rounded, with deep furrows. Grayish-red pale surface with areas of capsular thickening. *Fibrocongestive splenomegaly probable*

grayish and its surface is very *irregular* because of retraction (Fig. 4.10). In these uncertain situations laparoscopy can provide some important indirect diagnostic elements through, for example, *examination of the liver* and *the study of portal hypertension.* In isolated splenomegaly, a reliable impression of the condition of the liver is very important. Laparoscopy can in fact evidence liver cirrhosis even where there are no clinical or bio-humoral signs of liver disease. We are dealing here with those forms that we call "anatomical cirrhosis" [17], the assessment of which may provide a satisfactory explanation for the splenomegaly. On the other hand, if the liver is found to be normal, the splenomegaly can be considered primary and autonomous, and independent of a liver disease.

Garcia Molinero et al. [16] hold that liver exploration is often the "key" when diagnosing splenomegaly. The finding of any collateral circulation from portal hypertension allows us fairly reliably to assume that the spleen enlargement has a hemodynamic origin. Now that collateral circulations can be studied sonographically, here laparoscopy has lost much of its value. We must, however, bear in mind that with endoscopy the small veins can be examined with greater accuracy; these veins are not revealed sonographically. So endoscopic findings are much more accurate and important, above all when searching for small initial collateral circulations limited to particular sectors. Where there is manifest cirrhosis, it is less important to demonstrate collateral circulations because the hepatopathy itself explains the etiopathogenesis of the spleen enlargement. But if the liver is intact, signs of portal hypertension play a decisive role because they allow us to establish that the splenomegaly is due to prehepatic portal hypertension. As these signs of portal hypertension are not always evident, they should be searched for thoroughly in some key spots. In splenomegalies, in particular, the vessels on the phrenocholic ligament should be studied as there are natural connexions between the portal and caval circulations. If dilated and turgid veins are found in this site, indicating the presence of a collateral portacaval circulation, then the splenomegaly is almost certainly due to prehepatic portal hypertension (see Sect. 6.3).

Laparoscopic biopsy moreover allows a diagnosis to be made also in a number of these types of splenomegaly. Any biopsies are blind because there are no visible lesions from which to take the sample and so there is less likelihood of encountering diseased tissue. Nevertheless, if multiple biopsies are taken (at least three from different parts of the spleen), the probability of making a diagnosis is increased.

In 190 cases of splenomegaly without significant macroscopic alterations, which amounted to 86% of all the uncertain nature splenomegalies studied by us laparoscopically [15], a certain diagnosis was made in 40 cases, in which the splenomegaly depended upon diffuse infiltration of productive processes, the nature of which varied, without macroscopically perceptible lesions (16 Hodgkin's disease lymphomas, 10 non-Hodgkin's disease lymphomas, 6 sarcoidoses, 3 tuberculoses, 5 others). In 20 cases the histological finding was normal, although we should always be aware of the danger of false negatives.

Finally, in the large majority (130 cases, 68%) of splenomegalies that could be interpreted macroscopically, biopsy demonstrated only a "congestion of sinuses," "splenic pulp hyperplasia," "fibrosis," "follicular hyperplasia," etc. These findings are not useless because they enable us to rule out true splenopathy. They do not always allow a clinical diagnosis to be made, but they fairly reliably rule out a granulomatous or neoplastic organic disease.

Laparoscopy therefore enables us to make an otherwise impossible diagnosis in some cases of splenomegaly with insignificant sonographic and macroscopic findings. It certainly provides us with useful orientation.

4.3.3 Conclusions

1. Laparoscopy, above all if it is systematically associated with biopsy, was, in the presonographic era, the most effective means for the study of splenomegalies that had not been diagnosed on a clinical basis.

2. Imaging techniques, and mainly the more widespread use of sonography, have reduced the number of undiagnosed splenomegalies and so the indications for laparoscopy have diminished.

3. Laparoscopy, however, is still of considerable value in this field in inverse proportion to the diagnostic efficacy of sonography. The latter is (a) *very high* when the splenomegaly is sustained by focal lesions with a liquid content, and therefore the indications for laparoscopy

are few and far between; (b) *moderate* in solid lesions of an appreciable size, so here laparoscopy is quite frequently used; and (c) *slight* in splenomegaly with diffuse alterations – in these cases the indications for laparoscopy with biopsy are still almost total. (d) We must bear in mind, however, that also with laparoscopy and biopsy an accurate, clinically useful, diagnosis can be obtained in only about 25% of patients with splenomegaly.

4.4 Abdominal Masses

When an abdominal mass is palpated, we must always consider a large number of diagnostic hypotheses because of its different possible origins and natures. However, the following are useful clues: site, size, shape, consistency, surface characteristics, relationship with other abdominal organs, immobility or mobility, and any pain to the patient at palpation.

However, further investigations are almost always required to make a reliable clinical diagnosis of a mass that is the main symptom in a generally insignificant picture, whether it is an isolated or accidental finding. In the presonographic era, despite its limitations, above all its inability to study the retroperitoneal formations, laparsocopy was the most valuable available diagnostic tool for abdominal masses. Until 1979, in our center laparoscopy was performed to diagnose a clinically undiagnosed abdominal mass in 203 (3.2%) cases in a total of 6230 examinations [18]. In this series, laparoscopy, integrated where possible with biopsy, was found to be of definite diagnostic use. In 98 cases (almost 50%), a certain diagnosis was obtained, and this was confirmed or clarified by the histological examination. In another 60 cases in which it was not possible to take a biopsy, a fairly reliable macroscopic diagnosis was made. In only about 20% was it impossible to make a diagnosis at all.

However, if we consider the different laparoscopic diagnoses of these patients, it emerges that in the majority a laparoscopy would now no longer be performed. These diagnoses were: (a) hypertrophic cirrhosis, severe steatosis, primary or secondary liver carcinoma, cysts, angiomas, etc.; (b) gallbladder hydrops; (c) neoplastic spread to the omentum and mesentery; and (d) cysts of the mesentery, intestine, etc.

4.4.1 Present Indications for Laparoscopy

At present sonography and, where necessary, echoguided biopsy have enabled us to make a diagnosis satisfactorily in the great majority of patients with abdominal masses. The indications for laparoscopy have diminished. Gandolfi et al. [19] report that in the presonographic era, from 1973 to 1974, they performed laparoscopy in 3.1% of a total of 667 patients, whereas in 1980–1981 it was performed in only 1.1% of 769 patients with clinically undiagnosed palpable abdominal masses. In our center in 1986 the indications for laparoscopy to diagnose abdominal masses fell to about 1% in a total of 768 laparoscopies performed.

With sonography palpable abdominal masses are almost always identified and we can also detect masses that fail to have clinical manifestations and that cannot be detected at the clinical examination.

Masses with a liquid content are easily recognized and their characteristics are distinct enough for a good diagnostic picture: thin-needle puncture and an examination of the aspirated liquid enables the diagnosis to be clarified in a very high percentage of cases.

Solid masses are also easily identified but there may be diagnostic doubts as to the origin and nature of the disease, above all when a mass is so large that it comprises other nearby organs without there being a recognizable cleavage plane. An uncertain echographic picture is, however, clarified with thin-needle biopsy, which in such cases is easily performed because the target is large.

In this field, the results obtained with echography and fine-needle biopsy are 98% specificity and about 90% diagnostic accuracy. The percentages for the diagnoses obtained are therefore much higher than those obtained with laparoscopy and biopsy.

Radiologists believe that sonography has completely replaced laparoscopy. Yet, although this technique has certainly lost many of its indications, our experience of echography combined with laparoscopy has demonstrated that there are cases in which only laparoscopy can provide further insight when the sonographic diagnosis is either doubtful or unobtainable.

The diseases that can cause a clinically undiagnosable abdominal mass for which imaging techniques fail to provide a satisfactory picture and call for laparoscopic clarification can be summarized as follows: (a) *neoplasms* and *chronic phlogosis of the gallbladder* (cholecystitis and pericholecystitis) and (b) *tumors and chronic phlogosis of the large intestine and peritoneum*.

4.4.1.1 Neoplasms and Chronic Inflammation of the Gallbladder

Sonography usually demonstrates whether or not a mass in the right hypochondrium has a cholecystic origin, although sometimes this is difficult to establish because the gallbladder is surrounded by diseased tissue. A sonographic diagnosis of gallbladder carcinoma is based upon a rational assumption, which in turn is based upon the following data: (a) the site of the mass seems to replace the gallbladder, (b) formations entering the lumen are present, (c) irregular thickening of the wall is observed at the site of the mass, and (d) there may be spread to the liver – this may be in an adjacent area or it may be a distant metastasis.

The above elements are not always certain and some may be overlooked; fine-needle biopsy may, moreover, be unobtainable or may fail to provide useful clues. There are therefore many obstacles to overcome, above all when a differential diagnosis is to be made between a neoplastic gallbladder mass and chronic cholecystitis, sometimes with calculosis in which an important and diffuse pericholecystitis has developed. Nor is the finding of stones in or near the mass decisive because associated stones and tumors are frequent.

In these particular situations laparoscopy is certainly indicated. However, this technique is also limited by the following: (a) the gallbladder is not always visible – in 70% of a series of ours of 98 laparoscopically studied patients [20, 21] it was possible to explore the gallbladder directly and in the remaining patients thick adhesions fixed the omental fat and hid the organ; (b) the diagnosis is almost always based on the macroscopic finding because it is impossible to take a biopsy from the wall.

Notwithstanding the above shortcomings, laparoscopy is of considerable value in the diagnosis of neoplastic masses sustained by a gallbladder tumor that was not revealed sonographically; the diagnosis is based on macroscopic findings demonstrating the following alterations, alterations that

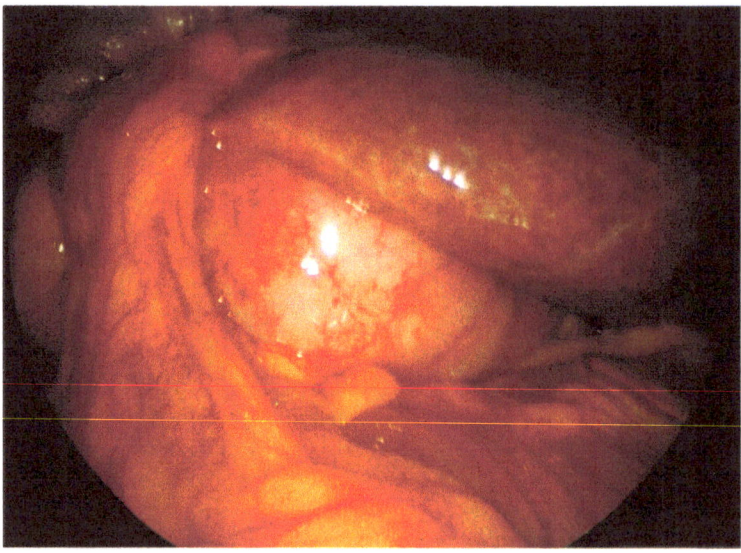

Fig. 4.11. Mass in the right hypochondrium. The gall-bladder, which is enlarged and has wall thickening, shifts the right lobe of the liver upwards; some omental adipose tissue adheres to the gallbladder. *Carcinoma of the gallbladder and pericholecystitis*

are not always shown by sonography: (a) considerable increase in volume and great tension and rigidity, which raise the gallbladder so it appears to project under the lobe of the liver; (b) thickening of the wall, which appears regular, smooth, and flattened or also has raised plaques or nodules; (c) a whitish glazed aspect, or slight congestion; and (d) extremely hard and woody at palpation with the probe. These clues strongly suggest gallbladder carcinoma. In particular, if the organ is extraordinarily hard, this hardness, impossible to detect with other techniques, is a characteristic of definite value, for a diagnosis of carcinoma is highly probable and no other technique reveals this aspect. In other cases, laparoscopy demonstrates that the palpable mass consists of an enlarged gallbladder enclosed by thick omental tissue overlying the adhesion (Fig. 4.11). Macroscopically, the differential diagnosis between tumor and subacute-cholecistitis with pericholecystitis is not easy to make. Often, however, satisfactory clarification is provided by the finding of focuses of proximal spread to the liver of a neoplastic process from which biopsies can be taken, and these completely resolve any doubts. With laparoscopy, in fact, the finding of small metastases to the liver or peritoneum that cannot be detected with so-

nography enables a certain diagnosis to be made, also when the gallbladder is completely covered or hidden by adhesions. This occurs frequently because in carcinoma of the gallbladder metastatization occurs early and in a high percentage of cases (89.7% in our series) [21].

4.4.1.2 Tumors of the Large Intestine and Peritoneum

There are other situations in which sonography can detect the mass, classify it as a solid formation, define its dimensions, shape, and relationship to the surrounding organs but cannot clarify its nature, partly because the echographic finding is not specific enough and, above all, because echo-guided biopsy is either unsuccessful or fails to give a significant finding. In these situations laparoscopy still has an absolute indication because in many cases the macroscopic finding and, where possible, target biopsy enable a diagnosis to be made.

Laparoscopy can demonstrate that the mass consists of so-called *plastic exudations*, i.e., dense, semi-solid, or solid fibrous collections that engulf adjacent organs and that have a neoplastiform mass arrangement that is, however, clearly inflammatory. These findings were once frequent in peritoneal tuberculosis, but they are no longer encountered. We are mainly concerned here with chronic circumscribed nonspecific peritonitis secondary to appendicitis, diverticulitis, or perforation of a diverticulum, etc.

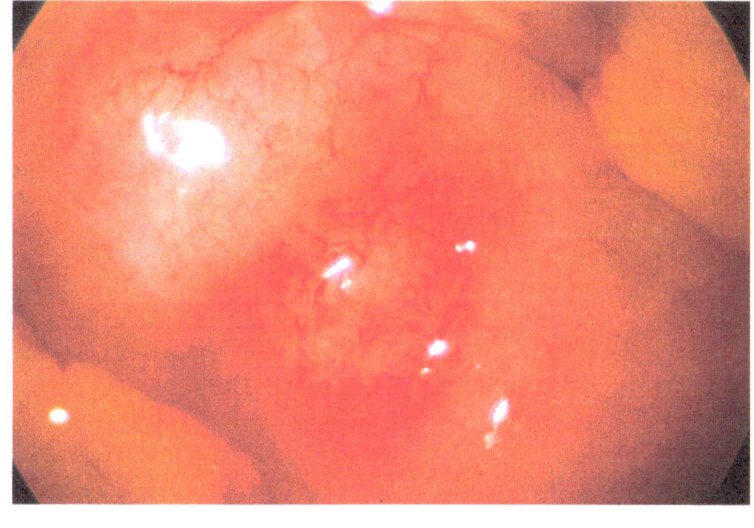

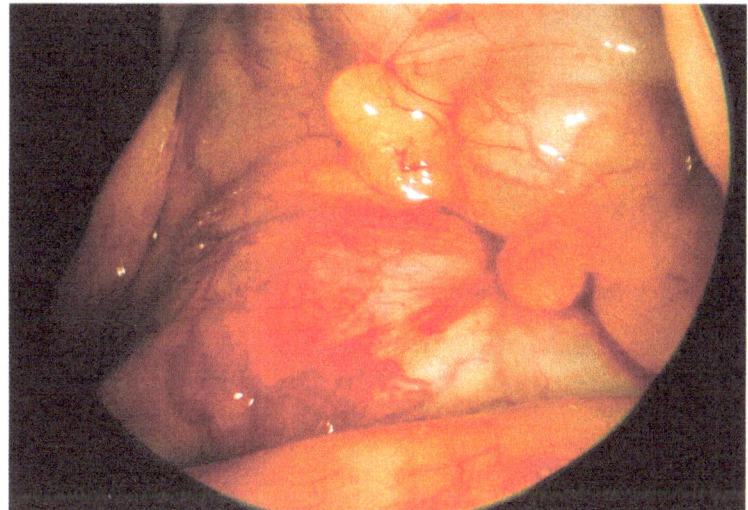

With laparoscopy we can discover whether the mass originates in the *small intestine*: in almost all cases it is due to benign or malignant neoplasms that are pushed out toward the exterior, leaving the intestinal lumen free. The appearance of the small instestine loop involved can vary: its volume may be increased, it may be smooth or congested, and it may have a very thick and hard wall. Or the wall may have a large plaque with thickening that is hard and retracted; the intestinal segment may be fixed to the strata underlying it. The macroscopic evaluation usually indicates a primary neoplasm, and this can occur in cases of malignant lymphoma (Fig. 4.12); sometimes the diagnosis is clarified by taking a biopsy from an enlarged lymph node or, where there is, for example, a lymphomatous infiltration, by taking a spleen biopsy.

Fig. 4.12. Abdominal mass. Small intestine loop enlarged and tumid; the surface is taut and smooth with a central retracted plaque. *Lymphoma of the small intestine? Histological confirmation with lymph node biopsy*

Fig. 4.13. Abdominal mass. From the mesentery fat protrudes an irregular mass enveloped in a thick fibrous capsule with signs of passive congestion. *Fibroleiomyoma of the small intestine*

If we consider the morphological characteristics of these lesions involving the intestinal wall and the compact nature of the tissue, it is evident that fine-needle biopsy is unlikely to be of use. With laparoscopy we can, moreover, reveal whether the undiagnosed mass is a parenchymatous formation, with a fleshy appearance; we can see whether it is large, whether its shape is irregular, and, if the probe is used to make the appropriate maneuvers, we can demonstrate whether it is connected to a loop of small intestine. A deep red color, a characteristic consistency, and the presence of a capsule enable us to diagnose macroscopically a benign neoplasm and define it as a fibroleiomyoma of the small intestine (Fig. 4.13). This evidence also allows us to predict that fine-needle biopsy would be futile because this benign tumor tissue allows only small, insignificant fragments to be obtained.

4.4.1.3 Malignant Peritoneal Neoplasm

Finally, we must consider the masses sustained by a malignant peritoneal neoplasm, above all of the mesentery and omentum. Echoguided fine-needle biopsy guarantees an extremely high diagnostic accuracy in forms due to a secondary carcinomatous infiltration, and these are the most frequent type. For the mesothelium, however, the histological examination of the small sample obtained with fine-needle biopsy does not appear to provide a satisfactory diagnosis. A malignancy can be reliably diagnosed but we cannot reliably establish whether it is a primary or secondary malignancy. Therefore laparoscopy is required to

make as accurate a diagnosis as possible – not because there are valid macroscopic criteria that enable us to distinguish between a mesothelioma and a metastatic tumor of the peritoneum, but because it is very difficult to make a histological diagnosis of a mesothelioma and a histochemical and immunohistochemical study is required, so plenty of tissue must be obtained, and fine-needle biopsy fails to provide it.

So laparoscopy is indispensable in these cases because it allows us to take multiple biopsies, thus providing enough tissue for a complete study (Fig. 4.14).

4.4.2 Conclusions

1. In the presonographic era, laparoscopy with biopsy was the most effective means for diagnosing an abdominal mass of an uncertain nature.

2. With the advent of imaging techniques the indications for laparoscopy have diminished enormously.

3. Laparoscopy is, however, still useful when the sonographic finding is not significant and, above all, when echoguided fine-needle biopsy is unsuccessful or fails to provide a solution, in particular for masses due to neoplastic or inflammatory diseases of the gallbladder and intestine and peritoneal mesothelioma.

Fig. 4.14. Mass of the upper abdominal wall. Marked diffuse thickening of the wall due to the presence of fleshy, compact, tissue. *Mesothelioma of the peritoneum probable*. Histological confirmation

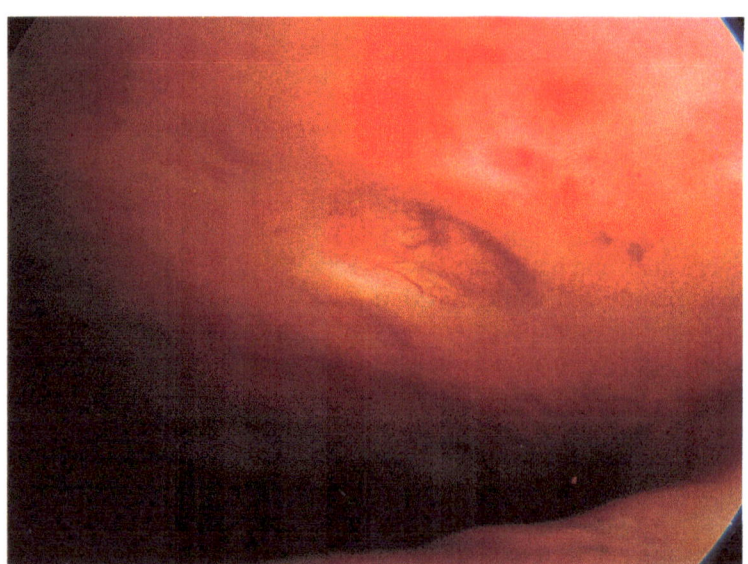

4.5 Jaundice

A diagnosis of jaundice depends mainly upon a distinction being made between "intrahepatic cholestasis" and "mechanical jaundice." The latter is due to a bile flow blockage from, for example, a tumor, a stone, or stenosis of the extrahepatic bile ducts. The main conditions giving rise to intrahepatic cholestasis are: *liver disease from drugs* or other toxic substances, *recurrent gravidic jaundice, benign recurrent cholestasis*, certain forms of *chronic active hepatitis, hepatocholangitis, primary or secondary biliary cirrhosis, common liver cirrhosis*, and *systemic* diseases such as Hodgkin's disease and non-Hodgkin's disease lymphoma or Besnier's granuloma. It is difficult to make a differential diagnosis between mechanical jaundice and intrahepatic cholestases, which have an etiopathogenesis that is completely different from that of mechanical jaundice, but which can give rise to a picture that is identical to that of mechanical jaundice from an extrahepatic obstacle. Moreover, the clinical and laboratory data and traditional radiology only rarely enable a reliable differentiation to be made between the two types of jaundice. On the other hand, from the practical viewpoint an accurate diagnosis is indispensable because the therapeutic approach can only be chosen after the differential diagnosis has been made. We must decide whether to initiate medical therapy for intrahepatic cholestasis or to refer the patient for surgery if the jaundice is mechanical.

For several years before sonography became available, laparoscopy was the best available means for making a differential diagnosis between mechanical and cholestatic jaundice. So laparoscopy was indicated whenever complete clinical, biological, and traditional radiological studies failed to allow a diagnosis to be made. A laparoscopic diagnosis is based on a series of possible macroscopic findings that appear in all treatises and that make up the classical "endoscopic semeiology of jaundice." The following provide useful

diagnostic clues: alterations of (a) the liver (surface characteristics, color, acinous pattern, consistency, etc.); (b) the gallbladder (form, volume, tension, wall characteristics, etc.); and (c) other nearby structures and areas (peritoneum and omentum, pancreatic region, venous circulation, etc.). The overall assessment is made by pooling the different findings and the likelihood of an accurate diagnosis is directly proportional to the quantity and clarity of the findings themselves. Biopsy, when possible, can make an important contribution.

From 1967 to 1981, in a total of 8483 laparoscopic examinations we performed 389 laparoscopies to diagnose jaundice; these amounted to 4.58% [22]. In over 67% of these cases, laparoscopy allowed us to make a certain distinction between intrahepatic cholestasis and mechanical jaundice while in 18% the diagnosis was considered "probable." In 14% laparoscopy did not allow a diagnosis to be made (Table 4.2).

In 135 (88%) of our 153 cases of intrahepatic cholestases, laparoscopy and biopsy enabled us to ascertain the nature of the conditions causing the jaundice; in the remaining 18% the diagnosis made was probable.

In about two-thirds of our cases of cholestatic jaundice we found chronic cholestatic hepatitis and different forms of cirrhosis (biliary, primary, and secondary, as well as common forms) and therefore the hepatocholangitis diffuse neoplastic infiltrations (primary carcinoma with cirrhosis, malignant lymphoma) and others. An exact diagnosis was made by Fassler in 128 cases of intrahepatic cholestases in a percentage identical to ours (88%) [23]. In cases of mechanical jaundice laparoscopy enabled an almost certain diagnosis to be made for the site of the obstruction in 60% of cases. It is more difficult to establish the type of obstacle: in a little over 14% a certain diagnosis was made, and in 13% the diagnosis was "probable" [22]. Therefore, like Marti Vicente [24], we may say that the diagnostic potential of laparoscopy in the differential diagnosis of cholestatic jaundice is overall

Table 4.2. Differential laparoscopic diagnosis between mechanical jaundice and intrahepatic cholestasis

Laparoscopic diagnosis	Certain (No. of cases)	Probable (No. of cases)	Uncertain (No. of cases)
Mechanical jaundice	140 (36.1%)	41 (10.5%)	55 (14.1%)
Intrahepatic cholestasis	123 (31.6%)	30 (7.7%)	
Total	263 (67.7%)	71 (18.2%)	55 (14.1%)

very high. An endoscopic retrograde cholangiopancreatographic examination (ERCP) or a percutaneous transhepatic cholangiogram (PTC), performed before or after the laparoscopy, confirmed the diagnosis in a very high percentage of cases.

4.5.1 Present Indications for Laparoscopy

With the advent of imaging techniques, the approach to jaundice was radically changed and the indications for diagnostic laparoscopy were greatly reduced. In their series, Gandolfi et al. [19] found that the percentage fell from 3.6% in the presonographic era to 0.8% after the advent of sonography. We also observed a considerable reduction – from 3.99% to 1.04%. Of course the reduction depends on the fact that when *dilated biliary ducts* are found with sonography it is easy to diagnose mechanical jaundice due to an extrahepatic obstruction with an accuracy universally reported as almost 100%. So sonographic results here are superior to those obtained laparoscopically. Moreover, sonography is a noninvasive technique.

Sonography is also more effective in detecting the site of the obstacle, with an accuracy ranging from 65% to 95%. Laparoscopy, as mentioned above, in our experience has an accuracy which normally never exceeds 60%, but can reach a maximum of 82% [24]. Finally, unlike laparoscopy, sonography enables us to establish the nature of the obstacle in an extremely high percentage of cases, whether dealing with stones, which are revealed extremely well by sonography, or with neoplasms – particularly if a fine-needle biopsy can be taken.

Finally, in cases that remain doubtful the invasive techniques of choice are ERCP – which allows a direct examination of Vater's papilla and any biopsies – and PTC.

So laparoscopy is not indicated when sonographically the bile ducts appear dilated. In our opinion laparoscopy is indicated only in cases of mechanical jaundice from malignant tumors without clinical or sonographic signs of metastasis for which a therapeutic program must be decided upon. It is important always to bear in mind that any negative sonographic finding may be a "false negative," so laparoscopy is the only available means for (a) demonstrating any liver metastases that have escaped detection by imaging techniques, either because they are small or because of their particular localization (Sect. 5.3) and (b) discovering neoplastic peritoneal localizations. This laparoscopic staging is invaluable because it allows us to choose the most appropriate approach such as curative or palliative surgery or other procedures, such as placement of temporary or permanent biliary drainages without surgery.

The problem is quite different in *cholestatic jaundice*, for which sonography reveals *undilated biliary ducts*. This occurs frequently: in our series, about 40% of patients with jaundice had laparoscopically diagnosed intrahepatic cholestasis. Sonography has a much lower diagnostic efficacy in these cases than in cases of mechanical jaundice. Using our "sonography for laparoscopy" technique, we compared and cross-checked the echographic and laparoscopic findings made in 58 patients with marked clinically undiagnosed cholestatic jaundice with undilated bile ducts at echography [25].

Echography provided clues for a good diagnostic orientation in only 15% of these cases, whereas laparoscopy with biopsy allowed a *certain* diagnosis to be made in 45 cases (75%), a diagnostic orientation in 6, and was inconclusive in another 7. It is easy to explain these results if we consider each particular disease recognized as causing the jaundice in each particular case: different types of cirrhosis (14 cases), hepatocholangites (8 cases), acute cholestatic hepatites (7 cases), diffuse neoplastic infiltrations (malignant lymphoma, hepatocarcinoma, etc.) (3 cases), etc. In all these processes, sonography integrated with thin-needle biopsy has a poor diagnostic efficacy. Yet nowadays it appears that many tend to be against the use of laparoscopy in the diagnosis of jaundice. We agree that laparoscopy is useless when echography can provide the diagnosis and, of course, when it is already known that the jaundice is mechanical. But when sonography can indicate only that there is an intrahepatic cholestasis, the case is not clear enough. In a study published in 1983, Etienne et al. [26] stated: "when echography demonstrates an intrahepatic cholestasis and the other data support this hypothesis, an aspiration blind biopsy is usually sufficient." We, however, disagree with this for the following reasons: (a) in cholestasis blind liver biopsy is risky because it can give rise to bile leakage from the biopsy hole – it is therefore contraindicated; the cholorrhea cannot be revealed and is uncontrollable, giving rise to choleperitoneum, which is always severe, and often fatal if steps are not taken promptly; (b) we, like many others, have found that liver biopsy is often inadequate for a diagnosis in such situations and it is futile unless supported by a macroscopic anatomical finding. Moreover, in 1987 Schiff stated that "laparoscopy is particularly valuable in the diagnosis of cirrhosis missed in blind biopsy specimens" [27].

We have already discussed the diagnostic value of laparoscopy in the diagnosis of different types of jaundice. But above all it should be stressed that: (a) the laparoscopic semeiology for jaundice is rich and significant enough to enable a very reliable macroscopic diagnosis to be made in the vast majority of cases and (b) biopsy during laparoscopy is not contraindicated even in the presence of cholestasis (because any cholorrhea can be detected easily and early and the Bio-Plug used to plug the biopsy hole (see Figs. 1.9, 1.10); it can therefore make a valid contribution by confirming the diagnosis and enhancing the diagnostic accuracy.

It is therefore reasonable to consider laparoscopy the most valid technique for the investigation of jaundice in which sonography shows undilated bile ducts without a reliable diagnosis being possible.

4.5.2 Main Laparoscopic Findings

As laparoscopy is still necessary in this field, it is opportune here to outline the fundamental elements of laparoscopic semeiology on which we base a diagnosis of cholestatic jaundice. The liver

diseases that most frequently give rise to intra-hepatic cholestasis are: cholestatic hepatitis, toxic hepatitis, hepatocholangitis, common and biliary cirrhosis, and diffuse neoplastic infiltration.

4.5.2.1 Cholestatic Hepatitis

In order to gain a good understanding of the macroscopic characteristics significant in making a differential diagnosis, reference must be made to Kalk's description: in *acute hepatitis* (for which, as is well known, neither biopsy nor laparoscopy are indicated) the surface of the liver is smooth, polished, tumid, and bright red (Fig. 4.15) and its lobular pattern has disappeared. In *jaundice from obstruction*, on the other hand, the organ is different shades of green depending on the specific case, and its lobular pattern is clear because there is no inflammation; the superficial lymphatic network is turgid because of stasis (Fig. 4.16). In practice, these criteria cannot always be strictly applied, although the color of the organ always provides important indications.

Cholestatic hepatitis can present a dramatic clinical picture which is sometimes identical to that of mechanical jaundice; laparoscopically the liver always has a particular color: only rarely is it the green that the high bilirubinemia values might suggest, nor is it the bright red found in the common forms of acute hepatitis. Its color may

Fig. 4.15. Kalk's "bright red liver" compatible with acute hepatitis. Marked congestion and edema; lobular pattern has disappeared

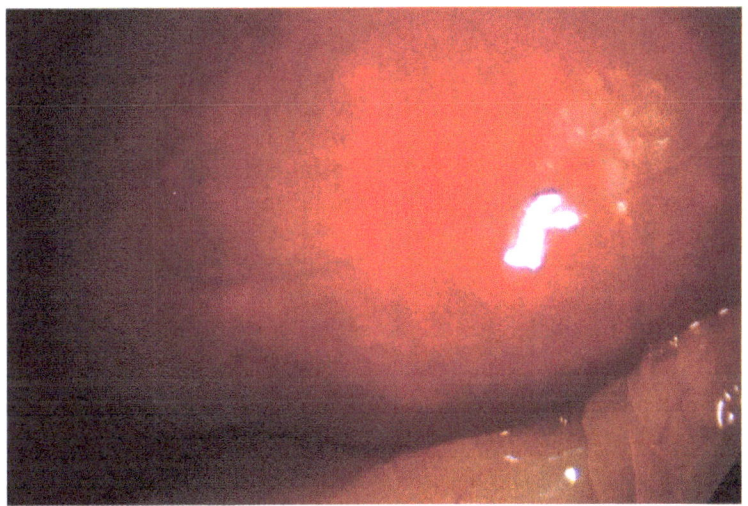

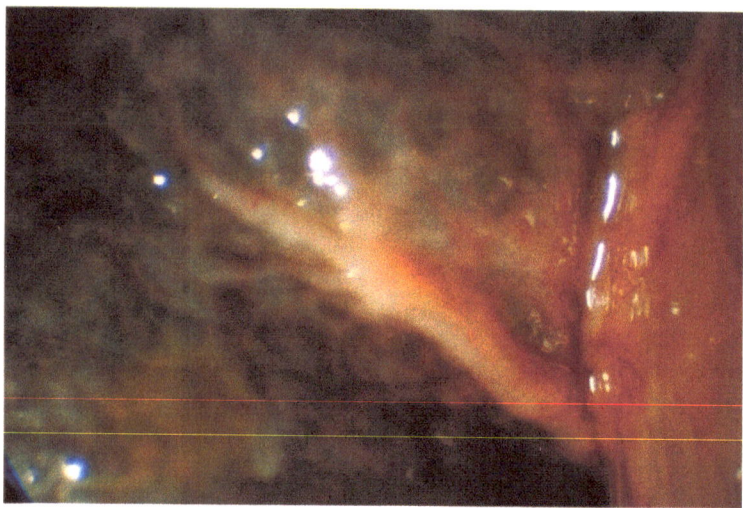

Fig. 4.16. Green liver, compatible with obstructive jaundice. Marked turgor of the lymphatics

seem almost normal; otherwise it may be red or, more often, coppercolored and slightly streaked, or with dark tattooing when the bilirubinemia is over 20 mg%. Moreover, the lobular pattern is usually quite difficult to discern (Fig. 4.17). Although modified, the inflammatory process char-

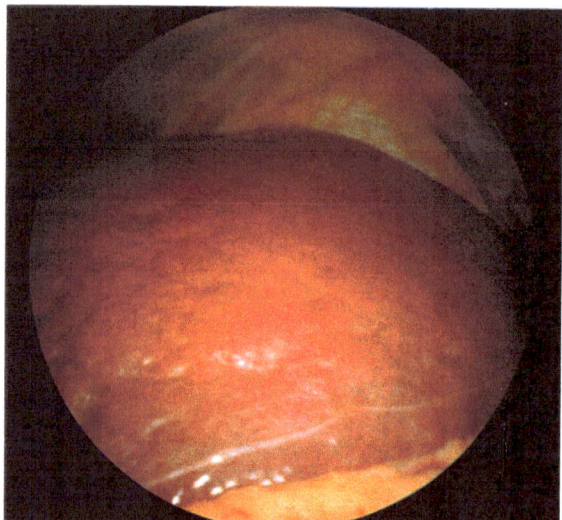

Fig. 4.17. *Intrahepatic cholestasis* (cholestatic hepatitis). Brownish-red notwithstanding the bilirubinemia of 25 mg%. Irregular surface with green tattooing. The degree of jaundice is revealed by the color of the fibrous part of the diaphragm that can be seen in the background

acteristics can be recognized, and this suggests hepatitis. Biopsy is certainly useful, although in our experience it is not always decisive.

4.5.2.2 Toxic Liver Diseases

In these forms the appearance of the liver can vary, so it is even more difficult to make a diagnosis. In severe icterogenic alcoholic hepatitis, the liver becomes enlarged and its margins rounded and the surface appears taut and smooth. The lobular pattern has disappeared and the color ranges from brown to yellow with a marked bluish-gray hue. In such cases the biopsy findings are usually significant. In toxicosis from drugs the liver examination does not provide specific enough findings, so it is difficult to make a reliable macroscopic diagnosis. The organ may be dark green, just as it is in the presence of severe extrahepatic stasis (Fig. 4.18). If the gallbladder is half empty as in the example given, mechanical jaundice cannot be ruled out because it might be caused by a "high" obstacle. Also the lobular pattern may be recognizable as in extrahepatic cholestasis (Fig. 4.19). In such cases the sonographic finding of undilated

———————————————→

Fig. 4.18. *Intrahepatic cholestasis* (hepatopathy from drugs). Bright green, lobular design has disappeared. Flaccid gallbladder

Fig. 4.19. *Intrahepatic cholestasis* (hepatopathy from drugs). Pronounced lobular pattern

Fig. 4.20. Intrahepatic cholestasis (hepatopathy from drugs). Liver variegated with red and green

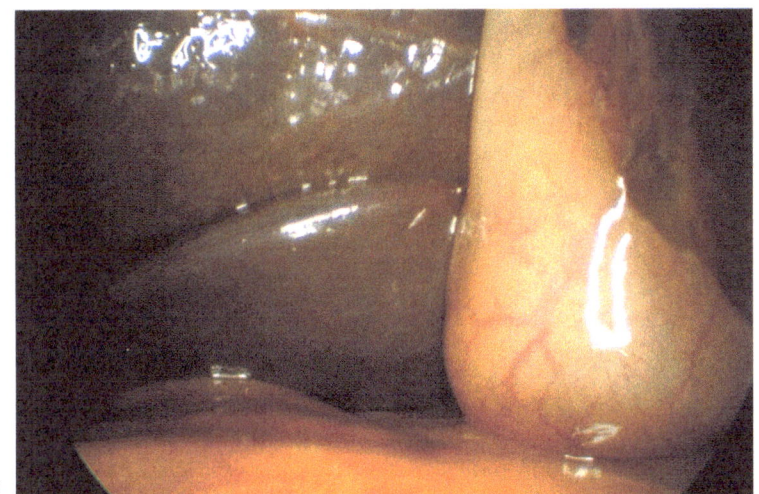

4.18

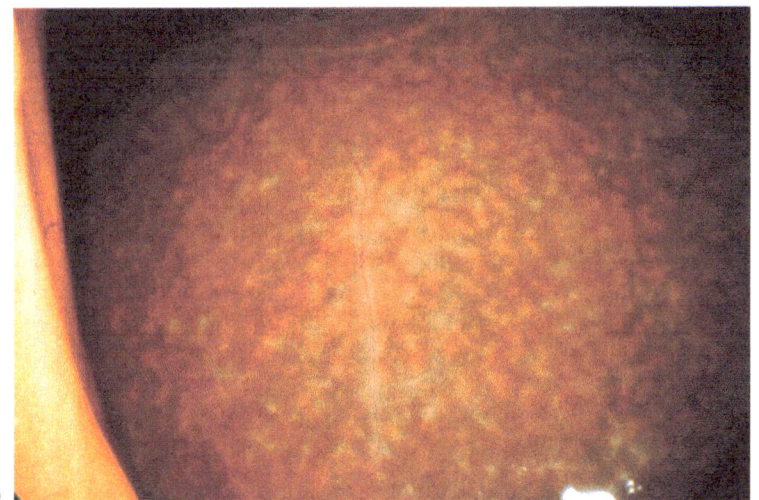

4.19

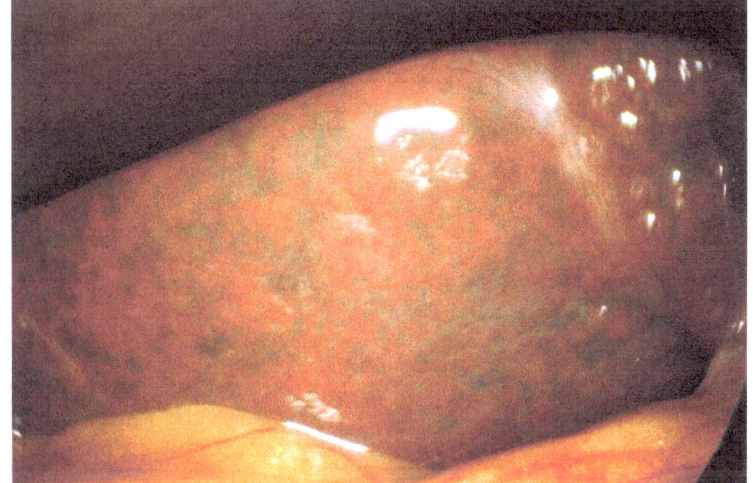

4.20

bile ducts alone suggests a parenchymal disease. It is thus demonstrated that it is important to integrate the two techniques. On other occasions the color of the liver is not uniform, because of the presence of extensive, slightly raised, irregular red areas, which alternate with clearly green areas (Fig. 4.20). These findings may suggest through exclusion a toxic liver disease, and usually the diagnosis is clarified by biopsy.

4.5.2.3 Hepatocholangitis

In *hepatocholangitis*, as in cholestatic hepatitis, the liver, even if the bilirubinemia values are very high, is never green and it has features typical of hepatitis: red, with branched colorations and an unclear lobular pattern. In long-standing forms, the surface may be slightly rough and the lobular pattern appears quite clear. These forms, however, often have a particular characteristic that enables a reliable diagnosis to be made: linear retracted streaks are visualized or slight grooves with a grayish-green background can be seen – these correspond to biliary vessels with inflammatory changes at different stages (Fig. 4.21). Under high magnification, we can detect the extremities of the smaller branches, which demonstrates cholangitis.

Target biopsies at these points confirm hepatocholangitis and provide an interesting insight, above all on how long-standing the disease is. Laparoscopy also allows us to complete the picture

with an examination of the gallbladder, which is often the focus of the origin of the disease and which can present different types of alteration (modification in size, active congestion, edema, wall-thickening, etc.) that both demonstrate whether there is subacute or chronic inflammation and enable us to make an accurate diagnosis.

4.5.2.4 Liver Cirrhosis

In most cases of cirrhosis, a slight subicterus is found with slight hyperbilirubinemia; sometimes an intense cholestatic jaundice is found and this may be the dominant symptom: the disease is either *common cirrhosis* or *primary* or *secondary biliary cirrhosis*.

In many cases, laparoscopy provides useful clues. In common cirrhosis with cholestatic jaundice, the appearance of the liver is typical of sectal cirrhosis or, more frequently, postnecrotic cirrhosis; it has a brownish surface, from which protrude some nodules that are "tattooed" dark green. In these cases, the laparoscopic picture clearly indicates cirrhosis and the diagnosis is therefore easy to make. Other forms are also of great interest – those in which the liver appear slightly enlarged, has round margins and a smooth surface, and is brownish red with a markedly green hue (Fig. 4.22). These findisngs do not permit the diagnosis to be made easily: the biopsy reveals liver cirrhosis with marked cholestasis, which is not suspected macroscopically. These forms are not nodular and their nature is only revealed by histology; because of this we call them "histological cirrhoses."

Secondary biliary cirrhosis can be diagnosed laparoscopically if the liver is found to be hard and green and its surface nodular. In the cholangitic forms, the liver often has a grayish hue due to capsule thickening, with surface streaks and bands that are retracted and embedded; these indicate persistent, repeated inflammation of the superficial bile ducts and of the surrounding hepatic parenchyma and show postnecrotic scar repair.

4.5.2.5 Diffuse Neoplastic Infiltrations

These are rare and depend mainly on malignant lymphoma. The macroscopic picture has no specific features; the liver characteristics vary – they may simulate steatosis or may appear normal, except for a certain enlargement or a greenish hue. The diagnosis can only be made with biopsy.

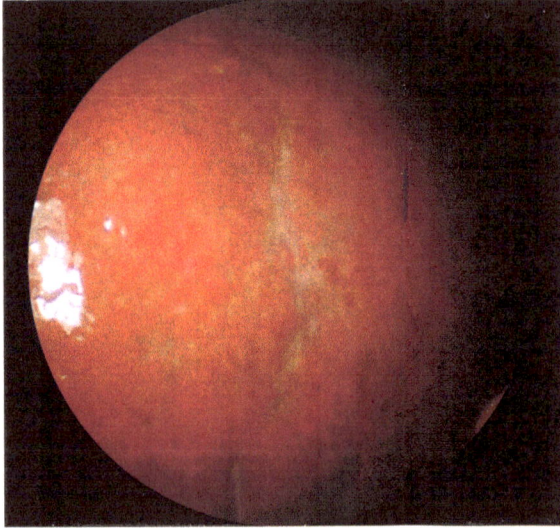

Fig. 4.21. Intrahepatic cholestasis (hepatocholangitis). Grayish-green grooves

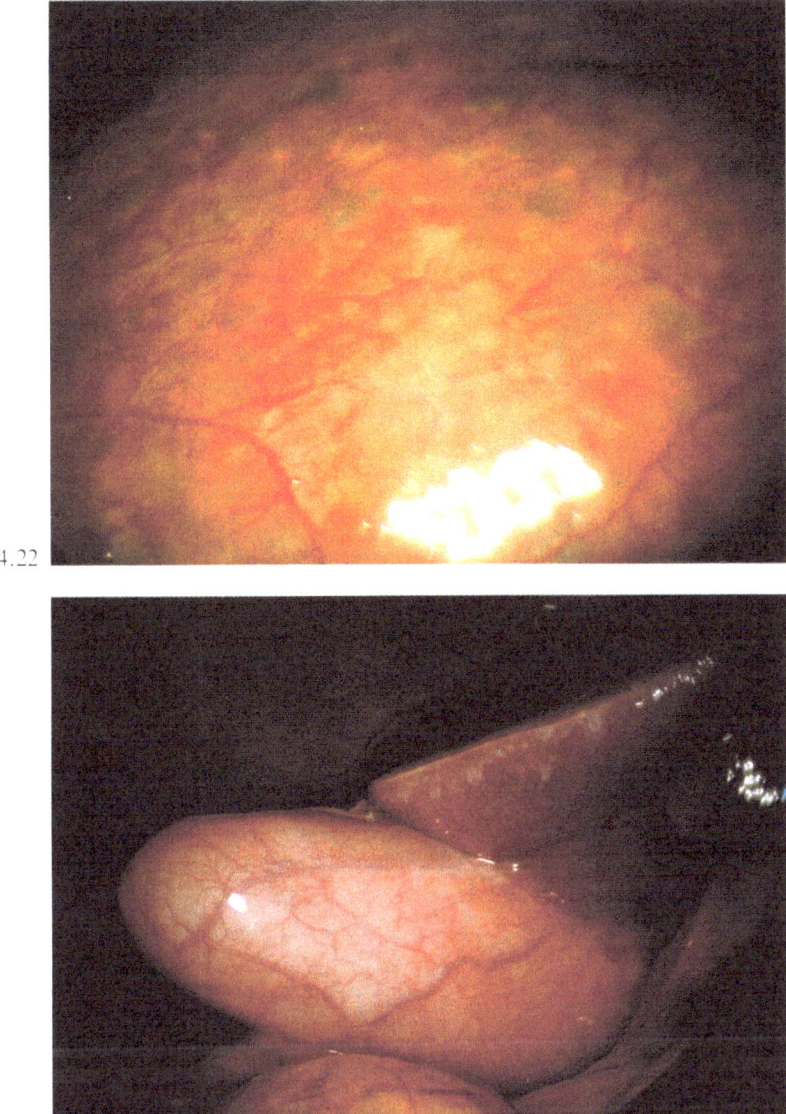

4.22

4.23

Fig. 4.22. *Intrahepatic cholestasis.* Smooth pale brown surface with green, hazy patches. Alcoholic hepatopathy? Biopsy: *cirrhosis of the liver with cholestasis*

Fig. 4.23. Brownish-red liver. Slightly enlarged gallbladder, taut, with an erectile appearance (laparoscopic Courvoiser-Terrier's sign). *Initial obstructive jaundice from undetected tumor of the head of the pancreas*

Finally, we cannot rule out mechanical jaundice if nondilated bile ducts are found sonographically, because, in some situations, although there is an obstacle to bile flow, the biliary tree seems normal. This is the case for: (a) the initial forms, in which direct bilirubin values indicate mild jaundice and the biliary tree tension has not caused sonographically detectable modifications and (b) cases in which the bile ducts and the gallbladder cannot be dilated because there is diffuse hardening of the liver or because there is a systematic endocanalicular gallbladder carcinoma spread. In these cases the validity of the indication for laparoscopy is confirmed: it indicates whether the jaundice is mechanical.

In initial jaundice, the liver appears normal and the gallbladder is not enlarged sonographically; it is, however, very taut and hard at palpation with the probe, and in this way we can recognize the Courvoisier-Terrier's sign, which is pathognomonic for the presence of a "low" obstacle (Fig. 4.23).

Morphological findings on liver status can provide exhaustive explanations for the lack of bile duct dilation (cirrhosis, signs of near spread, etc.).

4.5.3 Conclusions

1. In almost all cases echography enables us to distinguish between mechanical jaundice and intrahepatic cholestasis thanks to the finding of dilated bile ducts; it also allows us to establish the site and nature of the obstacle with greater precision than with laparoscopy.

2. Consequently, laparoscopy is no longer used for the differential diagnosis in cholestatic jaundice. It is now only indicated to detect any signs of spread of a known tumor to the liver, and, above all, the peritoneum, because these cannot be revealed sonographically.

3. When, however, sonography demonstrates that the bile ducts are not dilated, laparoscopy is still indicated. Traditional laparoscopic semeiology and biopsy (which unlike transcutaneous blind biopsy carries no risk) allow an accurate diagnosis of the nature of the disease to be made in a high percentage of cases.

4.6 Abdominal Pain

The nature of the numerous abdominal diseases characterized by pain varies considerably. It is therefore both impossible and useless to consider them one by one. We are interested here in the pathological conditions that are not diagnosed even after a thorough analysis has been made, the clinical and laboratory data evaluated and a complete instrumental study carried out.

In most of these cases explorative laparotomy is performed. Then laparoscopy is found to be an effective diagnostic tool in: (a) cases of persistent or critical abdominal pain that is long-standing or that is the only or the dominant symptom in a pathological picture that still cannot be explained after a complete study has been made; and (b) clearly ascertained diseases in which the presence of pain cannot be due to the disease itself and that must therefore be investigated in order to discover any other process that might accompany or overlie the known disease.

Laparoscopy has always been used occasionally for the diagnosis of abdominal pain, but only fairly recently has it been used systematically [28].

Given the great variety of possible situations in this field, the results obtained with laparoscopy vary greatly from case to case and therefore sometimes are difficult to understand. In other words, we may have different results with different values.

1. Certain diagnoses are made when the endoscopic examination enables us to detect a pathological process capable of causing abdominal pain. The diagnosis is certain when the macroscopic finding is significant and a biopsy can also be taken for a histological confirmation and clarification of the diagnosis. A definite answer to the diagnostic question was obtained in 32% of cases in our series of 285 laparoscopies performed to diagnose abdominal pain [29]. The main conditions for which the laparoscopic and biopsy findings enabled us to detect a lesion certainly responsible for the pain reported are in order of frequency: metastatic liver neoplasms (about 60% in our series), liver carcinomas (25%), and then peritoneal affections, etc.

2. Fairly reliable diagnoses are made when the impression is based on the macroscopic picture alone. The finding is significant and therefore the pain can be satisfactorily interpreted. However, the site, type, and characteristics of the lesion preclude a biopsy; or, otherwise, if a biopsy is taken, its findings are inconclusive. These diagnoses account for another 4% of cases, which are mainly: (a) subacute and chronic cholecystitis and pericholecystitis with evident signs of phlogosis; (b) taut adhesions between the parietal peritoneum and the organs – if put in traction with forceps, the pain increases or is triggered off in the same site and has the same characteristics as the spontaneous pain experienced by the patient; and (c) malignant neoplasm of the gallbladder.

3. Uncertain diagnosis when the laparoscopic findings are not decisive but provide some indications that may be of use. Here the findings are not clearly connected with the pain itself: (a) different types of adhesion which do not affect the parietal peritoneum and which, when in traction, do not provoke pain (33 cases among 73 incomplete diagnoses); (b) cholecystitis, adnexitis, chronic perivisceritis without signs of inflammation; and (c) "indirect signs" that may lead us to presume that there is a deep-seated lesion without allowing us to clarify its site and nature. These "uncertain" diagnoses account for 35% of the total.

4. No diagnosis. In 30% of cases laparoscopy fails to explain the pain experienced by the patient. Often the endoscopic picture is normal or lesions are found in the abdominal organs, but the lesions found cannot cause pain. Although this finding is not positive, it does allow us to rule out an organic lesion, at least in the explorable areas, and this is important because exclusively functional abdominal pain is very frequent.

Of course these "negative" findings may be false if there is a deep-seated lesion or if a lesion is hidden and cannot therefore be detected laparoscopically. So in the presonographic era, laparoscopy provided results that were decisive in diagnosing 36% of cases and it gave useful information in the remaining ones; this is no mean feat because it is extremely difficult to detect the cause of pain, which can depend on numerous different pathological abdominal conditions.

4.6.1 Present Indications for Laparoscopy

Now there are fewer cases of undiagnosed abdominal pain thanks to sonography which, above all in cases of malignant tumor, enables us to resolve diagnostic problems by detecting the lesion and, where necessary, taking a fine-needle biopsy. So there are now fewer indications for laparoscopy. In particular, when abdominal pain is caused by pancreatic or any other retroperitoneal tumors sonography is far more effective than any other technique, allowing a diagnosis to be made in cases that once would have been laparoscopic failures. Also in diagnosing pain we can use sonography, thereby avoiding a large number of superfluous or unfruitful laparoscopies.

However, we are of the opinion that when abdominal pain is a *single or dominant symptom* in the picture, there are still several indications for laparoscopy, and this belief is not based upon causal factors, but upon specific factors demonstrated by laparoscopy itself. Pain, whether accessional or continuous, of varying intensity, blunt or penetrating, is almost always experienced because there is a primary or secondary *participation* of the parietal or visceral *peritoneum*. For this reason with sonography it is difficult to detect any process that does not present parenchymal lesions but that mainly or exclusively affects the serous membrane. Any abdominal pain that is not clarified by a rigorous echographic study should still today constitute a definite indication for laparoscopy, and laparoscopy should certainly still be used as a diagnostic technique for pain.

4.6.2 Main Laparoscopic Findings

We cite here as examples some of the more frequent situations in which laparoscopy is a useful diagnostic tool:

When pain is localized at the *right or left hypochondrium* sometimes with a lateral and posterior irradiation, and for which any extraabdominal genesis can be ruled out; a pain that is not diagnosed sonographically may be due to a *subacute or chronic inflammatory process* affecting the serous membrane of the liver, gallbladder, or spleen.

"Perivisceritis" may be suspected on the basis of clinical findings, but is difficult to demonstrate and does not give a specific echographic finding.

Laparoscopy can give a tangible image and provide elements for the interpretation of the particular form of pain. It is, however, always difficult to define the etiology of this form because usually the macroscopic and bioptic findings only indicate an aspecific inflammation.

Of course the pictures vary considerably: in *perihepatitis* the serosa of the organs seems to have a diffuse thickening and congestion. Often the liver is fixed to the abdominal wall by an extensive and intricate adhesional network. These clearly phlogistic pictures allow us satisfactorily to explain the pain. Here we must also bear in mind that when adhesions are fixed to the parietal peritoneum, traction to the abdominal wall plays an important role in causing pain.

In certain cases the finding allows us also to establish the nature of the perivisceritis, with the presence of, sometimes numerous, small pinkish-white nodules. Macroscopically, these nodules may resemble a tubercular process, but, although they may appear inflammatory, a carcinomatous spread should always be considered. If a biopsy of these nodules is taken, the problem is easily resolved.

Pericholecystitis can be diagnosed by means of laparoscopy, but often the adhesions hide the gallbladder; and therefore the endoscopic diagnosis, which is based on indirect signs, depends only upon an impression, especially where the nature and activity of the process are concerned.

Malignant tumors, particularly those of the liver and gallbladder, frequently cause pain that presents as a single or a predominant symptom and that can remain undiagnosed even after a sonographic examination has been made. Echographic failure often depends on the fact that these neoplasms give a clinical picture that has pain as the only symptom, and this is because at an early stage they give rise to an important involvement of the local serous membrane and are therefore superficial, small and thin. Their characteristics often escape echographic detection but are easily recognized at laparoscopic examination. In cases of cirrhosis, it is more difficult to detect liver tumors echographically. We cite here a patient that presented clinically with intense pain to the right hypochondrium; with echography only signs of cirrhosis were detected, whereas with laparoscopy a primary tumor was found with a superficial plaque on the tip of the right lobe; there was also an intense peritoneal reaction that was circumscribed by thin adhesions that were stretched between the tumor and superior abdominal wall (Fig. 4.24). This picture clearly explains both the pain, caused by neoplastic circumscribed perihepatitis, and the reasons why echography failed to detect the neoplasia. The cirrhosis is confirmed and the tumor clearly consists of a flat thin plaque whose tissue merges with that of the liver parenchyma. The pain may also be due to a primary liver tumor without cirrhosis: the false echographic negative is made because the lesion is superficial and, although not small, it is flat and thin (Fig. 4.25).

A pain in the upper right abdomen due to a malignant tumor can be left undiagnosed after echography and can be clarified only with laparoscopy. We report here an example of liver metastasis to show how sometimes a false negative may depend on the site of the tumor itself. Neoplastic localizations in the vicinity of the gallbladder can in fact escape sonographic exploration while they are revealed easily with laparoscopy (Fig. 4.26). In the case presented here an echographic examination made immediately after laparoscopy, with a thorough exploration of the pericholecystic area indicated by the prior endoscopic examination, enabled us to detect, and ascertain the gravity of, a small hypodense area corresponding to the one seen macroscopically (Fig. 4.27) but that was not revealed by prelaparoscopic echography.

Isolated pain is a nonspecific, but important, sign of primary carcinoma of the gallbladder; in our series of 98 laparoscopically studied cases pain,

whether continual or accessional, was present in 61 cases and in 21 it was the only symptom [20, 21]. We have already outlined the difficulties involved in any attempt to make a sonographic diagnosis of this tumor, above all in its initial forms, which partially involve the organ wall and which can give rise to "false negatives." Laparoscopy can provide a good diagnostic orientation if a slightly raised, pale, and hard plaque is found, typical enough of the tumor. However, as it is often impossible to take a biopsy, no definite judgment can be made (Fig. 4.28). In cases of right hypochondrium pain with normal echographic findings, greater difficulty is encountered when the gallbladder has normal dimensions and has a diffusely thickened, very congested wall, sometimes with considerable lymphatic vessel turgidity. It may be impossible to make a differential diagnosis between cholecystitis and a tumor, and this situation is the most frequent cause of diagnostic pitfalls in this field.

Abdominal pain, in either the upper or the lower quadrant, can be caused by adhesions between organs and the abdominal wall secondary either to chronic circumscribed peritonitis or surgery. In these forms there is no inflammation, and the pain is entirely "mechanical," being due to traction of the wall on the peritoneum that occurs above all in relation to the different types of decubitus. This has already been discussed in operative laparoscopy. We can confirm that the adhesion is responsible for the pain by pulling the adhesions with the forceps to trigger the pain itself.

These adhesions can sometimes be resected endoscopically. Therefore laparoscopy can establish the cause of the pain and resolve the therapeutic

---

Fig. 4.24. Tip of the right lobe of the liver with cirrhotic nodules; pink plaque *at center.* Between this and the upper abdominal wall can be seen transparent fibrous fimbriae that pull the wall itself downwards. *Hepatocarcinoma on cirrhosis*; adhesions to the wall

Fig. 4.25. Lower surface of the right lobe of the liver. Numerous pinkish-white plaques. *Primary neoplasia of the liver?* Or *secondary neoplasia?* Biopsy: *cholangiocarcinoma*

Fig. 4.26. Upper surface of the right lobe of the liver. Proximal to the gallbladder a whitish nodule with a deep central crater can be seen. *Liver metastatic cancer*

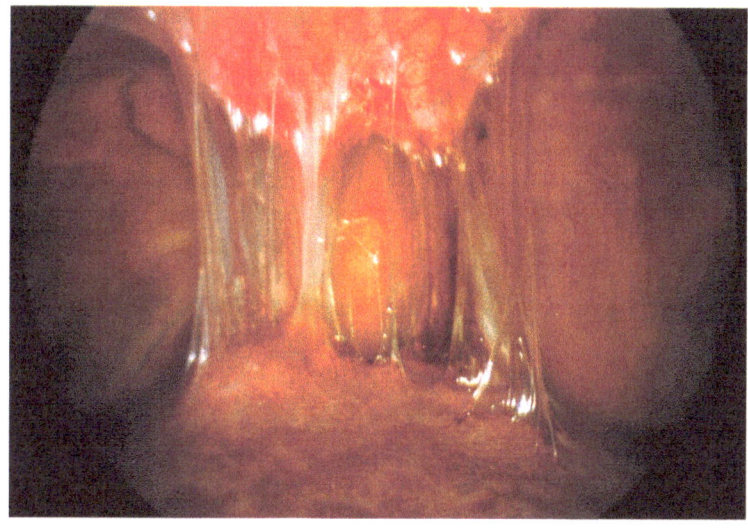

4.24

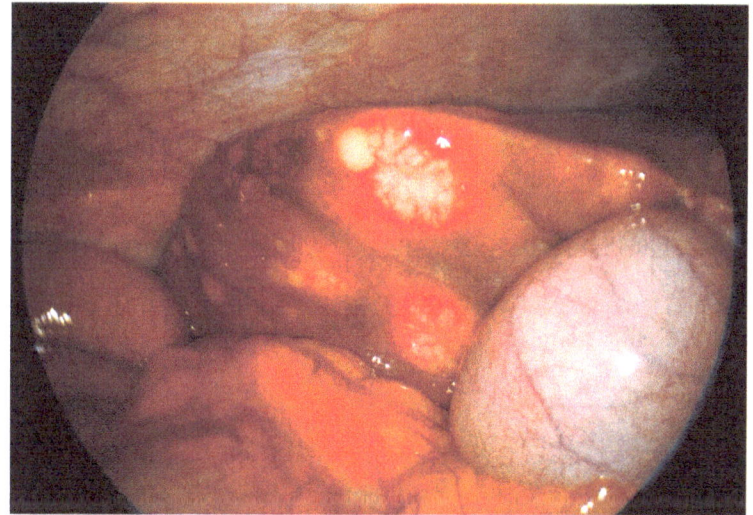

4.25

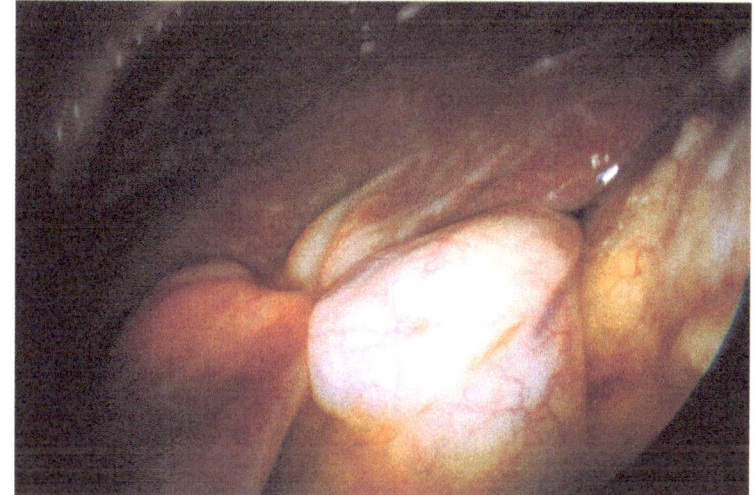

4.26

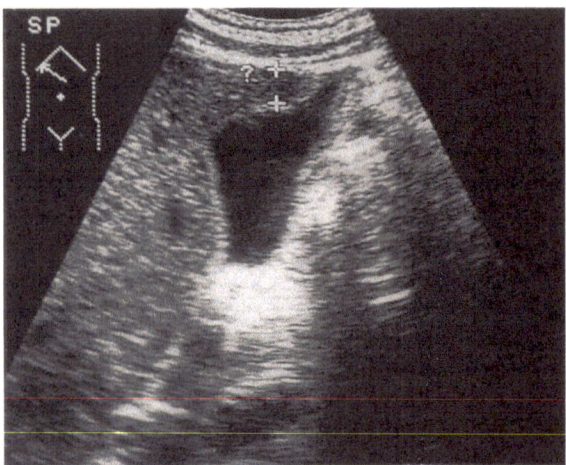

Fig. 4.27. Same case as in Fig. 4.26. Echography performed after laparoscopy. Guided by the endoscopic finding, a hypoechogenic area can be seen, and evaluated, above the gallbladder

problem. In other cases, however, a diagnosis alone can be made and resection cannot be performed because the adhesions: (a) are too thick and extensive; (b) are highly vascularized, with large, turgid, blood vessels, and there may therefore be a risk of intractable hemorrhage or, sometimes, (c) involve the intestine by directly fixing a loop to its wall (Fig. 4.29).

Fig. 4.28. Distended gallbladder; there is partial thickening of the wall and a small, irregular whitish plaque. *Carcinoma of the gallbladder*

Laparoscopy can moreover clarify the cause of upper abdominal accessional pain still undiagnosed after a negative clinical study, after laboratory studies fail to show any appreciable or specific alterations, and after sonography fails to indicate a particular disease. The endoscopic picture shows a series of small whitish-yellow plaques with irregular margins on the omental fat; these can be recognized as cytosteatonecrosis. We can confirm by biopsy that these are significant indirect signs of pancreatitis; the lack of congestion, of edema, or of any hemorrhage attests to the insidious nature of the form and its incomplete symptomatology.

In the great majority of cases, pain in the lower abdominal quadrants depends on affections of the female genitalia. Often the disease is on the border between internal and gynecological medicine, but the problem prevalently concerns *gynecological laparoscopy*. This has many indications and in cases of pelvic pain the findings include acute, subacute, and chronic adnexitis, benign and malignant uterine and ovarian neoplasms, postural habits and positional anomalies, and endometriosis. It is important to stress the fact that in gynecology lower abdominal pain accounts for the highest percentage (about 30%) of the negative laparoscopic findings: this demonstrates that isolated pain with a negative clinical and sonographic picture often depends upon a functional disturbance for which laparoscopy evidently can prove nothing.

From an internistic viewpoint, some pictures are dominated by progressive pain at the low abdomen that can persist for weeks, that can be

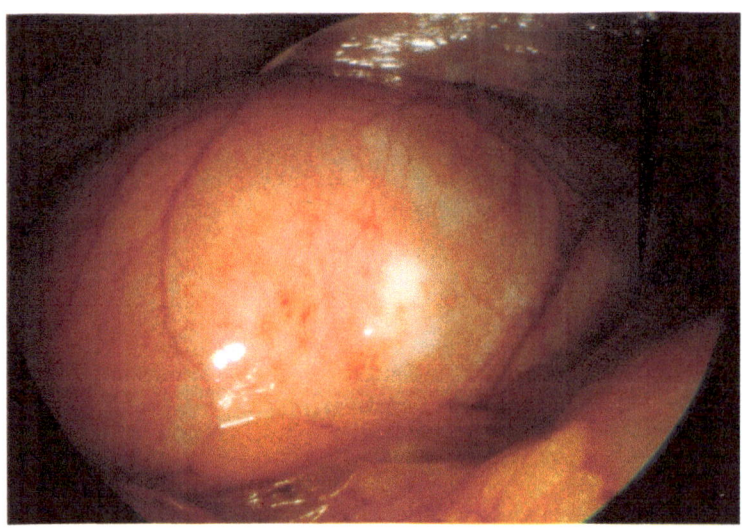

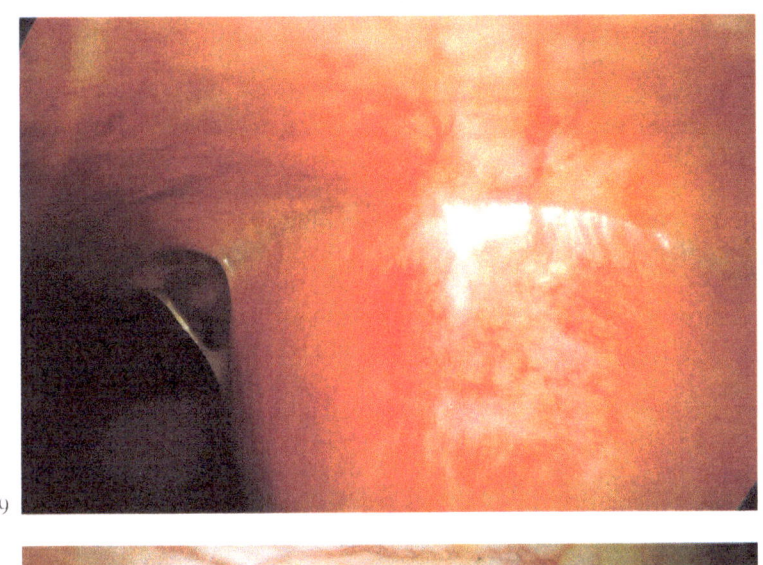

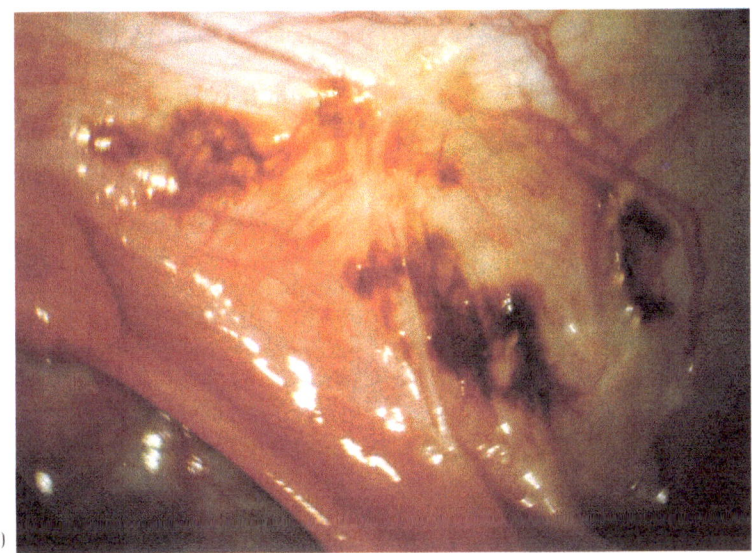

Fig. 4.29. Loop of the small intestine adheres to the upper abdominal wall

Fig. 4.30. Detail of the wall of the left hemidiaphragm on which can be seen deposits of an amorphous bright brown substance. *Diaphragmatic localization of endometriosis*

accompanied by biological signs of phlogosis, with a negative echographic picture, and in which laparoscopy demonstrates a slight congestion and a nodular spread with small miliary nodes. Here we are dealing with "discrete" peritoneal tuberculosis, without the leakage that characterizes most of these peritoneal diseases, the diagnosis of which, possible only with laparoscopy and biopsy, is of

extraordinary practical value because it enables us to initiate effective therapy immediately.

Finally, particularly worthy of mention is a disease that is strictly gynecological but capable of giving rise to, in its polymorphism, pictures that are of internistic interest.

This occurred in one of my patients [30] and in another patient observed by Llanio (Llanio 1984, personal communication). These two young women complained of only one symptom: pain. This was experienced in bands, was subcontinuous, and had a violent onset, radiating from the epigastric region to the sides and then posteriorly. There was a correlation between the pain and the premenstrual period; complete clinical examination and laboratory as well as instrumental studies, which included echography and CT, were negative.

Laparoscopy was therefore performed and it provided a clear picture of endometriosis with modest localizations on the parietal pelvic peritoneum, but above all with an important spread to both the hemidiaphragms (Fig. 4.30).

Such cases are rare, but they are still cases in which laparoscopy is the only technique that allows a reliable diagnosis to be made.

4.6.3 Conclusions

1. In the presonographic era laparoscopy clarified the cause of undiagnosed abdominal pain in 36% of cases.

2. Now sonography has enabled us to make a larger number of diagnoses and therefore the indications for laparoscopy in tumors, particularly those of the pancreas, have diminished accordingly.

3. Abdominal pain, as a single or predominant symptom is, however, very often due to peritoneal involvement, and peritoneal lesions are difficult to detect with sonography, and quite a few false echographic negatives are therefore made; so there are still a number of valid indications for laparoscopy.

4.7 Fever

It is always difficult to make a diagnosis when fever is the only, or the dominant, symptom in a disease. The conventional criteria accepted in the past to define "fever of unknown origin" were (a) the illness must have lasted at least 3 weeks; (b) the fever must have been over 38.3°C on several occasions; and (c) the diagnosis must still be uncertain despite a week of intensive investigation during hospitalization.

In the above cases even if there were no signs of abdominal disease, explorative laparotomy was performed, and it led to a certain diagnosis in about 60% of cases and nearly always provided useful information. Later, laparoscopy was successfully introduced as an alternative to laparotomy.

We were among the first to use laparoscopy systematically to discover the cause of an undiagnosed fever. In each case, the indication for laparoscopy depended upon the particular clinical hypothesis, which in turn was based on an awareness of the different abdominal diseases that can cause a fever, and also on an evaluation of the capacity of laparoscopy to detect and identify these particular diseases. Our experience in the presonographic era demonstrated that laparoscopy, associated with biopsy, enables an exact diagnosis to be made in over 60% of cases, the following findings being the most frequent: (a) *granulomas* (tuberculosis, sarcoidosis, brucellosis, etc.) to the liver and spleen; (b) *malignant lymphomas* localized in the spleen, liver, etc.; (c) *malignant primary tumors* of the liver; and, finally, (d) different types of abscess *collections* with different localizations.

Laparoscopy is unsuccessful when the lesions are situated deep, are inside the hepatic or splenic parenchyma, are in the retroperitoneum or are hidden. However, negative findings are of value because they allow us to establish reliably that the fever is not due to an abdominal lesion.

4.7.1 Present Indications for Laparoscopy

The number of cases of undiagnosed fever has diminished, thanks to imaging techniques, in particular sonography, so in certain situations laparoscopy is now useless. Where fever is due to *malignant neoplasm of the liver* or to an *abscess collection*, the echographic diagnosis, integrated with fine-needle, echoguided biopsy, is usually simple and sure. Moreover, liver tumors that cause a fever rarely escape sonographic detection because they are usually large, and often contain areas of necrosis and colliquation. In fact there is only a very slight risk of making a "false echographic negative" in cases of liver neoplasms with the clinical symptom of a fever.

Abscesses are clearly evidenced by sonography and transcutaneous puncture; and the study of aspirated material provides a clear definition, also from the etiological viewpoint. It is important to stress the fact that here sonography is again complementary to laparoscopy. Liquid collections, whether from abscesses or pseudoabscesses, are usually deep seated and either fail to appear on the organ surface or present only part of their wall. So laparoscopy in these cases either fails to allow a diagnosis to be made, or, if a diagnosis is made, it is unreliable because it is almost always based solely upon incomplete findings or indirect signs. So sonography is preferred to laparoscopy in cases in which the latter is unlikely to provide a reliable diagnosis. However, while sonography can detect collections and malignant tumors, it rarely detects other processes that often cause fever. Laparoscopy can therefore still be considered a valid method for the diagnosis of a temperature of uncertain nature.

In 1981, Solis-Herruzo et al. reached the above conclusion after performing a laparoscopic examination in 70 patients who had fevers that could not be diagnosed even after a very thorough clinical examination had been made [31]. Sonography then was less efficient than it is now and fine-needle echoguided biopsies were not taken. The series was, however, "filtered" by CT scan and the rigorous criteria used to decide upon whether or not laparoscopy was indicated is reflected indirectly, by the endoscopic findings themselves (Table 4.3). In fact in only two of the laparoscopically diagnosed cases was the fever caused by liver neoplasms (one primary and the other secondary); in another case the cause was an abscess and in another a hydatid cyst. It is evident that in the great majority of these cases TAC had provided the diagnosis and so laparoscopy was not performed because it would have been useless. The most frequent laparoscopic findings were granulomatous diseases, malignant lymphomas, collagen diseases, etc. Presumably laparoscopy

Table 4.3. Laparoscopy in fever of unknown origin (70 cases). [34]

True diagnosis by laparoscopy	
Category	Number of cases
Infectious (5 cases)	
Tuberculosis	3
Chronic cholecystitis	1
Pyogenic liver abscess	1
Neoplastic diseases (7 cases)	
Lymphoma	4
Primary liver cancer	1
Cancer of the gallbladder	1
Secondary liver cancer	1
Collagen diseases (4 cases)	
Necrotizing angitis	4
Other causes (16 cases)	
Chronic active hepatitis	3
Granulomatous diseases	10
Sarcoidosis	1
Hydatid cyst	1
Total	31 (44.2%)

had been indicated in these cases because TAC had failed to provide a diagnosis.

According to Solis-Herruzo et al. laparoscopy is still a valid means for diagnosing a fever: in 44% of cases a certain diagnosis was made, in 17% no diagnosis was made, although significant diagnotic indications were given, and 22% had no diagnosis.

Laparoscopy is particularly valuable when the clinical examination or biological tests show signs of an abdominal disease [32].

4.7.2 Main Laparoscopic Findings

Our results, obtained by systematically comparing the echographic with the laparoscopic study, fully confirm that some indications for endoscopy are still valid. Moreover, the type of disease and the characteristics of the different laparoscopic findings can satisfactorily explain why the imaging techniques had given a negative or insignificant finding in the cases selected for laparoscopy. Now in series of patients undergoing laparoscopy, *abscess collections* are no longer found and *liver tumors* are hardly ever found because they have already been detected by ultrasound, and therefore diagnosed, making laparoscopy superfluous. *Liver carcinoma* has become a rare laparoscopic finding, as is *metastatic tumor*.

Melanoblastoma can give rise to a diffuse febrile metastatic spread, characterized by small lesions of the liver and peritoneum that escape detection by noninvasive techniques, but that can be diagnosed laparoscopically (Fig. 4.31). In these cases it is often very difficult to establish where the tumor originates.

Primary carcinoma of the gallbladder may also cause fever, which is usually associated with other symptoms. Sometimes, however, although this is rare (1% in our series) it may be the only sign of the disease and may therefore preclude a diagnosis. In such cases, the diagnostic problem can be solved by laparoscopy. However, most of the diseases that can cause fever that is not diagnosed are *granulomatous processes* and *malignant lymphomas*. If localized in the liver, spleen, and peritoneum, these diseases have features that are difficult to identify with imaging techniques.

Tuberculosis is fairly frequent, and can cause symptoms that are mainly febrile, above all when the lesions affect the liver and spleen. The laparoscopic findings are of lesions that are usually extremely small, which may be numerous and

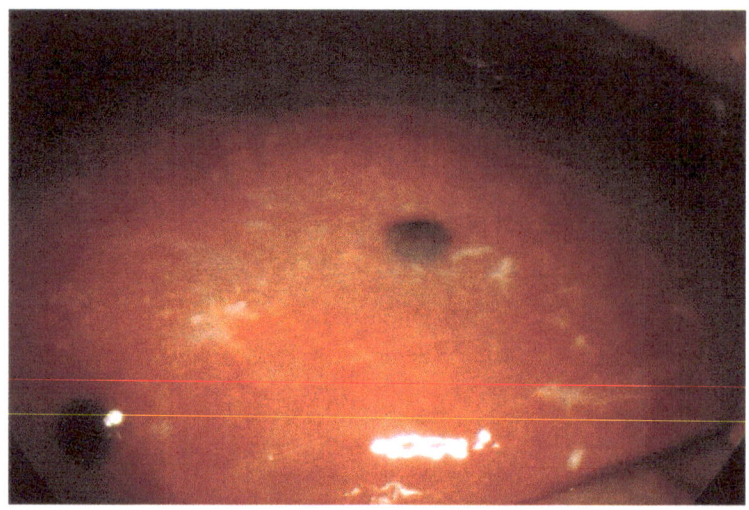

4.31

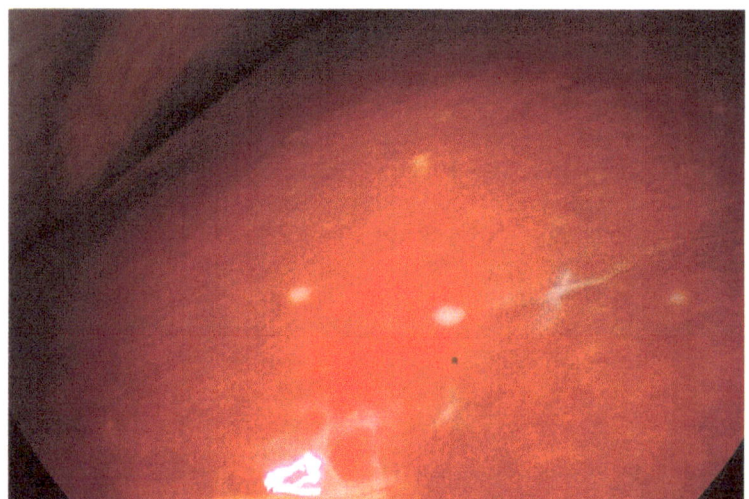

4.32

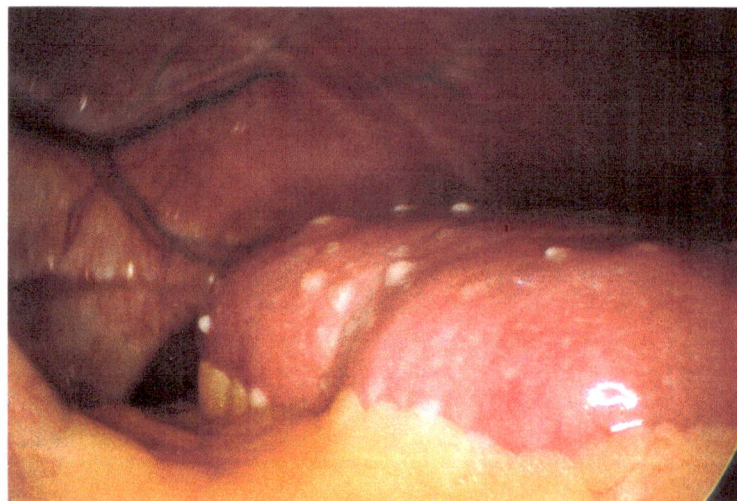

4.33

diffuse, and which appear on the surface of the liver (Fig. 4.32) or spleen (Fig. 4.33) as points, spots, or miliary-form granules with a whitish or yellowy-white hue. Because they are so small, these lesions give false-negative findings at CT and ultrasound. On the other hand, no reliable differential diagnosis can be made macroscopically, but, with target biopsy of the liver and spleen, the nature of the lesions can be established, especially if muliple biopsies are taken. When fever is the only symptom of abdominal tuberculosis, the granulomatous lesions are found only in the hepatic and splenic parenchyma and usually the peritoneum is not affected. When the latter is involved the main symptom is ascites.

Splenic and hepatic *brucelloses* may have fever as their only symptom and may be impossible to diagnose with noninvasive techniques. As the laparoscopic finding is similar to those for other types of granuloma, the diagnosis must be made by means of biopsy.

As well as giving rise to negative sonographic findings, some granulomas can give rise to "uncertain" pictures. These pictures are very important because they allow us to guess that the fever may be caused by an abdominal disease, but they do not help us make the diagnosis, especially if the fine-needle echoguided biopsy findings are not significant. In such cases, the sonographic examination itself points to the need for laparoscopy. In one of our cases of fever with moderate hepatomegaly, the sonographic finding was compatible with both diffuse liver disease and malignant neoplastic infiltration (Fig. 4.34). Echoguided fine-needle biopsy gave no reliable findings. Laparoscopy clearly demonstrated alterations, but the picture was difficult to interpret (Fig. 4.35). The histological examination made with several laparoscopic biopsy samples eventually allowed a diagnosis of liver *sarcoidosis* to be made. Figure 4.36 gives a further example of the value of lap-

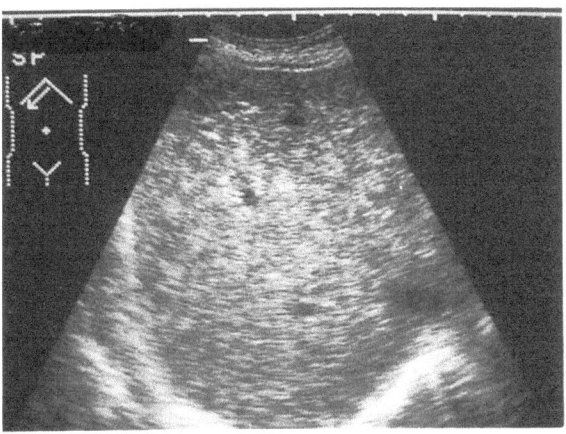

Fig. 4.34. Echographic oblique subcostal scan. Right lobe of the liver has a markedly dishomogeneous echostructure due to diffuse hyperechogenic granulation? *Diffuse hepatopathy? Granulomatosis? Lymphomatous infiltration?*

aroscopy in the diagnosis of fever when the echographic finding is uncertain. Sonography demonstrated that on the liver a small hyperechogenic areas was present with blurred contours; its nature was uncertain. The finding with fine-needle echoguided biopsy suggested malignant lymphoma. As the diagnosis was not satisfactory, laparoscopy was performed: on the right lobe of the liver, near to the point indicated at sonography, there was a single round lesion with features suggesting lymphoma. Biopsy, however, demonstrated *leishmaniosis*.

Finally, of particular importance is fever that is a dominant symptom of a *malignant lymphoma* and, above all, of a Hodgkin's disease lymphoma. In these cases splenomegaly is frequent and it is an important datum for diagnostic orientation. It must always be kept in mind, however, that in the initial stages, which can last up to 3 months, the spleen may not be enlarged and the blood test results may be normal. There is a period in its evolution that the disease has fever as its main symptom.

The above notion is important because in cases of undiagnosed temperature it suggests a malignant lymphoma, even if there are no signs of it and, even if, in particular the spleen is not enlarged. In these cases, the sonographic finding is negative and laparoscopy is clearly indicated. In the majority of cases the spleen may not be enlarged, but does present different-sized macroscopic lesions with features that suggest a lymp-

◀━━━━━━━━━━━━━━━

Fig. 4.31. Upper surface of the left lobe of the liver: some small shiny black, slightly raised, nodules are seen. *Metastasis to the liver from melanoblastoma*

Fig. 4.32. Upper surface of right lobe of the liver; small whitish spots. *Malignant lymphoma? Granuloma?* Biopsy: *tuberculosis of the liver*

Fig. 4.33. Upper surface of the right lobe of the liver: small rounded, whitish spots. *Malignant lymphoma? Granuloma?* Biopsy: *tuberculosis of the spleen*

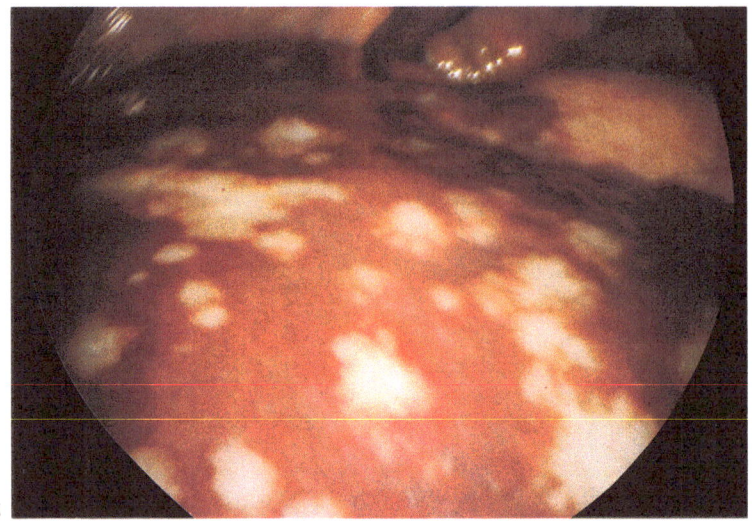

4.35

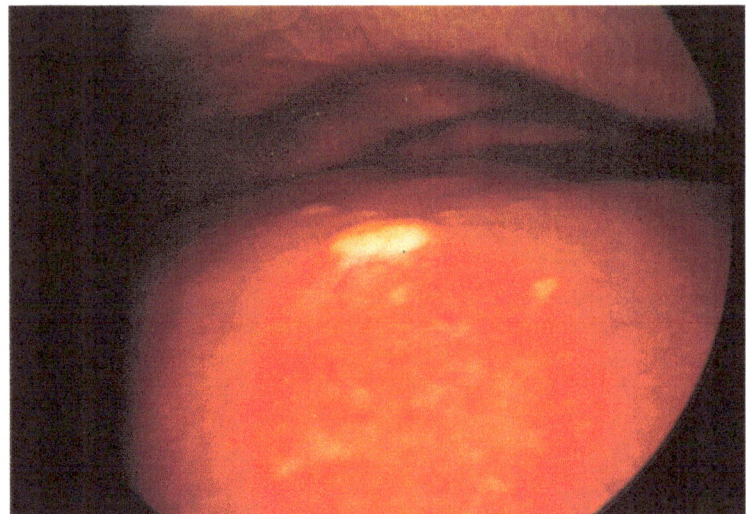

4.36

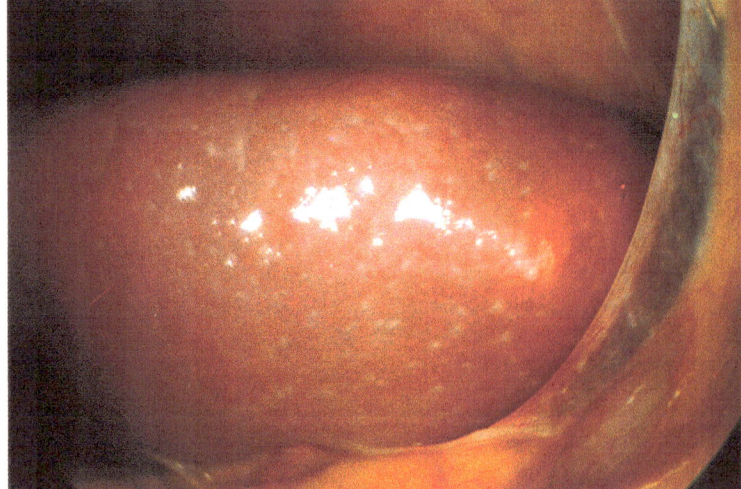

4.37

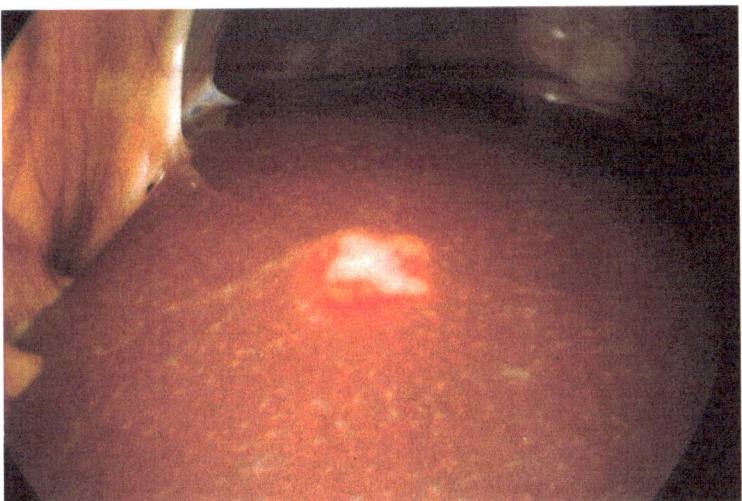

Fig. 4.38. Upper surface of the left lobe of the liver. Flat whitish-pink "quadrifoglio" formation. Malignant lymphoma? Biopsy: *Hodgkin's disease lymphoma*

homatous process and that are a good target for biopsy (Fig. 4.37). In other cases, the spleen is not enlarged and it has no visible lesions; here it is necessary to take multiple biopsies (no less than four) from different points of the organ. We can thus sometimes collect lymphomatous tissue and make a diagnosis that would otherwise be impossible. In about 5% of our series biopsy was taken in cases of suspected splenopathy from a normal-sized spleen without apparent lesions.

On other occasions laparoscopy demonstrated hepatic lesions from which it is easy to take a biopsy, and the biopsy itself allows an accurate diagnosis to be made (Fig. 4.38). In such cases it is superfluous to study the spleen.

Fig. 4.35. Same case as in Fig. 4.34. Numerous flat, round, whitish plaques, some with irregular margins, isolated or confluent. *Malignant lymphoma? Cholangio-carcinoma? Metastatic neoplasia?* Biopsy: *sarcoidosis of the liver*

Fig. 4.36. Upper surface of the right lobe of the liver. Whitish-yellow raised nodule surrounded by other smaller nodules. *Malignant lymphoma? Granuloma?* Biopsy: *leishmaniosis of the liver*

Fig. 4.37. Spleen normal size, contained in the phrenocholic ligament. Detail of the lower pole where a small slightly protruding nodule can be seen; its color is slightly lighter than that of the surrounding parenchyma. *Malignant lymphoma?* Biopsy: *Hodgkin's disease lymphoma*

4.7.3 Conclusions

1. Laparoscopy, widely used in the presonographic era for the diagnosis of so-called "fevers of unknown origin," has proved to be a highly effective method, enabling us to detect the disease causing the fever in about 60% of cases.

2. At present sonography can detect some of these processes, mainly abscess collections and malignant tumors of the liver and spleen, thus making laparoscopy superfluous.

3. There are, however, many diseases (granuloma, malignant lymphoma, etc.) that can cause fever and their localization within abdominal organs cannot be detected or clarified by noninvasive techniques.

4. Therefore, laparoscopy is still often indicated in the diagnosis of "fever of unknown origin."

References

1. Dagnini G, Bergamo S, Caldironi MW, Marin G, Patella M (1980) La laparoscopia nella diagnosi di situazioni cliniche incerte caratterizzate da un versamento addominale. G Gastroenterol Endosc 3: 39–46
2. Geasce TM, Spitaels JM, Moshal MG, Simjee AE (1981) Peritoneoscopy in the diagnosis of tubercolous peritonitis. Gastrointest Endosc 2:66–68
3. Henning H, Look D (1985) Peritoneum. In: Henning H, Look D: Laparoskopie. Thieme, Stuttgart
4. Dagnini G (1980) Ascites. In: Clinical laparoscopy. Piccin Medical, Padua

5. Salky BA (1983) Laparoscopic diagnosis of peritoneal mesothelioma. Gastrointest Endosc 1:65
6. Piccigallo E, Jeffers LJ, Reddy KR, Caldironi MW, Parenti A, Schiff ER (1988) Malignant peritoneal mesothelioma. A clinical and laparoscopic study of ten cases. Dig Dis Sci 33:633–639
7. Rodriguez de Lope C, San Miguel Joglar G, Pons Romeo F (1982) Laparoscopic diagnosis of tuberculous ascites. Endoscopy 14:178–179
8. Jorge AD (1984) Peritoneal tuberculosis. Endoscopy 16:10–12
9. Alberti-Flor J, Vaughan S, Dewey Dunn G (1985) Laparoscopy and tuberculous peritonitis. Gastrointest Endosc 31(2):106–107
10. Boyd WP (1987) Laparoscopy in ascites and peritoneal diseases. In: Sivak MV (ed) Gastroenterologic endoscopy. Saunders Philadelphia
11. Babando MG, Lombardo L (1985) False asciti: bilancio dell'esperienza laparoscopica in 10 anni (1975–1985). G Ital Endosc Dig 3:381
12. Beck K (1980) Farbatlas der Laparoskopie. Schattauer, Stuttgart
13. Dagnini G (1980) Hepatomegaly. In: Dagnini G (ed) Clinical laparoscopy. Piccin Medical, Padua
14. Henning H, Look D (1985) Laparoskopie. Thieme, Stuttgart
15. Dagnini G, Caldironi MW, Marin G, Patella M (1984) Laparoscopic splenic biopsy. Endoscopy 2(16):43–84
16. Garcia Molinero MJ, Solis Herruzo JA, Munoz Yagüe MT (1981) La laparoscopia en el estudio de las esplenomegalias. Gastroenterol Hepatol 4(10):515–519
17. Dagnini G (1987) Laparoscopy in cirrhosis and portal hypertension. In: Sivak MV (ed) Gastroenterologic endoscopy. Saunders, Philadelphia
18. Dagnini G, Marin G, Patella M, Bergamo S, Caldironi MW (1980) Masse dell'addome superiore: laparoscopia. In: Aggiornamenti in epatologia. Compositori, Bologna
19. Gandolfi L, Rossi A, Leo P, Solmi L, Muratori R (1985) Indications for laparoscopy before and after the introduction of ultrasonography. Gastrointest Endosc 31(1):1–3
20. Dagnini G, Marin G, Patella M, Tufano A (1983) La diagnosi laparoscopica di carcinoma primitivo della colecisti. Studio su 98 casi. Gastroenterologo 5(2):63–67
21. Dagnini G, Marin G, Patella M, Zotti S (1984) Laparoscopy in the diagnosis of primary carcinoma of the gallbladder. Gastrointest Endosc 30(5):289–291
22. Dagnini G, Marin G, Patella M, Zotti S (1983) La place de la laparoscopie dans le diagnostic différentiel des ictères cholestatiques. Med Chir Dig 12:195–199
23. Fassler S (1980) The exploration techniques of jaundice. Acta Endoscopia 10(1):53–55
24. Marti Vicente A (1981) La laparoscopia en la colostasis. Acta Med Port [Suppl] 3:17–22
25. Patella M, Frizzarin M, Sonzin M, Paccagnella P (1985) La posizione attuale della laparoscopia nella diagnosi degli itteri colestatici. G Ital Endosc Dig 3:376
26. Buffet C, Pelletier G, Etienne JP (1983) Que reste-t-il de la laparoscopie en 1983? Clin Biol 7:134–140
27. Schiff L (1987) Jaundice. Clinical pearls and series revisited. J Clin Gastroenterol 9(4):383–385
28. Dagnini G (1980) Clinical laparoscopy. Piccin Medical, Padua
29. Dagnini G (1980) La laparoscopia nella diagnosi del dolore addominale. G Gastroenterol End 3:15–19
30. Brigato G, Miola E (1987) Endometriosi diaframmatica. Ginecol Clin 7(1):52–55
31. Solis-Herruzo JA, Benita V, Morillas JD (1981) Laparoscopy in fever of unknown origin – study of seventy cases. Endoscopy 13:207–210
32. Rouge PE, Grasset J, Franco A, Aubert H, Massot C, Rachaie M (1981) La laparoscopie avec biopsie hépatique dans le diagnostic des fièvres prolongées inespliquées. Rev Med Interne 2:151–156

5 Liver Diseases

Laparoscopy has long been used for the study of the liver, and has long been of crucial importance in the diagnosis of liver diseases and also in the knowledge of the nature and natural history of some of the diseases themselves.

The macroscopic and bioptic findings made by means of laparoscopy enable us to clarify quite different diseases in a very high percentage of cases. So this technique has a wide range of indications. In 1979, before the boom in imaging techniques [1], I specified that laparoscopy could resolve two types of problem in (a) the diagnosis and (b) the clarification and classification of:

1. Diseases with symptoms that clearly, or presumably, involved the liver, diseases that were not diagnosed after a complete clinical, radiological, and laboratory examination: hepatomegaly, jaundice, pain to the right hypochondrium and fever with an unknown cause.

2. Diseases that were detected, but not studied in enough detail: (a) alcoholic liver disease, (b) chronic hepatitis, and (c) liver cirrhosis.

Imaging techniques have contributed to the diagnostic methods for the study of the liver and thanks to them the clinical picture in such cases can be clarified and improved upon. And now sonography, the noninvasive technique of choice, is a really valid filter for patients who would once have been submitted to laparoscopy.

Sonography can demonstrate: (a) an apparently *normal* liver, (b) a picture compatible with *diffuse liver disease*, and (c) *focal lesions*.

The decision to perform a laparoscopy is based upon these results in relation, above all, to whether or not they can provide the answers to the different diagnostic questions. The criteria once used to evaluate whether laparoscopy was indicated must now of course be modified.

It is opportune here to subdivide liver diseases into two groups. The sonographic findings indicate which category a particular case belongs to – *diffuse* or *characterized* by *focal lesions*.

We consider here problems related to the diagnosis and study of *diffuse noncirrhotic liver diseases* and *liver cirrhosis*. Of course these diseases are so closely related that they are considered separately only for the sake of clarity. It is important to remember that, while imaging techniques are very useful for screening, they do not have great diagnostic value.

In *liver steatosis* the organ appears enlarged and there is an increased echogenicity, its intensity depending upon the amount of accumulated fat. Ultrasonography is highly sensitive when the phenomenon is marked; the specificity is good, but there are pitfalls. *Chronic hepatitis* does not have a typical ultrasound picture. In most cases the liver appears normal; it may be slightly enlarged; and rough and irregular echoes and some intrahepatic vessel alterations may be observed, above all if there is coexisting fibrosis. In *cirrhosis* the echographic symptoms consist mainly of: (a) at-depth "attenuation sign," with an echo diminution, making it difficult to display the deeper area of the liver, and echo distortion; (b) an altered ratio between the caudate lobe and the right lobe volumes, the former predominating; (c) a diffuse diminution in echogenicity if there is a coexistent steatosis; (d) a nodular deformation of the margin, which appears mainly in large-nodule cirrhosis. The following signs of portal hypertension are also of value: dilation of the vena porta, splenic vein and superior mesenteric vein, any recanalization of the umbilical vein, splenomegaly and ascites – which can be demonstrated sonographically, even if it is limited.

In our view, the work by Vogel et al. [2] has greatly contributed toward an accurate understanding of the value of sonography in the diagnosis of diffuse liver disease. The aim of their prospective study was to establish simple criteria for the interpretation of sonographic findings in diffuse liver disease in patients for whom a diagnosis had already been made on the basis of laparoscopy and biopsy. The macroscopic and microscopic data were systematically documented using the semiquantative method and this facilitated a comparison with the sonographic pictures. The work is not recent (1980), but since then sonography does not appear to have undergone any important changes in this sector [3–6]. However, the strict methodological criteria used for surgery have made its conclusions highly reliable. It is stated that it is relatively *simple* to distinguish between a normal and a diseased liver in cases of alcoholic liver steatosis and of obvious cirrhosis; this is *possible* in chronic active hepatitis with an increase in fibrous tissue and *uncertain* in moderate chronic active hepatitis and in chronic persistent hepatitis. Echography does no more than this. Attention is drawn in particular to the fact that its negative predictive value is very low in the various forms of widespread liver disease; we cannot be sure that the liver is normal even if echography is negative. The ultrasounds show only slight sensitivity even in the presence of advanced liver lesions, like cirrhosis; a great many false negatives are therefore obtained. Moreover, fibrosis and fat give a highly similar attenuated echographic pattern. Therefore, since fat and fibrous tissue frequently coexist, it is very difficult to establish whether sonographic alterations are due to one or the other histological alteration [6]. Furthermore, it is impossible to distinguish between increased ultrasound brightness due to steatosis or to fibrosis and other possible causes of a "bright" liver. This lack of specificity greatly reduces the usefulness of sonography in the diagnosis of widespread disease.

So imaging techniques provide additional information, but this information is not decisive in solving the different clinical problems that emerge and there is wide agreement that the diagnosis can be made only on the basis of anatomohistological data. Therefore the status of laparoscopy in the study of diffuse liver disease has not changed. However, some interesting variations have been made to the classical treatises, and it is opportune to examine them here.

5.1 Diffuse Noncirrhotic Liver Diseases

5.1.1 Alcoholic Liver Disease

Alcoholic liver disease is usually long-standing, sometimes with acute episodes; it presents in various forms, which have the same etiology but which have different anatomoclinical characteristics, significance, and prognosis. They are clearly recognized and can be nosographically pictured in a satisfactory way. The pictures observed are, however, quite different, and the diagnostic problems involved are frequently difficult to overcome.

Some chronic alcoholics have mild, unclear symptoms, so the clinical picture is very vague. The patients complain of dyspepsia, which is sometimes mild, varying from a simple feeling of "heaviness" and tension to the epigastrium to a mild sensation, with complaints concerning loss of appetite and so forth. They may complain of asthenia, but feel that their general health is quite good. Objectively, the liver is usually enlarged, sometimes greatly so. The laboratory findings may be negative or show signs of a functional disorder.

Once, this type of picture suggested alcoholic liver disease of the steatotic type, but an anatomohistological study with blind biopsy or with laparoscopy was required in order to obtain a clearer picture. However, we used highly selective criteria for laparoscopic indications. We suggested that the patients with hepatomegaly and altered laboratory findings should be submitted to further examinations 2 months after ceasing alcohol consumption. In many cases, after this period of abstinence, the picture appeared to have normalized, as can happen in simple steatosis; any other investigation was therefore superfluous.

On the other hand, laparoscopy was performed when the hepatomegaly was constant and the functional picture continued to be altered. This selection was made to obviate a number of redundant invasive studies.

Now sonography has greatly increased the likelihood of clarifying the features of alcoholic liver disease at this stage because it enables us easily to detect the steatosis, which is the most significant lesion, and it also fairly accurately indicates the entity of the fatty infiltration. It is also useful to perform repeated echographies at intervals as these show whether or not there is regression. However, echography fails to distinguish between degenerative alcoholic liver disease (such as simple steatosis, which can regress until there is a total "restitutio ad integrum" and alcoholic hepatitis, whose evolutive features are well known. This differential diagnosis can only be made after a histological examination. Probably laparoscopy is not indispensable; blind biopsy can be sufficient. Of course the diagnostic accuracy depends on the histological finding.

The difference between pure steatosis and hepatitis is clear. Degenerative hepatitis is marked by a diffuse fatty infiltration with swelling, hepatocyte clarification, and, in some cases, the presence of Mallory's bodies. Hepatitis has the same picture, but it also has signs of necrotic and inflammatory lesions (polymorphonuclear and round cell infiltrates).

The macroscopic alterations visible laparoscopically to the naked eye are interesting and can enable us to distinguish between degenerative and phlogistic forms, but only if the picture is complete and significant. Some classical pictures should be kept in mind, for reference: an enlarged liver with rounded margins and a smooth taut pale yellow surface, with no lobular pattern, is typical of massive diffuse steatosis (Fig. 5.1). Zonular steatosis can be suspected if there is an accentuated pattern and dark-red areas of liver tissue that alternate with well-delineated yellow areas (Fig. 5.2). However, alcoholic hepatitis can be suspected if the liver is enlarged, has a smooth reddish orange surface (due to fatty infiltration and active congestion), and has no acinous design (due to congestion). Depending on the prevalence of active congestion and steatosis, different features can be observed, such as a "cinnabar" liver (Fig. 5.3) or "orange" liver. These are classical laparoscopic pictures, and they are equally significant (Fig. 5.4).

So laparoscopy allows us, when findings are somewhat unclear, to distinguish between degenerative and inflammatory alcoholic liver disease. It always gives interesting clues that enhance the diagnostic accuracy and reliability. However, biopsy always has the last word. As already mentioned, we as a rule prefer laparoscopic to blind transcutaneous biopsy. But in alcoholic liver disease, transcutaneous biopsy can also provide a satisfactory diagnosis. In fact Lindner, a great believer in the superiority of laparoscopic biopsy, said that liver steatosis was one of the few indications for blind biopsy [7].

It is important here to stress that the dividing line between chronic alcoholic hepatitis and cirrhosis is often unclear and so with blind biopsy there is always a risk of failing to diagnose initial

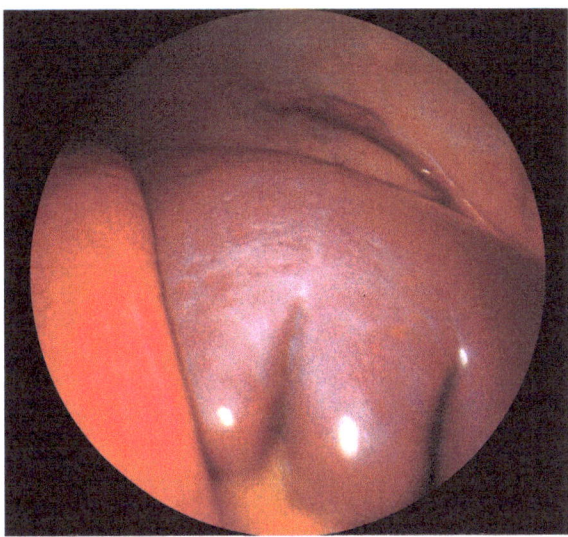

Fig. 5.1. The margin of the left lobe of the liver is yellow and has lost its lobular pattern. Large spleen of the congestive type and dilation of small peritoneal vessels. *Diffuse steatosis of the liver with secondary portal hypertension*

cirrhosis with a modest or incomplete picture. This aspect is further discussed in Sect. 5.2.

Finally, marked liver steatosis can give rise to portal hypertension. The sinusoidal lumen, compressed by hepatocytes that are swollen by lipid infiltration, is considered the most likely cause. The phenomenon can be very marked and, in the early literature, digestive hemorrhages from the rupture of esophageal varices are described. More frequently, however, it is moderate and can disappear completely when the steatosis has resolved. In these cases, a finding of hepatomegaly with splenomegaly, sometimes with slight alterations in the biochemical picture, is not easy to interpret clinically.

By demonstrating major steatosis, sonography can explain the liver enlargement and confirm the splenomegaly, the origin of which, however, is still unestablished. Blind biopsy partly resolves this problem because it can accurately reveal the steatosis, ruling out any phlogosis. But it does not allow us to either explain the splenomegaly or reliably rule out cirrhosis. Because of this, laparoscopy is definitely indicated; the questions are answered by macroscopic data, which demonstrate whether (a) the liver enlargement is really due to widespread steatosis and there is no cirrhosis; (b) the splenomegaly is congestive, and (c) there is portal hypertension, revealed by small veins that

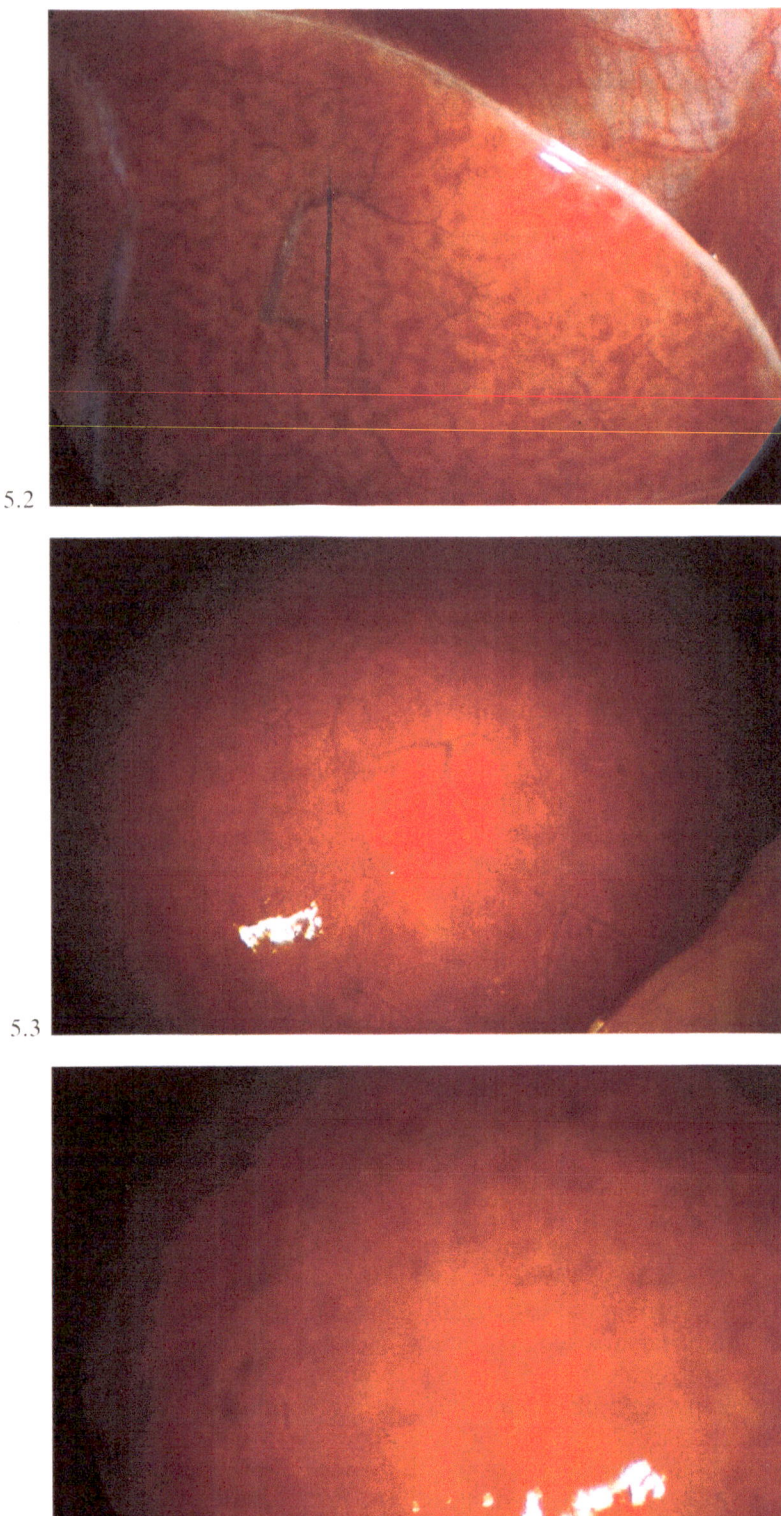

5.2

5.3

5.4

are enlarged and turgid, the expression of a portacaval collateral circulation. These vessels are too small to be detected by ultrasound (see Fig. 5.1).

Laparoscopy is not usually indicated in acute alcoholic hepatitis. The clinical picture is easily recognized and the histological lesions are clear and well defined. Blind biopsy is therefore sufficient for a good diagnostic clarification. On the other hand, different considerations must be made when the acute hepatitis is not an isolated episode but occurs repeatedly and is superimposed on pre-existing chronic hepatitis. In these cases the acute process is a complication of the liver disease itself and it can considerably modify the features of the liver disease. Laparoscopy is indicated because it can demonstrate fairly specific macroscopic lesions, with small excavations showing a loss of tissue from hepatocytolysis and circumscribed reddish areas that stand out against the smooth yellowish surface of the steatotic liver, typical of inflammation. As these alterations are often circumscribed, with blind biopsy they may be missed, so laparoscopic target biopsy is more reliable. In these cases the laparobioptic diagnosis is important because it enables us to detect the transformation from steatosis into chronic hepatitis, which can progressively become ingravescent, developing into cirrhosis.

Alcoholic cirrhosis and the problems connected with it are discussed more fully in Sect. 5.2.

5.1.2 Chronic Hepatitis

Noninvasive imaging techniques have a low diagnostic value in the study of hepatitis, so in this field the criteria for the use of laparoscopy have not undergone important changes. Anatomohistological data are still crucial to the diagnosis and clarification of these forms. In typical acute hepatitis with a normal course and complete resolution, laparoscopy, like blind liver biopsy, is not indicated.

◀――――――――――――

Fig. 5.2. Lower surface of the left lobe of the liver. *Zonal liver steatosis*

Fig. 5.3. Left lobe of the liver with rounded margin; smooth surface, steatosis, and active congestion: "cinnabar" liver. *Alcoholic hepatitis*? Confirmation with biopsy

Fig. 5.4. Surface of the liver is orange because of steatosis and active congestion. *Alcoholic hepatitis*? Confirmation with biopsy

The laparoscopic findings in acute hepatitis are well known and have been aptly summarized in Kalk's classical definition: "*large red liver*" (see Fig. 4.15). Of course a knowledge of these pictures was of great theoretical value for an exact interpretation of the process, but active hepatitis has been diagnosed on the basis of other information above all biochemical data, for quite some time. The only exception to this is acute cholestatic hepatitis because it can be very difficult to distinguish it from obstructive jaundice (see Sect. 4.5).

The case is different for chronic hepatitis. In chronicization several different clinical and histological alterations can be found; they correspond respectively to a picture of *chronic persistent hepatitis* and *chronic active hepatitis*.

Of course the differential diagnosis between these two forms is of great importance: the "persistent" form is of little clinical importance and eventually resolves spontaneously whereas "active" hepatitis tends to develop into cirrhosis.

5.1.2.1 Chronic Persistent Hepatitis

From the etiopathogenetic viewpoint, chronic hepatitis is the result of acute viral hepatitis or it has another unestablished etiology that may be overlooked; its clinical symptoms are scarce or are not particularly significant – sometimes they are nonexistent. Also the objectivity is modest and the main datum is alterations in the laboratory examinations. The exact diagnosis is, however, made on the basis of histological findings. The fundamental histological sign is an inflammatory lymphocytic infiltration of the portal space, which appears enlarged; the infiltration is strictly limited to this area and spares the lobules. Signs of necrosis of the surrounding lamina are either absent or minimal; sometimes balloon-shaped hepatocytes and small focal necroses are found. The macroscopic picture is very disappointing. The liver may in fact appear to be normal or may have an appearance resembling that of viral hepatitis [8]. It may be slightly enlarged and have a generally soft consistency. The surface is smooth, sometimes with small retractions from previous cytolysis; its color varies, from red, from slight congestion, to pale pink. The lobular pattern is usually unclear. This poor, aspecific outcome does not call for a laparoscopy, which is universally considered redundant in such cases.

We, too, have always been of the opinion that in the great majority of cases a blind biopsy is adequate for a first appraisal, and this should be followed by periodic clinical and biochemical control. We have also specified, however, that laparoscopy was indicated in certain cases, when the clinical picture shows any atypias that throw doubt upon the accuracy of a diagnosis of persistent hepatitis [9]. The symptoms for which we suggest a laparobioptical control are mainly: (a) hard hepatomegaly, sometimes with a slight spleen enlargement and (b) a prolonged course, with a deterioration in biochemical test findings, in particular with a gradual increase in gamma globulins.

I believe that this scheme is still valid, even if it does have the disadvantage of being controlled by criteria that are not very rigorous and that depend greatly upon a subjective interpretation. In this respect, however, sonography can provide some useful clues, in spite of the fact that its findings are not considered particularly valuable.

In cases of chronic persistent laparobioptically ascertained hepatitis, sonography is unlikely to distinguish between a normal and a diseased liver [2] and it gives rise to a high number of false negatives [10–12, 5, 6]. Its lack of specificity has also been stressed by all. Of course sonography does not enable us to diagnose persistent hepatitis and it can in no way replace laparobiopsy. It can, however, provide findings that indicate whether laparoscopy should be performed in a particular case. We have discussed indications in anomalies in the symptomatological picture of persistent hepatitis and, in particular, clinically revealed hepatomegaly. Here echography can provide interesting clues, clarifying the liver size and, above all, demonstrating any parenchymal alterations. In fact, sonography can detect liver fibrosis – with a good sensitivity. This echographic finding cannot be used on its own for diagnostic purposes because it has a low specificity, but it provides an important clue as to whether laparoscopy with biopsy should be performed so as to study further the features and define the type of liver disease. I am therefore of the opinion that laparoscopy is indicated when symptoms are compatible with chronic persistent hepatitis, but the echographic finding simply indicates a "disease." Other authors [13, 10] also believe that echographic screening is a useful indicator of whether or not laparoscopy should be performed [13].

The endoscopic findings can vary greatly and sometimes findings may be unexpected. The liver may appear only slightly enlarged but there may be no evident lesions: in these cases, multiple biopsies must be taken from different points of the organ. More often than not the picture that emerges corresponds to the so-called *simple hepatic fibrosis* that laparoscopy defines well, allowing us nosographically to picture these forms, which are the anatomical expression of so-called "chronic inactive hepatites." These findings are made during recovery from persistent or perhaps even moderately active hepatitis. The histological picture from multiple biopsies can confirm simple fibrosis or indicate whether the disease is active. In certain cases, different types of scar can be seen; sometimes very extensive, or retracted, they are the result of repair following previous hepatocytolysis (Fig. 5.5). The presence of these areas of total fibrosis further demonstrates the need, even in the so-called "diffuse" diseases, to decide where the biopsy should be taken from, because the finding can vary greatly, depending on the particular area from which it is taken. This decision can only be followed through if laparoscopy is used.

On other occasions the liver is enlarged and its surface is made uneven by deep grooves and areas of depression, but the parenchyma is normal and the surface smooth. These alterations are due to cytolysis. The biopsies can, however, demonstrate that although the macroscopic picture appears to be extremely serious, this is only persistent chronic hepatitis (Fig. 5.6). Other cases may be clinically similar and have analogous echographic findings, but laparoscopy confirms that the organ is enlarged, that there are deep grooves and macroscopic features typical of fibrosis. The liver surface is uneven because of obviously cirrhotic fine nodules (Fig. 5.7).

I am of the opinion that today, in view of the achievements with echographic screening, one should wait if findings are negative and that

Fig. 5.5. Detail of the surface of the liver which is grayish blue because of a slight capsular thickening. Scar craters. Biopsy: *chronic persistent hepatitis*

Fig. 5.6. Left lobe of the liver is very irregular because of extensive retracted areas. The remaining parenchyma is smooth and apparently unaltered. Biopsy: *chronic persistent hepatitis*

Fig. 5.7. Right lobe of the liver with deep grooves. The parenchyma appears stiff and the surface is nodulated. *Medionodular cirrhosis of the liver*

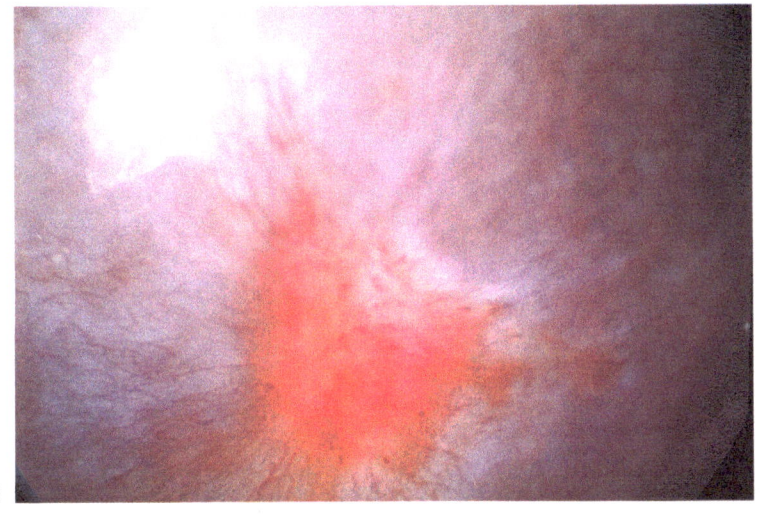

5.5

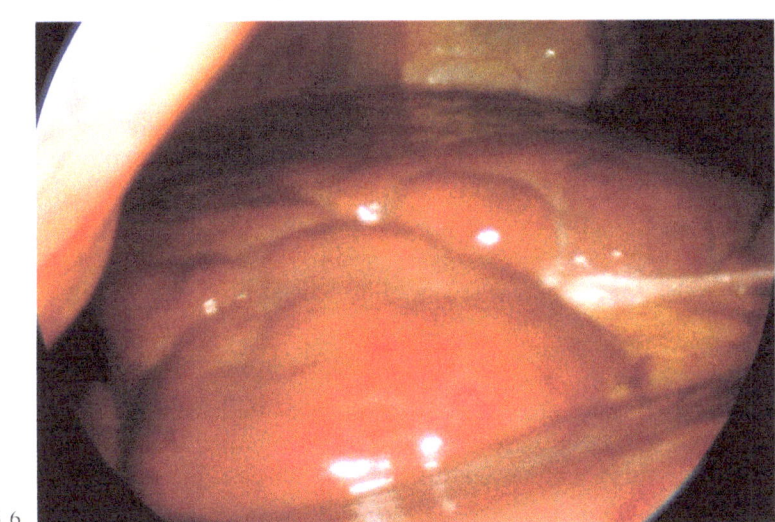

5.6

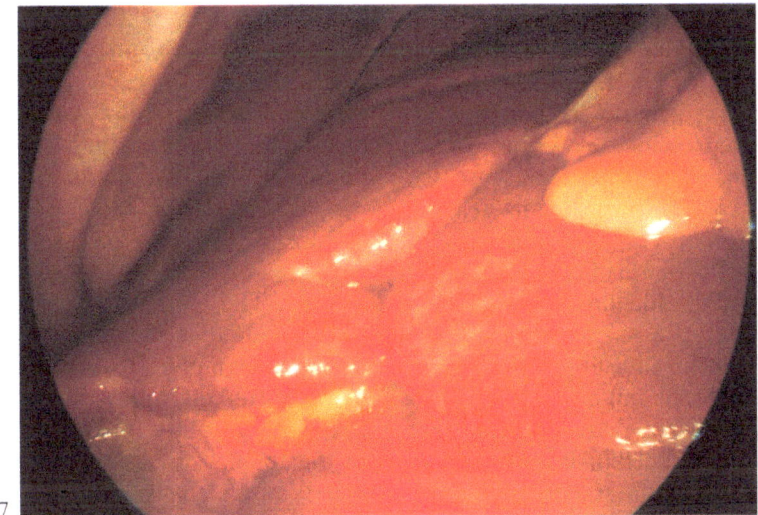

5.7

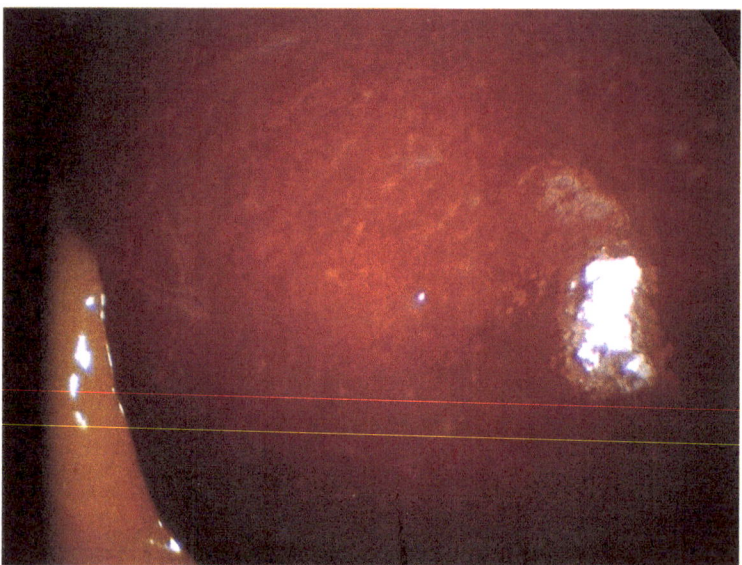

Fig. 5.8. Detail of the right lobe of the liver: the surface is smooth. Numerous small whitish areas with hazy borders can be seen. *Granulomatous hepatopathy*? Biopsy: *sarcoidosic hepatopathy*

laparoscopy is indicated when sonography indicates fibrosis. The examinations discussed here show how necessary it is to make an in-depth study of the diagnosis in cases of clinically diagnosed "persistent hepatitis." The principle remains that laparoscopy is useful in patients whose general picture is deteriorating and who have clinical and biochemical symptoms of persistent hepatitis with a prolonged course. This situation may be due above all to active hepatitis. The histological findings from a single-blind biopsy may be important, but it is not certain whether the sample itself represents the entire organ. Laparoscopy may not be decisive because frequently the macroscopic picture has no peculiar characteristics. But laparoscopy does allow us to take multiple biopsies, thus collecting plenty of tissue and increasing the likelihood of making a reliable diagnosis.

Furthermore, when the clinical picture is atypical, particularly when the initial acute hepatitis cannot be reliably detected, *chronic granulomatous hepatitis* may be suspected; it could be, for example, tubercular, brucellosic, or sarcoidosic.

Laparoscopy almost always enables us to make a diagnosis [14]. The macroscopic picture may suggest a general systemic granulomatous disease.

In most cases, the liver surface appears almost normal; it is smooth, and on it can be seen numerous small whitish points or granules (Fig. 5.8).

The liver may even appear normal. The bioptic results are decisive, above all if target biopsies are taken from the small lesions.

5.1.2.2 Chronic Active Hepatitis

According to the still valid document from Acapulco, chronic active hepatitis is a long-standing chronic disease of the liver that can develop into a more serious disease, such as cirrhosis; or it may persist without changing or disappear, either spontaneously or as a result of treatment.

The biochemical and clinical symptoms of chronic active hepatitis can vary greatly from case to case with respect to the quality and entity of the phenomena. This depends on the severity of the particular form and on the evolutive stage the disease has reached; the clues, however, allow the disease to be largely recognized and defined, but the final diagnosis is based on the histological picture. The sign of chronic active hepatitis in the long-standing forms is an inflammatory infiltration of lymphocytes, granulocytes, and histiocytes that involves the portal space. But in active hepatitis the infiltration extends beyond the space to the lobules, separating its cords. The hepatocytes, either singly or in groups, are then surrounded by infiltration cells and isolated from the rest of the parenchyma. In these areas can be found the so-called "piecemeal necrosis," which is typical of cellular necrosis. This histological sign is the precondition for the breakdown of the liver structure. The lesions can be divided into two categories on the basis of their features: the *moderately active* (type A) and *highly active* (type B) forms.

Imaging techniques provide inadequate information for the diagnosis of chronic active hepatitis. Sonography can provide exact information on the size of the liver, but this is not a particularly important datum. It may also detect a diffuse parenchymal abnormality with a sensitivity of up to 80%. All of these conditions can, however, have quite similar sonographic features with an overall increase in echogenicity, the so-called "bright" liver [11]. Furthermore, these signs are not specific and they appear at a relatively late stage. Echography in fact can give a pathological picture when the liver structure alterations give an intense and irregular parenchymal echogenicity, due to extensive areas of regeneration and an increase in fibrous tissue. This type of alteration is either absent or modest in chronic active hepatitis, so the ultrasound picture in such cases may appear normal or show only slight alterations [15], thus giving rise to a high number of false negatives. We must therefore stress the need for pathological data for a diagnosis to be made. The classical concepts have not changed: histology still allows a diagnosis of chronic hepatitis to be made, but with endoscopy extra, very important, information can be collected at the different pathological stages – and for this reason laparoscopy must always be performed. The great majority of those who, like us, have systematically compared echographic with laparobioptic results [13, 15, 16] still feel that it is inadvisable to rely only upon a histological examination, but prefer in all cases also to perform laparoscopy for a preliminary diagnosis.

Chronic active hepatitis causes macroscopically visible liver alterations, but this observation is not usually of diagnostic use. However, if pooled, the findings can be integrated with those from biopsy. Henning [8] recently stated that in his experience the "highest degree of reliability" is attained by combining a laparoscopic inspection with a histological evaluation through selective liver biopsy. He adds that, thanks to technological progress made, we can now see some surface details that were once impossible to observe, and this has improved the efficacy of endoscopic inspection. The macroscopic findings made later may then be a decisive contribution to a good diagnostic orientation. The liver surface may be quite bright red, and smooth; the lobular pattern may have disappeared (Fig. 5.9). In other cases there are also circumscribed, fairly deep, grooves, with no traces of scar tissue from loss of tissue due to recent cytolysis.

These findings must be confirmed histologically because they can also appear in persistent hepatitis: they are, however, very revealing. According to Mörl [3], in difficult cases the classification of hepatitis into persistent or aggressive is facilitated if one has a knowledge of the liver surface and the structure of the veins and lymphatics. Small lymphatic vessels indicate an increased lymph production, and this is a macroscopic sign of considerable diagnostic value. In chronic active hepatitis, the liver can also be paler because there is circumscribed dystrophy, flat scars, fibrotic processes, initial fibrosis, etc., and the color of the organ ranges from salmon pink to a pale muddy color that can give the liver a variegated appearance (Fig. 5.10). Here it is opportune to recall Kalk's classical description of a "large variegated liver."

Laparoscopy and biopsy are also the best available means for evaluating the activity of hepatitis. As is known, there are many discrepancies between the degree of enzyme increase and the histologically ascertainable inflammatory activity, but these discrepancies can be clarified after laparoscopy [12]. Here the macroscopic finding that most suggests an intense phlogistic activity appears to be red patches that are circumscribed but not sharply delimited or petechia-like hemorrhages. Under magnification these are identifiable, in part, as tufts of arterial vessels resembling spider nevi (Fig. 5.11).

The different ways in which chronic active hepatitis can present suggest that the likelihood of a reliable laparoscopic diagnosis is proportional to the number of findings made and their significance. But there is no doubt that if laparoscopy and biopsy are integrated they provide highly valuable information for, above all, the basic diagnosis.

Transcutaneous blind biopsy is useful, mainly for the follow-up. Now blind biopsy is being widely reintroduced. In fact recent improvements in our knowledge of chronic viral hepatitis have shown that in order to work out a therapy program and make a prognostic evaluation it is far more important to define the etiology and route of infection than the type and entity of the acute necrosis. It is therefore necessary to use histochemical

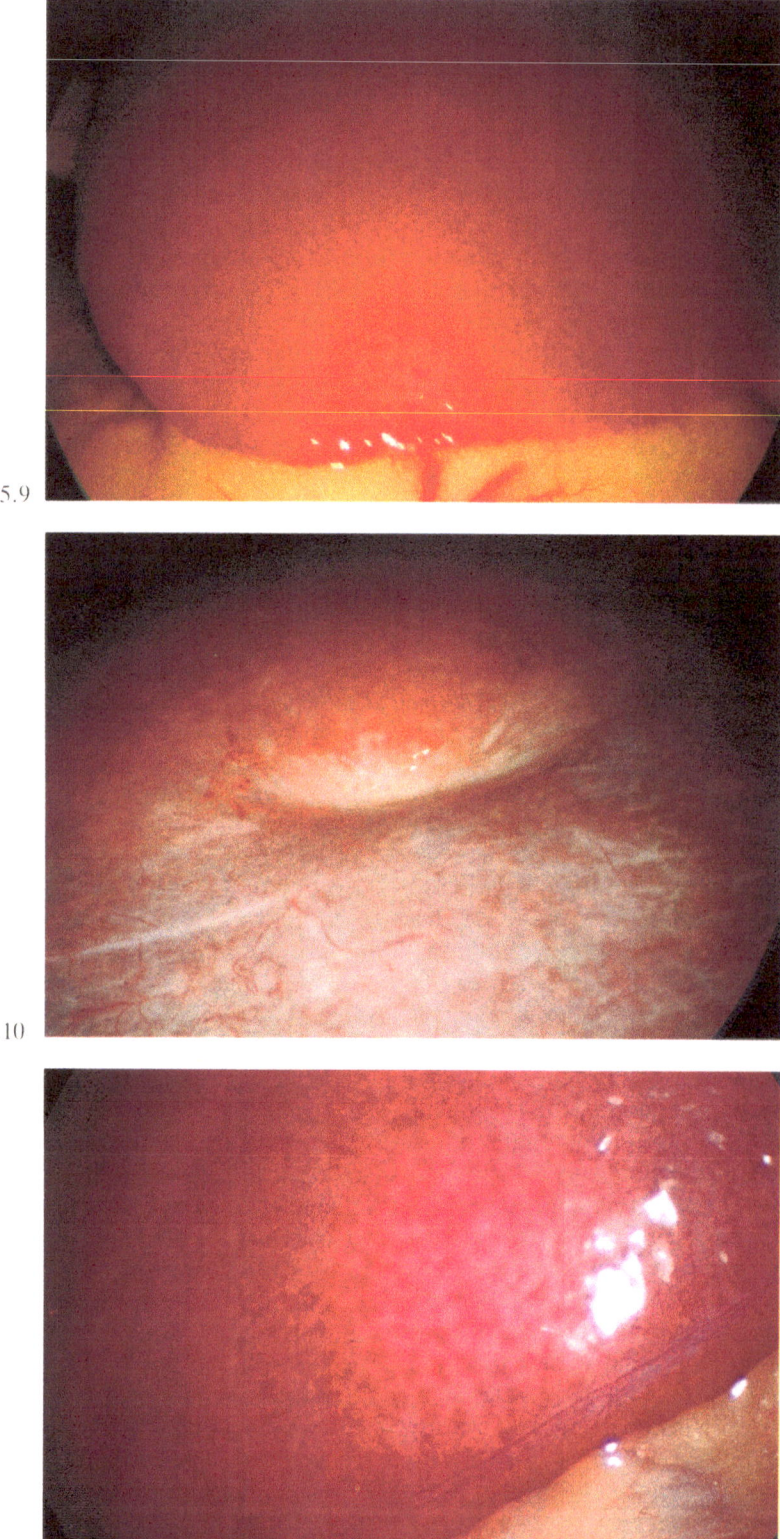

5.9

5.10

5.11

coloration techniques for viral liver antigens. For this type of investigation, transcutaneous puncture is the ideal method because it allows us to withdraw a large enough tissue sample (Verme G 1988, personal communication).

Finally, for the evolution of chronic hepatitis, which belongs to the vast and complex problem of the diagnosis of liver cirrhosis, see Sect. 5.2.

5.1.3 Conclusions

1. In alcoholic disease, sonography sufficiently clearly shows the presence of steatosis, which is the most characteristic lesion.

2. To distinguish between pure steatosis and alcoholic hepatitis, however, anatomical and histological clues are needed.

3. The macroscopic laparoscopic picture provides useful indications because for the degenerative and phlogistic forms there are fairly specific examples, but any diagnostic certainty depends on the biopsy.

4. In alcoholic liver disease blind biopsy may be enough for a diagnosis to be made. In some cases, however, laparoscopy is indicated and must be decided upon in each individual case.

5. Imaging techniques provide poor, and not very significant, findings for the diagnosis of hepatitis and also give rise to a high percentage of false negatives.

6. The distinctive feature enabling us to distinguish between the "persistent" and "aggressive" types of hepatitis is histological.

7. In patients with clinical and biohumoral pictures compatible with persistent hepatitis, echography can indicate those in which laparoscopy may be indicated.

8. Laparoscopy is always indicated in cases in which active chronic hepatitis may be suspected.

9. The macroscopic picture of active hepatitis can vary greatly and there are no absolutely specific findings. But a good diagnostic orientation can be made and these findings can be integrated with the histological study in order to make the most accurate possible diagnosis.

10. Blind biopsy is still useful, in particular for the follow-up, and in the near future it will probably be reintroduced on a large scale so that more histochemical investigations can be made.

5.2 Cirrhosis of the Liver

Liver cirrhosis is characterized by such evident and specific morphological changes that a quick and reliable diagnosis can be made through inspection alone. Therefore laparoscopy has long been considered the most suitable technique for diagnosing liver cirrhosis in living patients. When imaging techniques became available the situation did not change because, although echography can ascertain the presence of cirrhosis, it generally does so only when the disease is at a particularly advanced stage.

The ultrasound findings enabling a diagnosis of cirrhosis to be made, such as an increase in fine parenchymal echoes, "bright liver," nodular deformation of the margins and caudate lobe increase, depend upon echographic alterations that occur only when cirrhosis is severe. The most reliable findings for the diagnosis are signs of portal hypertension with collateral circulations consisting of large-caliber vessels. These findings are made when the disease is at an advanced stage. False negatives can also be made.

Echography is useful for screening but not for an accurate diagnosis. So laparoscopy is still the best available method for the study of cirrhosis, showing an enormous range of symptoms, which have already been exhaustively described elsewhere in great detail.

5.2.1 Main Laparoscopic Findings

The primary and specific laparoscopic finding in cirrhosis is the presence of "*regenerative nodules*"

Fig. 5.9. Surface of left lobe of the liver is red and its lobular pattern has disappeared. *Chronic hepatitis*? Biopsy: *chronic active hepatitis*

Fig. 5.10. Deep grooves from scars: the lower surface is not well visualized because of capsular thickening. *Chronic hepatitis*? Biopsy: *chronic active hepatitis*

Fig. 5.11. Margin of left lobe of the liver enlarged. Congested parenchyma with small bright red halos. *Probably chronic active hepatitis*. Confirmation with biopsy

on the liver surface. These may be *small*, ranging from the size of a grain of millet to a peppercorn. The *medium* nodules are pea-sized while the *large* ones range from the size of a walnut to that of a potato. The small and medium nodules are usually numerous, regular in shape, and surrounded by thin septa of light-gray fibrous tissue.

The shape and distribution of the larger nodules vary, making the liver surface very irregular. Although they can also be separated by thin and sometimes incomplete septa, more frequently they are isolated by wide, deep furrows of pale, retracted fibrous tissue. These areas of scarring are often deeply depressed, with a white background; they may be linear, simple or branched, polygonal or stellate. Postnecrotic scarring may be extensive and appears as vast, flat areas bordering a nodular zone.

Regenerative nodules may be markedly elevated [17] ("semispheral nodular type") or barely raised above the surface, although clearly evident.

Sometimes, however, the regenerative nodules are not very pronounced and therefore are barely perceptible to the laparoscopist. The diagnosis is tricky. If there are true nodules it is cirrhosis; otherwise it is only liver sclerosis, which can follow different diseases.

In these cases it is very useful to examine the organ surface with incident light. Nodules, even if not very elevated, reflect the light as numerous small luminous points. If, instead, the surface is rough but not nodular, the light is irregularly dispersed. In these circumstances a specific diagnosis can be made by obtaining a biopsy.

In some cases the liver surface is smooth at laparoscopy while the histological findings demonstrate cirrhosis. There are forms without nodules, i.e., the so-called smooth or glabrous cirrhoses. Although difficult to diagnose macroscopically, if the liver is carefully examined, sometimes slightly raised isolated nodules can be detected. If the liver surface is observed close-up by nearing the laparoscope, changes suggesting cirrhosis can be seen. The lobular pattern is not visible and in its place are small, flat, round redbrown areas that stand out against the pale background. Although they are not protuberant, they can still be regenerative nodules; we suggest calling them "flat cirrhotic lesions" (Fig. 5.12).

The shape of the liver is usually unaltered. The greatest changes in form can be observed in macronodular cirrhosis, in which one or both lobes can consist of a few regenerative nodules varying in size and shape, and that are separated by deep grooves or by extensive and retracted scar tissue. In these cases the liver appears grossly deformed, being referred to as Kalk's "potato liver". The *size* of a cirrhotic liver may be normal, increased, or decreased. Since laparoscopy enables us to ascertain the size of both lobes in relation to specific reference points and to the thickness of the lobes themselves, it gives us a fairly accurate idea of the exact liver volume.

An increase or reduction in the liver volume may be observed in both lobes. Sometimes, however, there is an asymmetrical volume increase, with one lobe enlarged or reduced while the other appears normal or, respectively, smaller or larger.

In cirrhosis the *consistency* of the liver is generally increased because of the presence of fibrous tissue. However, the consistency varies depending on the stage of the cirrhosis: in fully developed forms the liver is very hard. The firmer consistency is evident at simple inspection because the lobes no longer rest upon the underlying organs, but appear rigid and abnormally raised, so much so that often the posterior surface is visible.

This is particularly evident to the left, where the lobe, which is normally molded to the gastric surface, is almost suspended and barely touches the underlying stomach.

The increase in the consistency and hardness of the organ can be ascertained by direct palpation with the probe. The tissue firmness can also be judged by inserting the liver biopsy needle into the parenchyma and feeling any resistance.

A hard liver is therefore a typical feature of cirrhosis. Sometimes, however, even in the presence of a clear-cut surface nodulation, the changes in consistency may be slight. This finding is more likely to be obtained in the early stages of cirrhosis when the fibrosis is slight.

In cases of cirrhosis, an inspection of the anterior liver margins is of great importance. If these show changes, the changes occur, as mentioned above, in relation to the volume and consistency of the organ; but other types of change are also of importance.

The liver margin may be normal in cirrhosis: more often, however, it is fine and sharp, especially when the lobe is small and regularly shaped (Fig. 5.13). Sometimes it may be entirely bordered by a thin, continuous whitish shiny fibrous band. This feature is frequently observed, but it can also be found in chronic hepatitis. In other cases the liver margin may appear notched or scal-

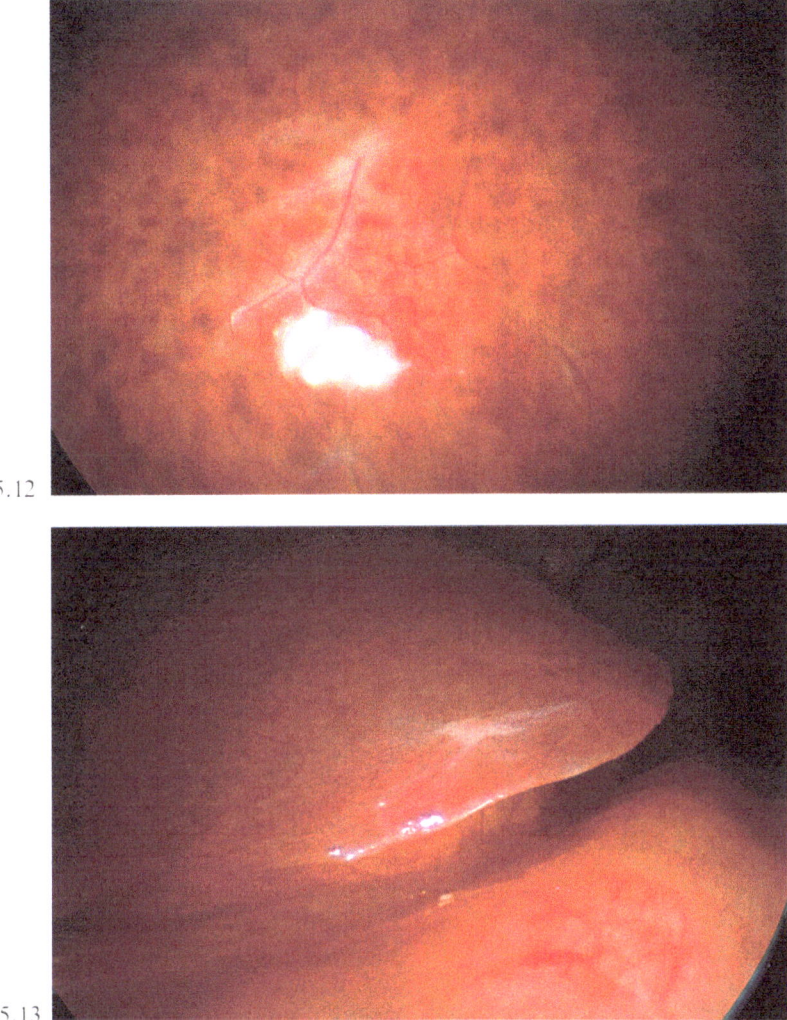

5.12

5.13

Fig. 5.12. *Histological cirrhosis* – smooth liver surface. Reddish brown patches against the yellowish parenchymal background. The macroscopic findings suggest a diagnosis of *non-cirrhotic alcoholic hepatopathy*. Biopsy: *cirrhosis of the liver*

Fig. 5.13. *Glabrous cirrhosis* – left lobe of the liver has nodule-free surface that is stiff, with clear margins, raised to the stomach, which is in the foreground. Biopsy: *cirrhosis of the liver*

loped, with indentations and protrusions of varying dimensions.

The liver margin may be thickened and rounded, as usually occurs when the entire lobe is enlarged. The outline of the edge may be regular or grossly irregular and can be bordered by the aforementioned fibrous bands.

It is important to study the liver surface. If the capsule is normal, and therefore completely transparent, all the features of the parenchyma can be observed. In cirrhosis the capsule is sometimes thickened and opaque because of previous inflammation. The thickening may be diffuse or circumscribed and varies in degree. Any examination of the parenchyma may therefore be hindered and sometimes the nodules are hidden.

Any color variations in cirrhosis are significant. These findings are discussed elsewhere. However, it is important to point out that the liver surface may be bright red, the intensity varying, the color being either diffuse or circumscribed. Close magnification reveals that the redness is due to an increased number of small capsular vessels of increased caliber as well as capsular capillaries that form a thick, hazy network. This is typical of "active" congestion. Analogous alterations can be observed in the small veins which, because of passive congestion, appear thickened and turgid, dark red, and well defined.

In cirrhosis the lymphatic vessels may also seem more numerous, enlarged and turgid, often branched, and translucent and shining. These changes may be isolated or associated with alterations in other small surface vessels and this may indicate either inflammation or stasis-congestion.

On the surface of a cirrhotic liver a quite frequent finding is small, whitish and glassy formations containing a liquid; similar to pinheads, they are often very numerous, being found mainly near the liver margins. These so-called *lymphatic microcysts* resemble miliary tuberculosis nodules and should therefore be carefully examined for differentiation. They are not found at autopsy and are therefore a laparoscopic finding only. They are a result of parenchyma induration blocking lymph drainage.

Lymphatic microcysts can be found in other forms of hepatosclerosis, although they do indicate cirrhosis and can therefore be used to confirm the diagnosis in uncertain cases.

5.2.2 Etiological Diagnosis

An etiological diagnosis of cirrhosis is made on the basis of a combination of epidemiological, clinical, and histological investigations [18]. Cirrhosis is the end stage of several different liver diseases, and, at this stage, more alterations lose any specific features that might have once made them recognizable. Furthermore, the morphological picture can also be greatly modified by diverse associated or superimposed cirrhogenic factors, as is frequently the case in, for example, alcoholic and viral hepatitis. The macroscopic findings can therefore pose problems, but certain laparoscopic findings may suggest an etiology. As a reference point we use the list of possible etiological factors in cirrhosis proposed by Anthony [18]. (Table 5.1).

Group A comprises established associations between etiological factors and cirrhosis; we consider here in particular the laparoscopic findings that concern: (a) *viral hepatitis*, (b) *alcoholism*, (c) *metabolic disorders*, and (d) *biliary diseases*.

Venous outflow obstruction (veno-occlusive disease, Budd-Chiari syndrome) and severe prolonged cardiac stasis result in progressive liver

Table 5.1. Etiological factors in cirrhosis (from [18])

A. Cirrhosis with established etiological associations:
   1. Viral hepatitis
   2. Alcoholism
   3. Metabolic disorders (e.g., hemochromatosis, Wilson's disease, α_1-antitrypsin deficiency, type IV glycogenosis, galactosemia)
   4. Biliary disease (intrahepatic and extrahepatic)
   5. Venous outflow obstruction (venoocclusive disease, Budd-Chiari syndrome)
   6. Toxins and therapeutic drugs (e.g., certain pyrrolizidine alkaloids with allyl side chains, methotrexate, oxyphenisatin, α-methyldopa)
   7. Intestinal bypass operations for obesity
   8. Other (e.g., sarcoidoses)
B. Debatable etiological factors:
   1. Autoimmunity
   2. Mycotoxins
   3. Schistosomiasis
   4. Malnutrition
   5. Others
C. Cirrhosis of unknown etiology:
   1. With well-defined pattern – Indian childhood cirrhosis
   2. Without well-defined pattern – "cryptogenic" cirrhosis

alterations, so-called cardiac cirrhosis. This form, however, also in my experience, does not have the features of true cirrhosis, but rather those of hepatic fibrosis. The liver is enlarged, the capsule thickened, and the surface wine red and irregular, but it lacks true regenerative nodules. In our opinion venous stasis alone does not cause cirrhosis; it must be associated with other factors to do so.

No link between cirrhosis, toxins, and therapeutic drugs has been demonstrated. We followed up many patients who had different forms of polychemotherapy for malignant tumors and, months or years after treatment, observed degenerative liver diseases and liver sclerosis, which was often severe, with extensive scarring and marked parenchymal atrophy. We never, however, identified regenerative nodules in these patients and therefore never found cirrhosis.

We have had no experience of laparoscopy in patients who have undergone intestinal bypass surgery for obesity. Lastly, in granulomatous sarcoidosic hepatitis, we have sometimes found that the liver is hard and its surface grossly altered by numerous deep scars. This picture, however, differs greatly from that of true cirrhosis which, in our experience and in that of others [19], does not

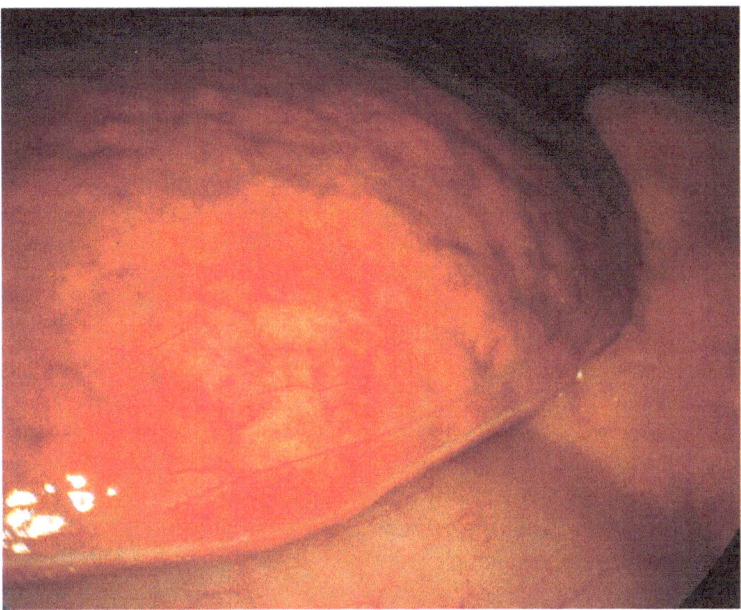

Fig. 5.14. *Fatty cirrhosis* – left lobe of the liver, yellowish thickening with medium nodules. Margin bordered by thin fibrous band. Biopsy: *fatty cirrhosis*

occur in sarcoidosis. In these forms signs of portal hypertension can also be found [20].

Group B comprises the questionable etiological factors. Malnutrition has been recognized as a cause of cirrhosis ("cirrhosis from inadequate nutrition"). Some aspects of these conditions may be associated with alcoholism.

Cirrhosis of unknown etiology, very frequent in our experience, cannot present characteristic laparoscopic findings.

Alcoholic cirrhosis usually presents in a micronodular form. Steatosis, usually present in alcoholic cirrhosis, gives the liver a yellow tone. Alcoholic cirrhosis is referred to as "micronodular," "septal," or "fatty," although the latter term is inappropriate because fatty accumulation is not always extensive. The distinctive feature of true *fatty cirrhosis* is enlargement of the liver, which appears hard, with small regular nodules. It is overtly yellow, often with pink or bright yellow-orange spots and variegations due to a combination of yellow nodules and the cinnabar-red background produced by inflammatory necrosis. Fatty cirrhosis is the most indicative finding for the diagnosis of alcoholic cirrhosis (Fig. 5.14).

A laparoscopic finding of cirrhosis without nodules can also be very important. These smooth or glabrous forms (see Fig. 5.12), which often have an important component of steatosis, are almost always the result of alcoholism, so in these cases an alcoholic etiology is highly probable.

Another feature that can suggest that alcoholism is the cause is increased iron accumulation, shown by a rust-brown hue. It is, however, important to distinguish between true cirrhosis with a *secondary hemosiderin accumulation* and *primary hemochromatosis*, which has different characteristics and, of course, a different significance.

Cirrhosis due to hepatitis is usually macronodular and easily recognized by direct observation. Large or enormous nodules and extensive scar tissue indicate that a massive hepatitis with extensive necrosis has evolved into cirrhosis. It is important to bear in mind that in pure forms of viral postnecrotic cirrhosis steatosis is absent.

The above-mentioned findings can be considered "theoretical." We cannot, however, state, as others have, that the form with "small and medium" or "septal" nodules is synonymous with nutritional alcoholic cirrhosis, while the "macronodular" form is the consequence of viral hepatitis. This is not necessarily true. Micronodular cirrhosis sometimes has a viral cause, whereas macronodular forms are sometimes due to alcoholism.

It is even more difficult to make an etiological diagnosis in cirrhosis with small and medium nodules surrounded by narrow septa and associated with large, irregular and retracted scars and large nodules that are clearly postnecrotic.

The systematic use of laparoscopy allows us to document numerous transitional stages of cirrhosis, which is the result of repeated extensive parenchymal necrosis against a background of micronodular cirrhosis due to recurrent alcoholic damage or episodes of hepatitis resulting in extensive scarring. These findings of "mixed" cirrhosis preclude any conclusions concerning the original cause. With laparoscopy it is possible reliably to diagnose forms of cirrhosis with specific macroscopic features.

Above all, *hemochromatosis* and *Wilson's disease cirrhosis* can be identified, although other varieties in this category do not have distinguishing macroscopic features. One form, which can develop into "porphyria cutanea tarda" is distinctive; it does not appear in Anthony's list.

Alcoholic cirrhosis may be accompanied by hemosiderin deposition in the liver cells. This presents as a classic cirrhosis, i.e., an atrophic or mildly hypertrophic liver which usually is the characteristic brown-rust color, with small and medium nodules. The color may vary toward yellow, red, or gray depending on the amount of iron and associated phenomena, such as steatosis, inflammation, and connective tissue proliferation.

A primary disorder in iron metabolism causes a liver disease with quite different features: always gross hepatomegaly with a markedly increased organ thickness. The surface is uniformly granular or rough, with fine nodules. It is brown with rust overtones. Sometimes a grayish connective tissue network can be seen without retraction being present.

Another differential finding revealed only laparoscopically is portal hypertension. In secondary iron deposition the disease is a true cirrhosis, and therefore often collateral circulations from portal hypertensions can be detected in the different sites. In primary hemochromatosis portal hypertension is found only in exceptional cases, even in the more severe or late stages.

Cirrhosis from *Wilson's* disease usually shows evident lesions that are easily recognized by laparoscopy, even in the initial stages [21]. However, as the disease evolves over a long period, the findings change. At first the liver is enlarged, its surface smooth and reddish with numerous spots with diameters ranging from 5 to 10 mm; they are dark bluish and flat or slightly raised (Fig. 5.15). In the later stages the spots become nodular, maintaining their dark coloration at their apices. The connective tissue component of the disease is not well developed, being shown by the brown-red color of the liver and an only slightly increased parenchymal consistency (Fig. 5.16).

In *late porphyria cutanea*, chronic hepatopathy is almost always observed. In about 30% of cases there is a laparoscopically diagnosable true cirrhosis. The appearance suggests micronodular cirrhosis that is distinguished by the gray-blue color of the nodules, particularly evident on their central, raised areas. Macroscopically they resemble cirrhosis from Wilson's disease. The differential diagnosis, however, is easy to make because, in porphyria, the liver tissue has a red fluorescence under ultraviolet light. This is shown by utilizing Wood's lamp on a biopsy tissue sample.

Biliary cirrhosis can have macroscopic features that allow the etiological diagnosis to be made. The main finding for cholestasis is the coloration, which ranges from gray to dark green, depending on the degree of stasis.

When this picture is observed, the following should be considered: (a) common cirrhosis in which the cholestasis is not the cause but occurs secondary to associated disease such as acute viral or alcoholic hepatitis, liver failure, or mechanical obstruction; (b) secondary biliary or pure cholestatic cirrhosis due, for example, to prolonged extrahepatic obstruction from calculi or biliary stricture; (c) cholangitic cirrhosis consequent to a chronic inflammatory process of the intrahepatic biliary tree; and/or (d) primary biliary cirrhosis.

In some cases laparoscopy provides useful, sometimes decisive diagnostic information, while in others it is not particularly advantageous or beneficial. *Common cirrhosis* with superimposed *cholestasis* can be diagnosed when the features typical of cirrhosis are present and the nodules are "tattooed" with green. However, if the cholestasis is obstructive it now can be demonstrated sonographically.

In *cholangitic biliary cirrhosis* the color of the liver varies, ranging from brown to green, but it often has a gray hue because of capsular thickening in wide bands or deep, retracted, and congested strips, sometimes with associated adhesions. These alterations are important for the diagnosis because they are the result of repeated and protracted inflammation of the superficial biliary canaliculi and the surrounding liver tissue with scar repair of the necrotic areas. Also of great importance are any alterations of the gallbladder

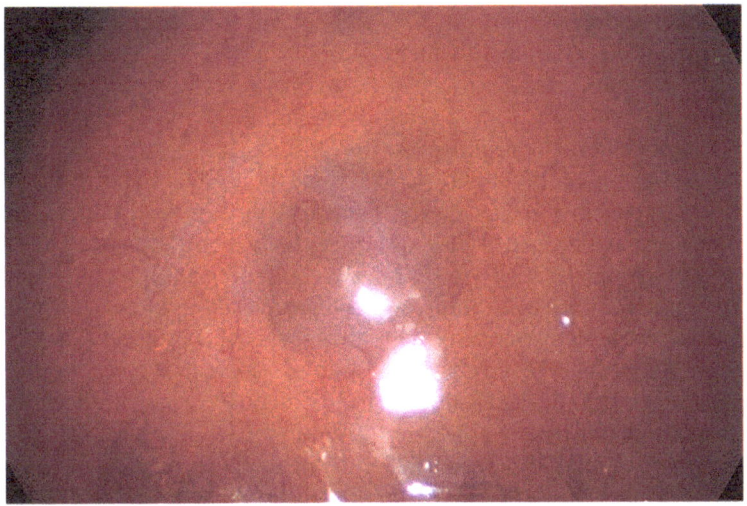

5.15

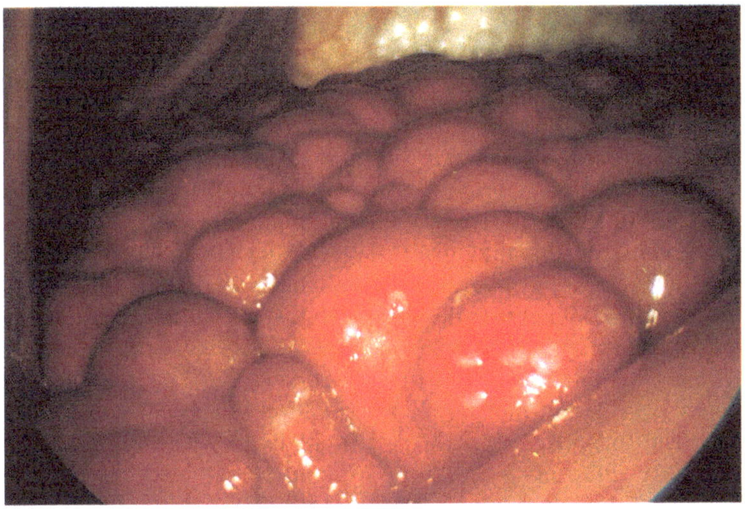

5.16

Fig. 5.15. *Wilson's disease* – initial stages. Detail of a slightly raised nodule

Fig. 5.16. *Wilson's disease* – advanced stage. Large spherical nodules give the liver surface a cobblestone appearance

– these demonstrate chronic inflammation, retraction, wall thickening, congestion and adhesions between the gallbladder and neighboring structures.

In *primary biliary cirrhosis* the appearance of the liver varies depending on the stage of the disease, although it has no specific signs that permit a laparoscopic diagnosis. The liver may be enlarged and hard with alterations suggesting congestive modifications: the surface may be slightly altered or have barely visible, or obvious, nodules. There may also be biliary tattooing. Recently significance was attributed to a finding of "*gentle undulation*" in the liver surface; this is the result of scarring and of chronic destructive nonsuppurative cholangitis of the portal space. This was observed laparoscopically in 11/13 cases of primary biliary cirrhosis [22].

5.2.3 Liver Biopsy

The histological confirmation of alterations in the hepatic architecture characterized by parenchymal destruction, fibrosis, and regenerative nodules is in theory the basis for the morphological diagnosis of cirrhosis, and it is therefore superfluous to stress the importance of biopsy.

A clear distinction, however, is important between the results of transcutaneous biopsy, which is more widely used, and those of laparoscopic biopsy.

In 1973 Lindner [7] stated that "percutaneous biopsy alone carries an unacceptably high risk of diagnostic error." This conclusion was based on his own considerable experience, a review of the literature, and a questionnaire sent in 1971 to German-speaking hepatologists. In a total of 33 372 blind biopsies an incomplete or mistaken diagnosis was made in 15%–50% of cases, depending on the cirrhosis; the highest error rate occurred in the macronodular forms.

There are explanations for the discrepancies between the results of percutaneous and those of laparoscopic biopsies. First, the sample obtained with blind biopsy is often too small and fragmented to enable a reliable study of its architecture to be carried out [23, 24]. Second, the sample may be taken from an area that is not involved, or from a regenerative nodule, so the sample appears to be normal (false negative). Otherwise, an area of trivial capsular fibrosis, the result of an irrelevant local process, may be taken, and this may give a false impression of cirrhosis (false positive).

It has also been observed that Menghini's needle tends preferentially to aspirate soft liver parenchyma, leaving the tougher connective tissue behind, and this problem is greater when nodules are large. The histological diagnosis of cirrhosis based on blind percutaneous biopsies is therefore not reliable enough. This has long been admitted, even by those who do not normally perform laparoscopy, i.e., the British. An editorial of 1971, entitled "Clarity and Confusion in Active Chronic Hepatitis," stated: "Cirrhosis is frequently already present at the time when active chronic hepatitis is diagnosed" [25]. In spite of this, several schools still use blind liver biopsy as the only basis for the morphological diagnosis of cirrhosis.

In view of the problems regarding biopsy in general (see Sect. 3.4.2), a more reliable histological investigation for the diagnosis of cirrhosis is required. So the biopsy simply must be taken under laparoscopic guidance. Laparoscopic biopsy in cirrhosis enables us to: (a) make, confirm, or clarify a diagnosis; (b) assess the disease activity; and (c) propose an etiological diagnosis.

To understand the meaning and value of biopsy in the diagnosis of cirrhosis, a comparison should always be made between the macroscopic findings. Errors can be made and/or the diagnosis based on the macroscopic finding may be uncertain. This is the case when it is difficult to establish whether the liver surface is scabrous or nodular, even more so when nodules are scarce or absent.

On the other hand, the pathologist may be faced with dubious pictures, and his or her diagnosis may contradict the macroscopic diagnosis. By combining the results of macroscopic and histological examinations, the most reliable possible diagnosis can be made [26, 27]. The macroscopic and histological findings must be complementary; agreement between the two parameters has been found in a range of 49%–89%. The discrepancies are probably linked to subjective judgment [28], which will never be overcome, but also to the precision of diagnostic criteria now used, in both histology and laparoscopy; they also depend on the degree of morphological evidence provided by the evolving cirrhosis. Ideally there should be agreement between the macroscopic and histological pictures: in such cases, the diagnosis is definite. But when the macroscopic and histological findings are not in agreement, we must decide which findings should be considered more reliable and this is a difficult task because the criteria change, depending on each particular case.

In our experience [29, 30], different types of situation emerge when laparoscopy is performed in patients with chronic liver disease in an attempt to establish whether cirrhosis is present (Fig. 5.17).

1. Cases with diffuse, evident nodulation on the surface of the liver: here the laparoscopist makes a diagnosis of cirrhosis, and the biopsy reveals at least one regenerative nodule surrounded by fibrous tissue and in about 80% confirms the diagnosis of cirrhosis. There is therefore agreement between the findings.

2. Cases with evident nodulation that is limited to one lobe or just a part of it: the histological examination, on tissue from this area, even in these cases demonstrates cirrhosis in over 80%.

3. The surface of the liver is smooth, regular, or with slight localized irregularities (scarring, roughness) or signs of steatosis for which a macroscopic diagnosis of cirrhosis cannot be made: histological examination demonstrates that cirrhosis is absent in 62%, gives an uncertain judgment (altered structure without evidence of nodules") in 27%, and indicates cirrhosis in the remaining 11%.

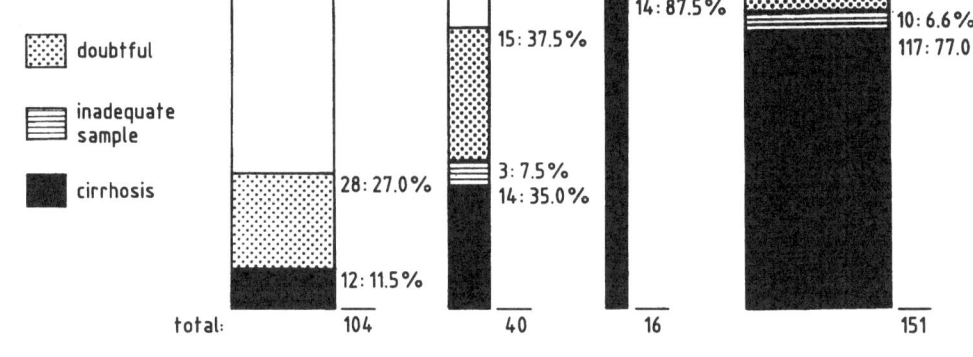

Fig. 5.17A–D. Comparison between laparoscopic and histological features in 311 cases. **A** No laparoscopic evidence of cirrhosis; **B** laparoscopic findings reveal "doubtful" or "uncertain" cirrhosis; **C** cirrhosis in a limited area of the liver; **D** generalized "diffuse cirrhosis"

4. When the liver surface is diffusely irregular (grooved, undulating, rough) or when nodules are not clearly evident, the laparoscopic diagnosis of liver sclerosis is "doubtful" or "uncertain." Biopsy is consistent with the doubtful findings in 45% of cases, demonstrates cirrhosis in 35%, and provides no evidence of cirrhosis in the remaining 20%.

In conclusion, the importance of the histological examination must be considered with respect to the general principle that when findings are contradictory the positive result (cirrhosis) should always be considered and the negative finding (no cirrhosis) ignored.

In my opinion therefore the importance of biopsy is inversely proportional to the significance of laparoscopic findings and vice versa. In fact the concordance between the laparoscopic and bioptic findings in cases in which the nodules are evident at laparoscopy practically negates the value of the histological examination [17, 30, 31]. If the biopsy result is negative, then one should consider a false negative. Therefore, when the macroscopic diagnosis of cirrhosis is certain biopsy may be superfluous, and if the coagulation parameters are markedly abnormal, biopsy should be avoided.

Conversely, the histological examination must be considered decisive when it demonstrates cir-

rhosis in a liver that laparoscopically appears to have no cirrhosis, with a smooth surface or with indefinite nodules. In the latter case multiple biopsies must always be taken from different points of the organ.

The activity of cirrhosis can be histologically ascertained by the extent and severity of necrosis and the consequent inflammatory reaction (round cell infiltration of the portal spaces, areas of fibrosis, etc.).

The histological signs of activity are certainly interesting but they do not have an absolute value. Often this does not correspond to the clinical and laboratory evaluation of disease activity. This is explained by the fact that the disease activity can vary from area to area and one small tissue sample is not necessarily representative.

Moreover, biopsy can reveal alterations due to secondary phenomena that appear in the course of cirrhosis such as infection, ischemic necrosis, and biliary obstruction. The histological study is important for the confirmation of some laparoscopic findings that suggest an *etiological diagnosis.* It may specify the type of lesion and show its nature, severity, and/or extent. It can add new information to that obtained laparoscopically, thus facilitating or clarifying the diagnosis, and also allowing an otherwise impossible etiological diagnosis to be made.

Supporting evidence for a laparoscopic diagnosis of alcoholic cirrhosis includes the micronodular pattern, steatosis, and any siderosis. More valuable than the histological picture in the diagnosis of alcoholic liver disease are features of alcoholic hepatitis, including hapatocyte swelling, focal neutrophil infiltration, and Mallory's hyalin bodies, although the latter are not always present in, nor are they specific for, an alcohol-induced disease.

The diagnosis of posthepatitic cirrhosis can be facilitated by the demonstration of hepatitis B surface antigen, by means of immunoperoxidases, although it is not invariably present. Other significant findings are ground-glass hepatocytes and intense inflammatory activity.

The laparoscopic features indicating a diagnosis of *primary hemochromatosis* are confirmed by the histological findings, with an increase in portal fibrosis and the formation of septa with hemosiderin in the hepatocytes and phagocytes. The parenchyma is almost unaltered and there is little inflammatory activity.

The characteristic histological feature of *Wilson's disease* is the demonstration of copper accumulation in the nodules.

Primary biliary cirrhosis has no specific laparoscopic findings and so its diagnosis depends on biopsy. The lesions, which vary during the course of the disease, affect the portal spaces. The bile ducts are hyperplastic or necrotic and are surrounded by a dense infiltration of lymphocytes, plasma cells, eosinophils, and granuloma-type epithelioid cells. Later, in the frankly cirrhotic stage, the space is replaced by connective tissue, the bile ducts disappear, and new perilobular ducts (Hering's ducts) are formed.

The histological picture is almost pathognomonic, but difficult to recognize with one fine-needle biopsy. Although laparoscopy is not particularly useful for the macroscopic diagnosis, it is still very important because it allows multiple biopsies to be taken and therefore increases the likelihood of the lesions being detected.

Histological findings do not add information to the diagnosis of *secondary biliary cirrhosis*.

5.2.4 Laparoscopic Classification

The different forms of cirrhosis have often been classified on the basis of their pathogenesis, morphology, and eponyms [31]. We propose here [37] a classification based on laparoscopic findings, a system similar to that used for a postmortem classification (Table 5.2). Laparoscopy, of course, can be performed repeatedly in live subjects and can therefore be used to follow the disease, from its earliest stages to the death of the patient. A

Table 5.2. Laparoscopic classification of liver cirrhosis (from [37])

Based on nodularity
  Size of the nodules
    Micro- and medionodular cirrhosis
    Macronodular cirrhosis
    Mixed cirrhosis
  Extent of nodule formation
    Diffuse nodulation
    Limited nodulation
  No evidence of nodules
    With other laparoscopic signs of cirrhosis:
      "Glabrous" cirrhosis
    Without other laparoscopic signs of cirrhosis:
      "Histological" cirrhosis
Based on liver size
  Hypertrophic cirrhosis
  Atrophic cirrhosis
  Atrophic-hypertrophic cirrhosis
Based on possible etiology
  Alcoholic cirrhosis
  Post-hepatitic cirrhosis
  Metabolic disorders
    Hemochromatosis
      Primary
      Secondary
    Wilson's disease
    Porphyria cutanea tarda
  Biliary disease
    Primary biliary cirrhosis
    Secondary biliary cirrhosis
      Cholestatic
      Cholangitic

cirrhotic liver undergoes many progressive morphological alterations, its shape, size, and characteristics changing radically with time. The morphological categories of cirrhosis do not represent specific diseases, but different stages and forms of a single process.

Laparoscopically, cirrhoses can be classified on the basis of: *nodulation, liver size,* and *etiology.*

The following classification for nodulation, which considers *nodule dimensions, nodule extent,* and *absence of nodules,* is based on the *dimensions of the nodules,* and is now almost universally accepted: (a) *micronodular,* when nodules have a diameter of less than 3 mm – this term has replaced all the synonyms, such as septal, portal, mononodular, and Laennec's; (b) *macronodular,* when the diameter is more than 3 mm, when nodules are irregular, with septa and large connectival areas – this term has replaced synonyms such as postnecrotic and irregular; and (c) nodules with a diameter of 3–6 mm may also be considered medium type.

Except for nodule diameter, the overall picture is similar to that of the micronodular forms. The term "mixed cirrhosis" applies to forms which have both small and large nodules in almost the same proportions. In mixed cirrhosis, as well as there being small and large nodules, there is also extensive deep scarring, a clear sign of prior massive necrosis.

An interesting attempt was made to relate the three different types of cirrhosis to the prognosis: 70% of patients with the micronodular form were alive after 5 years, 14% with the macronodular form and 42% with the mixed form. No patient with macronodular cirrhosis was alive 10 years after diagnosis [32]. The laparoscopic findings are therefore significant because, except for macronodular cirrhosis, these forms cannot be detected with needle biopsy alone. This classification requires a complete picture of the liver; it is based on information that, unless surgery is performed, can only be obtained with laparoscopy.

In theory there should be no argument as to whether the nodules have extended to the entire liver or only a part of it because cirrhosis by definition involves the entire organ. Anthony et al. [18] state that "focal lesions, e.g., focal nodular hyperplasia, do not constitute cirrhosis." However, they add that "the cirrhosis nodules do not develop simultaneously in all parts of the liver and the precise time of onset cannot be determined. The borderline between precirrhotic lesions and cirrhosis is not always sharp and is particularly difficult to establish in biopsy material." According to Scheuer [33], "An impression may be gained that cirrhosis is at an early stage of development on the one hand, or fully developed on the other."

These considerations appear logical without the help of laparoscopic findings and only with blind biopsy. In about 10% of all cases of cirrhosis, in our experience, the laparoscopic findings for the two lobes are quite different. For example, on the right the appearance may suggest simple chronic hepatitis (Fig. 5.18), while on the left there may be a clearly cirrhotic type of nodulation (Fig. 5.19). Biopsy findings also differ greatly, depending on the area from which the sample is taken, indicating chronic, or doubtful, hepatitis in the "smooth" areas and definite cirrhosis in the nodular zones. In one of our series, in over 87% of cases there was agreement between the laparoscopic and the histological diagnosis of cirrhosis [30].

These findings suggest the existence of another form of cirrhosis, which could be called "*limited nodulation*" in addition to the more common and classic "*diffuse form*" of nodulation. The former may represent one stage in the evolution of the disease [34]. These "incomplete" cirrhoses might correspond to an early stage of the disease and may therefore be valuable in indicating the prognosis.

The histological examination can demonstrate cirrhosis in a *smooth liver that appears to have no nodules*, and, according to the literature, this is found in percentages ranging from 0.5% to 10%. We are of the opinion, however, that when considering the forms without nodules, a distinction can be made between the following types.

1. Cases in which the nodules are not visualized or are occasional and hazy, but in which several other cirrhotic findings are present, such as parenchymal induration, thinning of margin, reduction in volume, lymphatic microcysts, and ascites. Here the expert laparoscopist can make the diagnosis: this is the so-called *glabrous cirrhosis* (see Fig. 5.13).
2. Cases in which the liver surface is smooth, sometimes even shiny, the only finding being flat parenchymal spots – frequently with steatosis (Figs. 5.12, 5.20). This picture is quite different from that of liver steatosis (Figs. 5.1, 5.2).

On other occasions, cirrhoses without nodules may have the "variegated" aspect that suggests chronic active hepatitis. Biopsy, however, demonstrates cirrhosis (Fig. 5.21). There are no other macroscopic signs except for liver enlargement and an increased consistency of the liver, findings that do not allow a diagnosis of cirrhosis to be made.

As biopsy provides the only data demonstrating cirrhosis, we suggested that these cases be named "*histological cirrhosis*" [29, 30]. We have observed 39 such cases in the past 3 years; they account for 10% of all the cirrhoses found in our center from 1985 to 1987. Their etiology, as indicated by the presence of steatosis, is often alcoholism.

By ascertaining *liver size* a distinction can be made between a *hypertrophic*, *atrophic*, and *normotrophic* liver. Some are of the opinion that the distinction between "atrophic" and "hypertrophic" is not of particular value, and that the atrophic form should be considered a particular type of evolution of the usual cirrhosis and so no classification based upon the volume of the organ can be of value. It is, however, important to as-

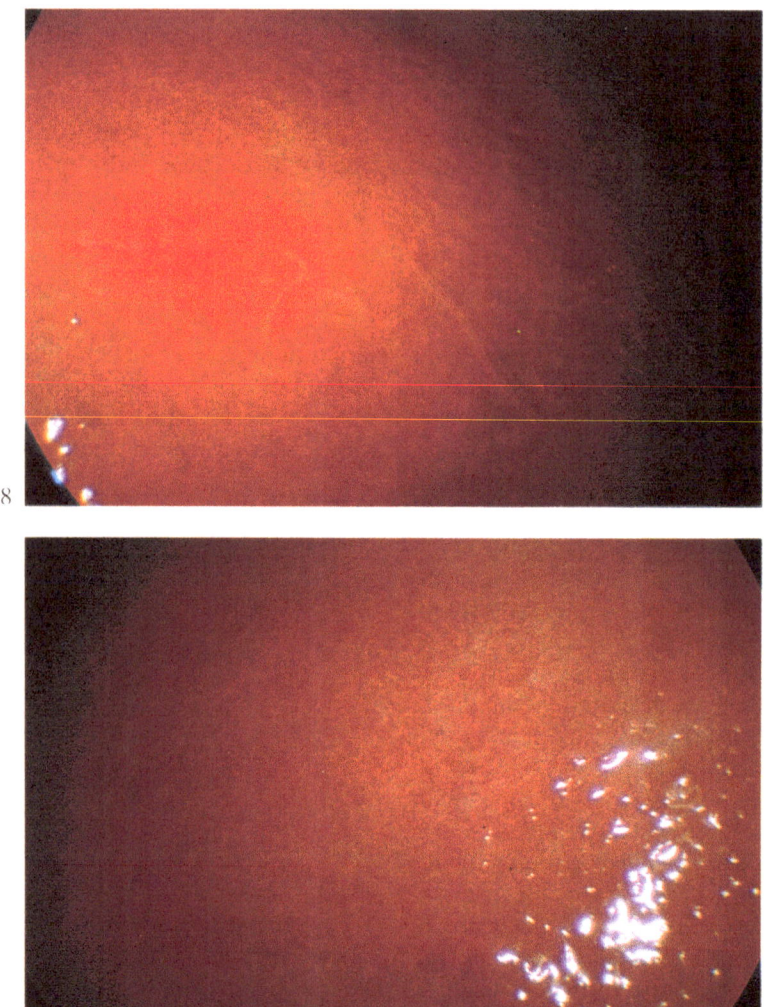

5.18

5.19

Fig. 5.18. *Limited cirrhosis* – Surface of the liver under high magnification: lobular pattern unrecognizable, slight dilation of the small lymphatic vessels. No nodules can be seen. Laparoscopic finding compatible with *chronic hepatitis*

Fig. 5.19. *Limited cirrhosis*. Same case as in Fig. 5.18. In another area of the organ can be seen numerous small nodules of the cirrhotic type. Biopsy: *micronodular cirrhosis*

certain the amount of parenchyma present and its functioning in order to gain an idea of the severity of cirrhosis.

The French School has always believed that it is of value to make a quantitative appraisal of the apparently functional liver parenchyma so as to establish the prognosis. Of course the quantity of liver tissue present is mainly proportional to the liver volume: it is important accurately to establish whether the particular form is hypertrophic or atrophic.

Apart from the overall atrophic or hypertrophic form, in some forms of cirrhosis one lobe is atrophic while the other is normal or hypertrophic; these are referred to as "atrophic-hypertrophic" (of the "right" or "left lobe" type).

There is a correlation between the volume of the cirrhotic liver and the prognosis. The usefulness of this classification should be borne out by the observation that 5 years after diagnosis 71% of the patients with a *hypertrophic* right lobe had survived while only 30% of those with an *atrophic*

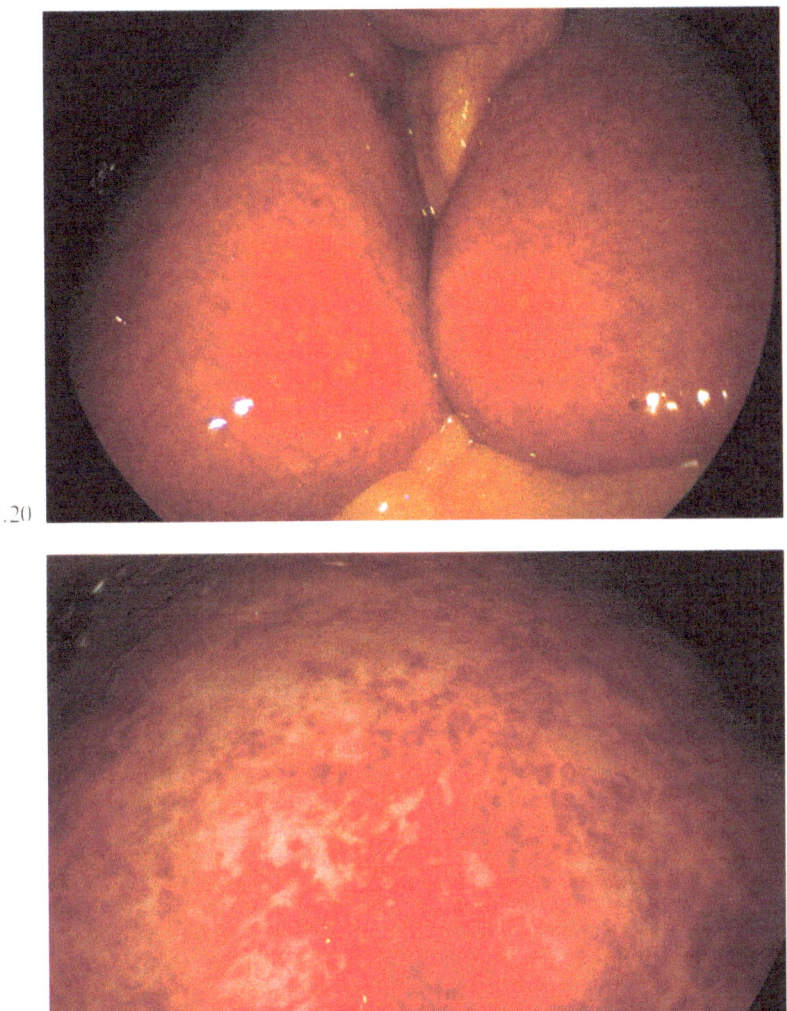

5.20

5.21

Fig. 5.20. *Histological cirrhosis.* Marked enlargement. Smooth surface with yellowish-brown background and reddish-brown spots (flat cirrhotic lesions). The macroscopic picture is compatible with a diagnosis of *alcoholic liver disease.* Biopsy: *cirrhosis of the liver*

Fig. 5.21. Histological cirrhosis. Detail of the liver surface: variegated liver. Chronic hepatitis? Biopsy: *cirrhosis of the liver*

right lobe were still alive; after 10 years, the figures are 53% and 12%, respectively [32].

Finally, if laparoscopic findings are integrated with those from biopsy, a "laparoscopic" classification based on the *etiology* can be made.

5.2.5 Cirrhosis and Liver Tumors

The use of laparoscopy in the diagnosis of liver tumors is discussed elsewhere. However, because of the relationship between malignant neoplasms and liver cirrhosis, it is opportune to mention them here. Frequently there is an association between cirrhosis and primary liver carcinoma, and this has been demonstrated both clinically and autopsically, the finding being made more and more often. Primary liver carcinoma has been found in 1%–1.6% of all laparoscopies, and in 66%–95% of cases it is associated with cirrhosis. More recently the association has been found in 76.1% [35]–81.7% of cases [36, 37] in Italy, 88% of cases in France [38], 46% [39]–63% of cases

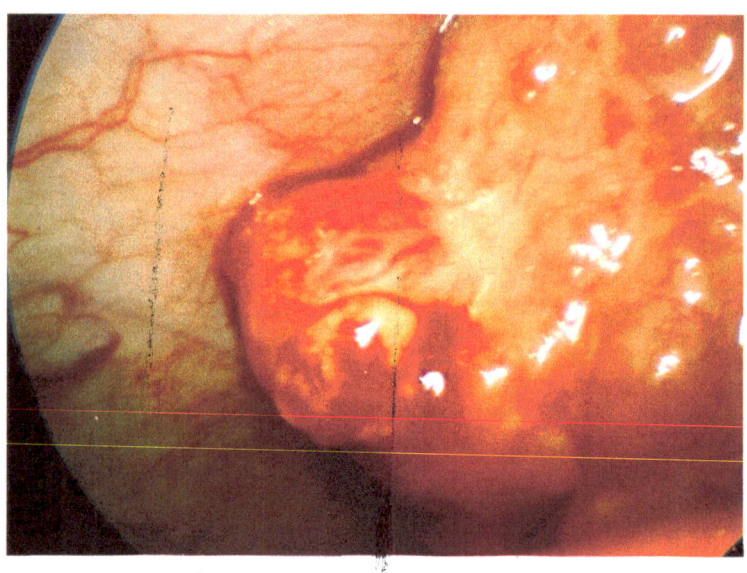

Fig. 5.22. *Nodular liver carcinoma overlying cirrhosis.* Small nodule, most of which is covered by liver tissue, protrudes at the lateral extremity of the right lobe, reaching the abdominal wall. Biopsy: *carcinoma of the liver*

[40] in the United States and 80.4% [41]–90% [42] of cases in Japan.

In our series of 10 000 laparoscopies we found 232 (2.3%) cases of primary carcinoma. One hundred and forty-six of these (63%) had cirrhosis and 86 (37%) had no cirrhosis. There was carcinoma with cirrhosis in about 5% of all the cases (2772) of cirrhosis we observed from 1968 to 1982.

Laparoscopic studies confirm that this tumor is becoming increasingly frequent, as has already been observed in autopsy material. In our series, the frequency was about 3.5% of all the cirrhoses in the two 5-year periods of 1968–1972 and 1973–1977, but was over 6% from 1982 to 1987.

The above observation is due in part to the fact that new screening methods are now available and they have made the indications for laparoscopy more accurate; progress has also been made in endoscopy and biopsy techniques and so a greater number of reliable diagnoses are now made.

However, there has been a real increase in the incidence of tumors. Unlike carcinoma without cirrhosis, cirrhotic carcinoma clearly predominates in males (a ratio of 5:1 in our series) and in the elderly.

In patients of 40–50 years of age, carcinomas were found in a little over 2% of all the cirrhoses;

this increases to over 10% in patients aged between 55 and 60 years and increases again in patients aged over 60 years [43]. In our experience there is no correlation between carcinoma and the type (either micro- or macronodular) of cirrhosis [44]. Although recently epidemiological, serological and tissue findings demonstrated a link with virus B infection, the role of this hepatitis virus in the genesis of primary liver carcinoma is controversial. In a prospective polycenter investigation made recently in Italy [35], a significant correlation was found between carcinoma and the serological markers of the B virus, but not between carcinoma and alcohol abuse. Similar results were reported in France [38]. Other authors failed to find a substantial link between carcinoma and the presence of hepatitis B virus [45, 46]. Yet, in our retrospective study, no significant correlation was found between the frequency of carcinoma and the cause of the cirrhosis [44].

From the histological viewpoint, in the tumors with cirrhosis hepatocarcinoma clearly prevails over cholangiocarcinoma, the frequencies being 93% and 7% respectively.

The laparoscopic findings, which are discussed again in Sect. 5.3, vary greatly. Liver carcinoma can give rise to the following pictures: (a) a single nodule (Fig. 5.22), (b) multiple nodules, and (c) diffuse infiltration. The laparoscopic examination usually shows whether the tumor is malignant, and also establishes its type, but a biopsy must also be taken as this is usually decisive.

It is well known that, unlike liver carcinomas, metastatic tumors in cirrhosis are rare, but the reason for this has yet to be understood. In our series of 2538 cases of laparoscopically observed cirrhosis, 167 presented as associated malignant primary tumor in an extrahepatic site, a tumor that could give metastasis to the liver. Liver metastases were, however, found in only 19 cases (see Fig. 5.41), making up about 11% of all the primary extrahepatic tumors, which in turn correspond to 0.75% of all the cases of cirrhosis [47].

In our series esophageal cancer was the tumor most frequently associated with cirrhosis (31.8%) but only in 3.7% of these cases were metastases found in the liver [48].

5.2.6 Present Indications for Laparoscopy

In cirrhosis laparoscopy is usually performed to confirm the diagnosis, elucidate the characteristics and type of cirrhosis, and, finally, study portal hypertension, which is discussed in Sect. 5.3. In order to confirm the diagnosis we believe it opportune to distinguish between (a) *cirrhosis with complete* and *typical clinical symptoms* and (b) *cirrhosis without a complete and typical picture*.

1. When the clinical picture is complete and typical the diagnosis is easy to make and laparoscopy might be considered superfluous. Yet if the "certain" clinical pictures are controlled laparoscopically, a percentage of diagnostic errors is discovered. We performed laparoscopy for diagnostic confirmation in a series of 1079 patients thought to have cirrhosis on the basis of clinical and laboratory data. The patients had been hospitalized and therefore presumably had been studied using the correct methods. The diagnosis was confirmed in 1015 patients. Thirty-eight of the remaining patients had chronic liver disease without cirrhosis, 6 had liver carcinoma, and 11 had abdominal diseases of organs other than the liver and peritoneum. In six patients the liver was practically normal. In the same period, we also discovered another 80 cases in which different diagnoses had been made (tumor of the liver and peritoneum, chronic peritonitis, etc.) but in which the laparoscopic diagnosis was cirrhosis. A fairly high number of "easily reached" diagnoses are therefore attained.

We are of the opinion that to have a certain macroscopic and histological diagnosis laparoscopy may be justified.

Some recognize that without laparoscopy diagnostic errors are made in 24% of cases [49], yet feel that this is of little importance. Although we do not share their opinion we do agree that the decision to perform laparoscopy should be made in each individual case.

2. However, laparoscopy is definitely indicated when the diagnosis of cirrhosis is uncertain because: (a) evidence necessary for the diagnosis is scarce and (b) there are atypical phenomena extraneous to a picture of cirrhosis, and they may be due to another disease.

Symptomatological atypia occurs in the *clinical* and *biochemical* pictures. Often in cirrhosis no causes can be found; but this is not true atypia – it is the so-called *cryptogenetic cirrhosis*.

The main and most important deviations from the clinical picture are: *abdominal pain, fever, jaundice, gross or irregular hepatomegaly*, and *modified ascitic characteristics*. When these atypical forms are found, other noninvasive investigations should be undertaken so as to establish whether there is an associated disease, above all a malignant tumor. In many cases, however, noninvasive techniques fail to resolve the problem and laparoscopy must be performed.

In the presonographic era we studied 139 patients with atypical forms of cirrhosis: laparoscopy demonstrated that about half had simple cirrhosis with atypical symptoms but that the other half had an associated or superimposed disease [1]. Table 5.3 shows the results of this research. Of course now the number of patients requiring laparoscopy would be smaller because the diagnosis would have been made beforehand using imaging techniques.

Pain that is spontaneous, accessional, continuous, or triggered by palpation is not a usual symptom of cirrhosis and should always lead to suspicion of neoplasm. So pain or its onset in a patient with suspected or confirmed liver cirrhosis should always be further investigated and, if a satisfactory diagnosis is not made, laparoscopy should be performed. In our series laparoscopy demonstrated hepatocarcinoma in 16 of the 28 patients who had pain. When *fever* is particularly severe and persistent, it cannot be due to simple cirrhosis. In 50% of the cases it depends upon associated gallbladder, peritoneal inflammation, or primary liver tumor. *Jaundice* associated with cirrhosis is usually mild and varies in intensity, being more marked during liver failure. However, deep, prolonged, noninflammatory jaundice that appears cholestatic is atypical and requires further investigation.

Table 5.3. Laparoscopic diagnosis of liver cirrhosis with atypical clinical symptoms; 139 cases (from [37])

Atypical symptom or finding	No.	Laparoscopic diagnosis	
		Simple cirrhosis	Cirrhosis complicated by
Pain	12	5	Hepatocarcinoma (6) Chronic cholecystitis (1)
Pain/jaundice	3	2	Chronic cholecystitis (1)
Pain/fever	4	–	Hepatocarcinoma (3) Gallbladder hydrops (1)
Pain/atypical ascites	4	–	Hepatocarcinoma (2) Subacute nonspecific peritonitis (1) Peritoneal tuberculosis (1)
Pain/hepatomegaly	5	–	Hepatocarcinoma (5)
Fever	9	5	Chronic cholecystitis (2) Hepatocarcinoma (1) Gallbladder hydrops (1)
Fever/jaundice	1	1	–
Fever/atypical ascites	3	2	Peritoneal tuberculosis (1)
Fever/hepatomegaly	1	1	–
Jaundice	12	3	Hepatocarcinoma (2) Cholangitis (4) Extrahepatic cholestasis (2) Chronic cholecystitis (1)
Jaundice/atypical ascites	2	2	–
Hepatomegaly	26	18	Hepatocarcinoma (8)
Hepatomegaly/atypical ascites	7	5	Hepatocarcinoma (2)
Atypical ascites	50	30	Subacute nonspecific peritonitis (8) Hepatocarcinoma (7) Peritoneal tuberculosis (2) Peritoneal carcinomatosis (1) Perihepatitis (2)
Total	139	74	(65)

In 3 out of 25 cases we found the jaundice was obstructive and sonography would have resolved the problem. But in the other cases laparoscopy would have been indispensable even now because the jaundice was due to simple cirrhosis with cholestasis or cholangitic cirrhosis.

When the liver is grossly enlarged, very hard and with surface irregularities, echography with fine-needle biopsy may not explain the picture, thus necessitating a laparoscopic investigation. These pictures can only be caused by cirrhosis, alcoholic cirrhosis in particular: in 63 patients with abnormal hepatomegaly, a simple cirrhosis was found in 39; in 15 cases laparoscopy demonstrated hepatocarcinoma.

Ascites which appears in cirrhosis is usually transudative. If, however, ascites is exudative, then laparoscopy is almost always indicated. In about 70% of such cases in our experience, however, simple cirrhosis was revealed by laparoscopy. But in other cases, laparoscopy demonstrated an associated disorder, which was frequently inflam-matory or neoplastic peritoneal disease. Sometimes laparoscopy does not allow a clear diagnosis to be made. There may be *serous* or *serofibrinous peritonitis* with an etiopathogenesis that is difficult to establish, the so-called *spontaneous bacterial peritonitis*, known to be an important complication of cirrhosis [50]. Or there may be a tubercular *exudative peritonitis* without visible lesions, in which laparoscopy demonstrates only a diffuse congestion of the serosa while biopsy findings are not significant.

Another complication is *peritoneal tuberculosis*, which is now rare, but very serious, because if it is not detected and treated promptly it is fatal. Guided biopsy samples can be taken from miliary or nodular lesions of the serosa so as to confirm the diagnosis. Finally, exudative ascites can be caused by *primary* or *secondary peritoneal tumor*; the diagnosis made with laparoscopy and biopsy is usually simple to establish.

When ascites is *hematic* or *serohematic*, the cirrhosis may be complicated by peritoneal tuberculosis, by a primary or secondary peritoneal tumor, or by a hepatocarcinoma. The percentage of laparobioptic diagnoses made in these cases is also very high.

Great attention should be paid to *atypical biochemical parameters*, i.e., the presence or appearance of clearly abnormal findings that are not entirely characteristic of cirrhosis. Particularly important are signs of "inflammation" (marked increase in the erythrocyte sedimentation rate, elevated alphaglobulin levels) or an increase in the serum enzyme levels [alkaline phosphatase, γ-glutamin-transpeptidase (γ-GT), lactatedehydrogenase, α-fetoprotein].

5.2.7 Conclusions

1. Noninvasive imaging techniques detect liver cirrhosis when lesions to the liver are pronounced and when signs of portal hypertension are present, but not in the initial stages or when lesions are less evident.

2. Laparoscopy is therefore still the most effective available means for a reliable and accurate diagnosis, and its indications have not changed. The classical laparoscopic findings are still valuable in the interpretation of different lesions and they often indicate their etiology.

3. If the laparoscopic picture is clear, laparoscopic biopsy is redundant, but it is necessary when the findings are unclear, especially where a distinction must be made between liver cirrhosis and chronic hepatitis. With biopsy useful information can be obtained on the inflammatory activity and on the etiology of the disease.

4. Cirrhosis is classified in a traditional way on the basis of the volume of the organ, nodule dimensions, etc. In some cases nodules are not diffuse but *sectorial* and in others no nodules can be detected (*smooth cirrhosis*); we call cirrhosis that can be demonstrated only with biopsy "*histological cirrhosis.*" A sound knowledge of these possibilities is of crucial importance in making the diagnosis.

5. In cirrhosis, laparoscopy is indicated: (a) to confirm the clinical diagnosis, in particular when symptoms are incomplete or present atypical clinical biochemical, radiological, and sonographic findings and (b) to study portal hypertension.

5.3 Focal Liver Lesions

Noninvasive imaging techniques facilitate the diagnosis of liver neoformations by revealing any "space-occupying lesions." Clinical pictures that once called for laparoscopy now call for sonography, which is of fundamental importance when: (a) the clinical picture suggests that a liver neoformation is probable or possible (hepatomegaly, pain, temperature, etc.) and (b) the laboratory picture reveals increased γ-GT, alkaline phosphatasis, and α-fetoprotein.

Echography is noninvasive, simple to perform, and relatively economical, now being used more and more often, also for prophylaxis, in patients at a high risk of developing a neoplasm (for example, cirrhotic patients, who have a systematic sonographic follow-up) and in the general population for screening. Imaging techniques have enormously increased our overall diagnostic potential in focal lesions of the liver, and this is of great importance when diagnosing malignant neoplasms.

As mentioned above, in *primary hepatocarcinoma* sonography in association with echoguided fine-needle biopsy has a high diagnostic specificity. Moreover, as patients at risk now have echographic checkups, highly accurate and early diagnoses are made and small, clinically obscure, neoplasms are identified and in a large number of cases the onset of clinical symptoms is predicted. In their famous work on the natural history of carcinoma of the liver, Okuda et al. [51] demonstrated that many echographically detectable liver carcinomas are clinically and biochemically hidden and moreover they can grow extremely slowly, originating even 2 years before any clinical symptoms appear. Now many such tumors are detected in their preclinical stages, and so fewer of them call for laparoscopy. Many small, deep, tumors that are diagnosed nowadays could not be detected laparoscopically.

Until about 10 years ago laparoscopy was the only available closed abdomen technique allowing a reliable and accurate diagnosis, but now it is rarely indicated. Data from the most important centers show that the reduction in the use of laparoscopy in focal lesions has been more marked than in any other field.

It is, however, opportune to make several considerations. Buscarini et al. [4] compared the indications for 100 laparoscopies performed consecutively before echoguided fine-needle biopsy insertion with another 100 laparoscopies performed after it. The number of liver metastases laparoscopically diagnosed fell from 27% in the first group to 8% in the second. The number of laparoscopies performed to diagnose primary carcinoma on the other hand failed to show any statistically significant variations. This suggests that the indication for laparoscopy in local diseases of the liver has certainly decreased, but that they still exist. In recent years the findings of the different noninvasive techniques were compared with those of laparoscopy, and it emerged that now the use of laparoscopy should be restricted to "particular cases." In the United States, however, where the use of laparoscopy is relatively recent, laparoscopy with target biopsy is still considered the most accurate available nonsurgical method for a reliable diagnosis [52–54]. In Italy in 1984, Spinelli et al. stressed the value of laparoscopy; they found no significant differences between the sensitivity of sonography and that of laparoscopy in the diagnosis of liver neoplasms, saying that, if associated, the techniques enabled a diagnosis to be made in a very high percentage of cases: 96.3% in liver carcinomas, 97.8% in metastases, 100% in angiomas [55].

These data confirm that sonography and laparoscopy should be considered complementary techniques: when used together they are an extremely effective diagnostic tool for liver tumors.

Echography and laparoscopy are well integrated in the "sonography for laparoscopy" combination we have proposed. This combination proved highly satisfactory in a recent study by Fornari et al. on 63 cases of focal liver lesions; the results obtained in the same patient with echography and fine-needle biopsy respectively were compared with those of laparoscopy and endoscopic target biopsy [56].

Fine-needle biopsy had a sensitivity of 76.5% and an overall accuracy of 84.1% while laparoscopy had a sensitivity of 74.3% and an overall accuracy of 82.7%, so being a little less effective. But when combined, the techniques attain a sensitivity of 97.5% and an overall accuracy of 98.4%. These data not only confirm that the techniques are complementary, but also show that the overall accuracy of 84.1% with echoguided biopsy alone is increased to 98.4% when laparoscopy is also used, so the latter increases the reliable diagnoses by 14%.

5.3.1 Present Indications for Laparoscopy

Laparoscopy is now indicated less often, but is still of great value in certain cases, the decision to perform it being made in each case on the basis of preliminary sonography results completed, where possible, by echoguided fine-needle biopsy.

Generally speaking, the need for laparoscopy is inversely proportional to the diagnostic value of the different echographic images, to the possibility of performing useful biopsies with a fine needle, and to the significance of the cytological and histological findings.

Many space-occupying lesions can be reliably diagnosed with sonography. Hepatic *cysts* and *abscesses* can easily be recognized because there is an optimal transmission of echoes through the liquid and they appear anechogenic or hypoechogenic, with a well-defined wall. Single or multiple cysts, which appear as echo-free smooth-walled masses, are diagnosed sonographically in 100% of cases.

It is usually easy to diagnose *hydatid* cysts, which have irregular echoes due to daughter cysts. *Abscesses* appear as masses that sometimes have cyst-like echoes that can most often be recognized through the presence of small intraluminal echoes from debris. Echo-guided puncture almost always confirms that there is an abscess, and shows whether it is, for example, pyogenic or amebic.

Of the benign tumors, *hemangiomas* can appear generally roundish and have varying sizes; they give high-pitched echoes and are distinct from their surrounding tissue. If these characteristics are observed, they are diagnosed (Fig. 5.23); on other occasions, hypoechogenic masses containing multiple low-pitch echoes are observed. Finally, an angioma may appear as a complex mass with a mainly hyperechogenic structure with small, irregular anechoic areas. This picture, which is frequently encountered, is typical of the larger forms (giant cavernous hemangiomas) (Fig. 5.24). It is important here to point out that these aspects can make it difficult to distinguish between them and malignant neoplasms.

The appearance of *primary malignant neoplasms* of the liver can vary, but some characteristics at least indicate malignancy. In most cases, the finding is quite distinctive, with a roundish markedly hyperechogenic mass that is clearly distinct from its surrounding tissue (Fig. 5.25); it may also be surrounded by a hyperechogenic halo. In some

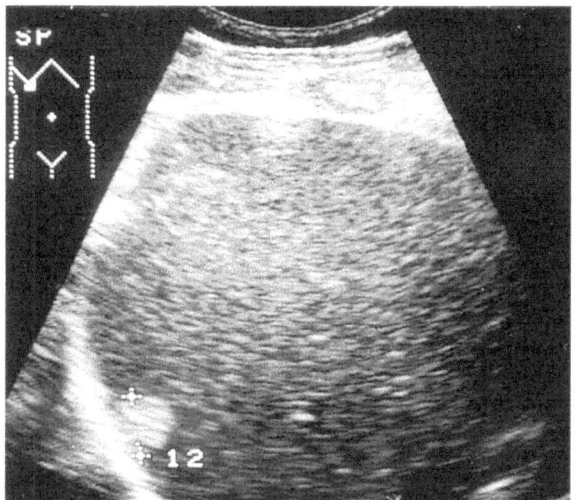

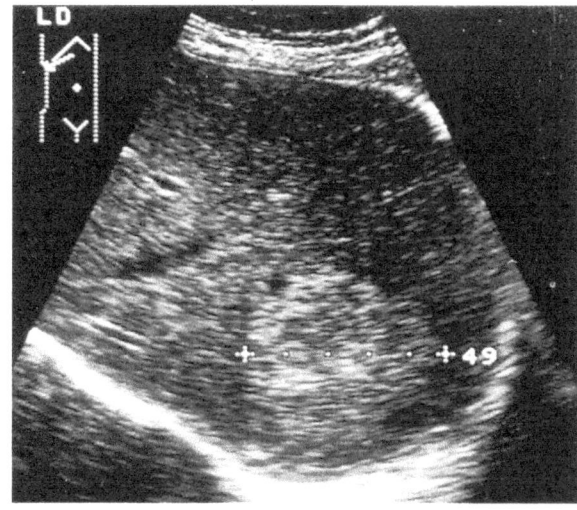

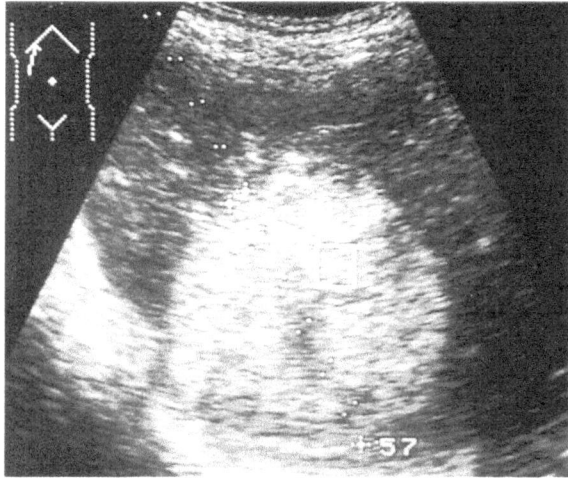

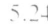

Fig. 5.23. Intercostal ultrasound oblique right scan. Small subdiaphragmatic hyperechogenic nodule with clear margins, spherical. Probably angioma. Laparoscopy useless. The US finding is uncertain, but laparoscopy is not indicated because, given its position, the lesion would be unlikely to be visualized with laparoscopy

Fig. 5.24. Intercostal ultrasound oblique right scan. Large round subdiaphragmatic hyperechogenic formations with clear margins without a peripheral halo. Surrounding liver tissue has a homogeneous isoechogenic structure. *Angioma? Adenoma? Malignant neoplasm?*

Fig. 5.25. Longitudinal echographic scan. Voluminous formation with a highly hyperechogenous echographic structure, clearly delimited except for the upper part, where the margin appears hazy. No peripheral halo. *Malignant neoplasm?*

cases the mass is hypoechoic, with an irregular and complex structure.

Other pictures show multiple nodules or a diffuse irregular echogenicity of the liver parenchyma. It is not always possible to diagnose a primary neoplasm or establish the tumor type. The images, however, enable fine-needle target biopsy to be performed; in a high percentage of cases it solves the diagnosis.

The appearance of metastatic liver tumors varies greatly, yet they can usually be recognized. The tumor may give rise to single or multiple hyperechogenic images or hyperechogenic areas. The so-called "*target-like*" or "*bull's eye*" images are highly typical; their center has a normal echogenicity surrounded by a hypoechogenic halo. Finally, the "heterogeneous mixed patterns" are characterized by diffuse and poorly delimited areas with irregular hyper- and hypoechoic areas that are

difficult to interpret. Any diagnostic difficulties are, however, usually overcome with echoguided biopsy.

However, it has yet to be established if and when laparoscopy is still indicated in the diagnosis of liver tumors. In our view, the systematic combined use of both techniques, "sonography for laparoscopy," enables us to establish in the most rational possible way what the present indications for laparoscopy are. To verify this we studied 260 patients with focal lesions of the liver. It is also important to stress that, when echographic, histological and cytological findings provide a "certain" diagnosis, laparoscopy is redundant. When these diagnoses are checked at a later date, a margin of error is found and this cannot be considered negligible. Some lesions that appear malignant at

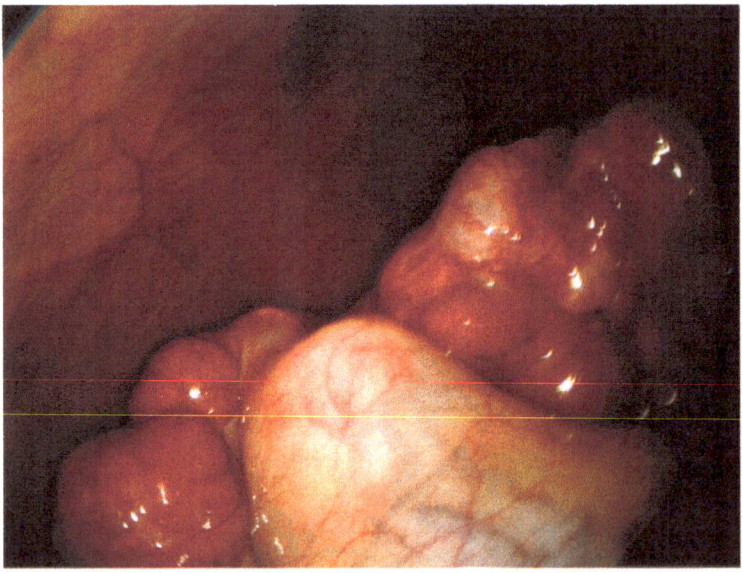

Fig. 5.26. Macronodular cirrhosis. On the right a rosy-white nodule already detected sonographically and diagnosed with fine-needle biopsy as a *hepatocarcinoma*. However, the nodule is not single: a small, pale nodule can be seen at the tip of the gallbladder

the microhistological or cytological examination are later discovered to be benign, and are therefore "false neoplastic positives." Inversely, with a fine-needle biopsy diagnosis a tumor may appear benign, but may later turn out to be malignant.

In 98 patients with focal lesions, for whom laparoscopy was not performed because it was considered superfluous, the diagnosis was later discovered to be inaccurate in 14 while in another 4 it was found that a malignant lesion had been overlooked.

It is clear that before considering the echographic and fine-needle biopsy diagnosis "definite," caution is necessary. When in doubt, laparoscopy should be performed. As is well known, this technique gives no "false positives" and, as recently observed [55, 4], it allows us to take tissue samples bioptically, which enable a very reliable histological examination to be made. Furthermore, in some patients with malignant tumors, laparoscopy may be indicated even if the diagnosis is certain because it can provide further insight, thus completing the diagnosis.

We performed laparoscopy as "a check" in 78 patients who had an echographic diagnosis of primary liver cancer and who therefore would not normally have undergone investigation. Thirty had a diagnosis of liver carcinoma. In 48, liver metastases from various tumors were found, 26 of which were known and 22 of which were an unexpected finding.

Laparoscopy provided the following additional information in 12 cases (15%):

1. In four cases liver carcinoma had been considered operable at sonography because only a small nodule was detected – laparoscopy showed further nodules (Fig. 5.26).
2. In two cases laparoscopy demonstrated that the neoplasm was far more extensive than indicated sonographically.
3. In five cases laparoscopy detected peritoneal and omental metastases that had been overlooked at the echographic exploration.
4. Finally, in one case a cytological diagnosis of metastatic cancer was changed into a diagnosis of malignant lymphoma.

It is obvious that this further information, provided only by laparoscopy, is of crucial importance because it can influence the therapeutic strategy chosen as well as the prognosis. In liver carcinoma considered operable on the basis of echography alone, laparoscopy may demonstrate that surgery is contraindicated. Furthermore, when ascertaining whether a liver carcinoma is operable, laparoscopy can show the status of the liver, particularly in cirrhosis, showing its severity, distribution, and localization as well as revealing any collateral circulations from portal hypertension. Laparoscopy is indicated in liver carcinoma for which clinical, biochemical, and echographic findings demonstrate that radical curative surgery is possible.

Finally, in metastatic liver tumors laparoscopy can improve upon the diagnosis made with echography and also on that made with fine-needle biopsy. The laparoscopic findings together with the results of guided multiple biopsies enable us to establish the site of origin and type of an unknown primary tumor responsible for the metastasis. This typification was successful in 90% of our cases of liver metastases for which the primary tumor was not known.

Echographic and echoguided fine-needle biopsy findings can be *doubtful*.

In an article published in 1981, Boyce and Nord [52] reviewed nodular lesions of the liver that can complicate the differential diagnosis. They pointed out that the "foci of metastatic carcinoma may be mimicked by a myriad of other abnormalities from congenital abnormalities to cirrhosis with regenerating nodules," and stated that laparoscopic and guided biopsy are the most accurate nonsurgical methods that can be used to provide a visual and histological diagnosis in such patients. Uncertain sonographic findings are certainly numerous [4, 57, 58]: some malignant tumors can simulate benign tumors or inflammatory masses. Sometimes small multiple abscesses are mistaken for metastases. It may be difficult to distinguish between primary and secondary liver neoplasms [59, 60].

It is of particular importance to make a differential diagnosis between malignant tumors and local benign lesions, above all with *liver cell adenoma, focal nodular hyperplasia*, and *hepatic angioma* [61–66]. Now, thanks to echoguided biopsy there are fewer uncertain cases, a reliable diagnosis being made in a very high percentage. In order to establish if and when laparoscopy might be useful, it is therefore necessary to use echoguided biopsy results as well as echographic images as a reference point.

Dubious sonographic findings that remain undiagnosed or uncertain despite the aid of fine-needle biopsy are frequently obtained when lesions are benign. Very often in such cases the histological picture is not significant and therefore does not allow us to establish the type of process or its nature. Moreover, even if it does not demonstrate malignancy, this does not mean that the process is benign. In such circumstances, if the echographically detected lesions are found in explor-

able areas of the liver, laparoscopy is indicated and it almost always solves the diagnostic doubts.

Focal hyperplasia and *adenoma* can create considerable diagnostic problems. Figure 5.27 shows an echographic finding with an uncertain hypoechogenic area. With echo-guided biopsy, scanty material is aspirated, consisting of some hepatocytes with no specific characteristics. Laparoscopy demonstrates two superficial protruding nodules that cannot easily be judged macroscopically (Fig. 5.28). The histological examination, made on abundant material taken using a cutting needle, demonstrates that this is a benign adenoma.

Irregular fatty infiltration of the liver was found in 7.5% of 3719 laparoscopies taken in the Mölln center [67], in the form of "yellow spots" on the organ surface.

When the phenomenon is particularly marked, the sonographic findings may be mistaken for those typical of liver metastasis [68]. Echography can demonstrate hypoechogenic areas that are suspicious (Fig. 5.29). Biopsy may reveal steatosis, but tends to give unreliable negative findings for neoplasms. Laparoscopy allows us to make a certain diagnosis by showing the presence of an area circumscribed by steatosis and, sometimes in a cirrhotic liver, a nodule that laparoscopically appears to be benign, consisting of adipose tissue.

It is difficult to distinguish between a malignant tumor and nodular focal hyperplasia associated with cirrhosis. Sonography may indicate suspect areas and, in these cases, malignancy cannot be ruled out on the basis of negative fine-needle biopsy. In such cases laparoscopy is indicated. With direct endoscopy marked diagnostic difficulty may also often be encountered because the macroscopic picture is often identical to that of cirrhosis. It is advisable always to take a biopsy even when the diagnosis of cirrhosis seems definite [69]. Moreover, sometimes the differential diagnosis is impossible to make even with liver carcinoma on cirrhosis because focal hyperplasia can give a similar picture. Diffuse liver carcinoma is sometimes characterized by a fairly uniform cirrhotic nodulation, some of the nodules being pale red, lard-like, and hard (Fig. 5.30). The diagnosis is therefore made with biopsy.

If echographic findings are doubtful and echoguided biopsy fails to indicate the diagnosis, there may be malignant, above all primary, neoplasms. An appropriate example of this is shown in Fig. 5.31. Echography detected a small hypoechogenic area in a deep site, suggesting a tumor. As echo-

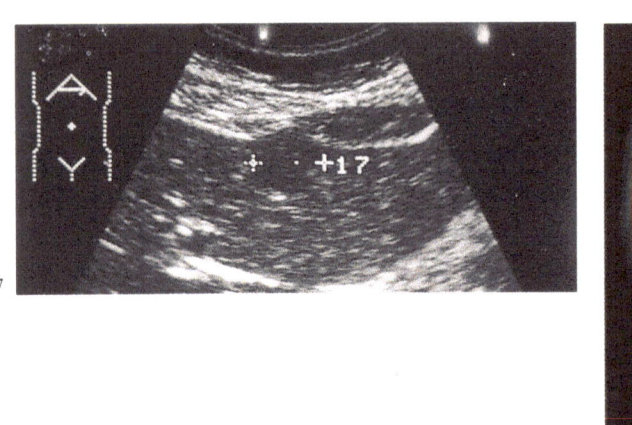

5.27

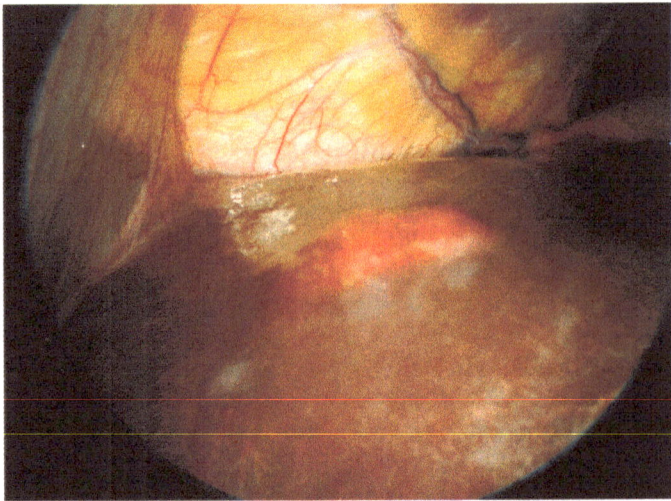

5.

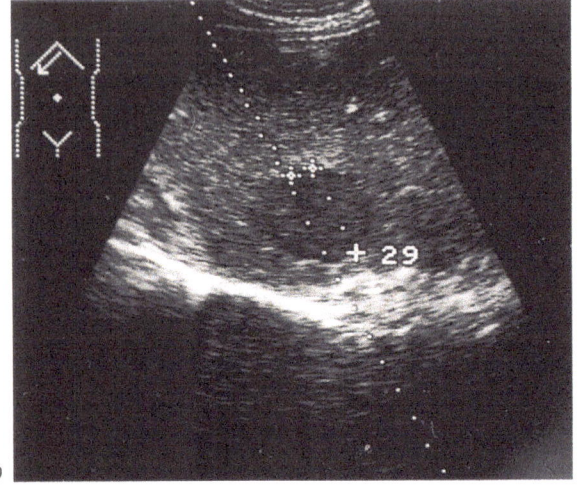

5.29

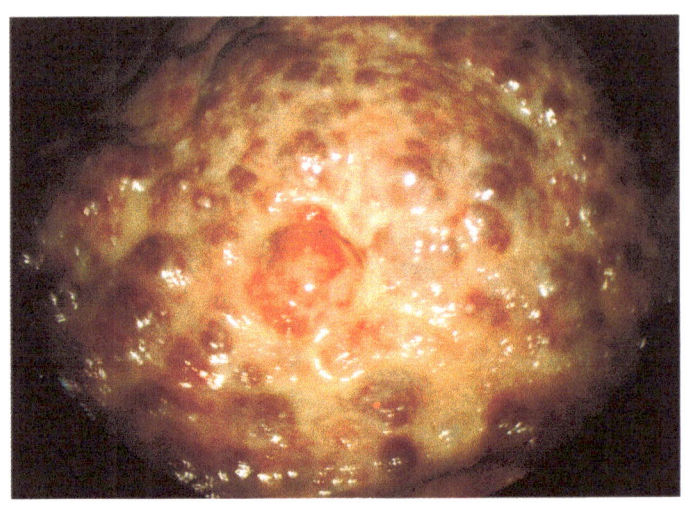

5

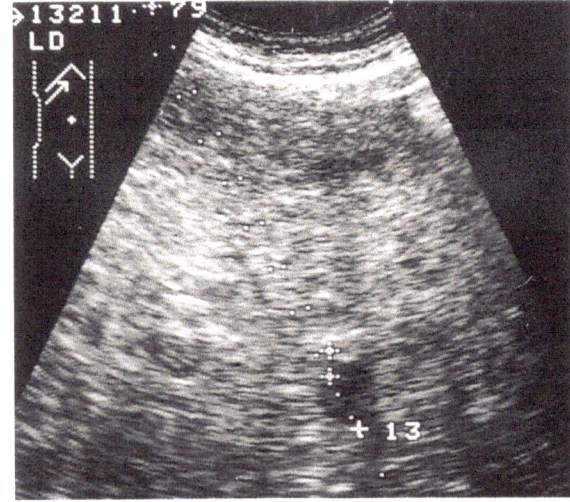

5.31

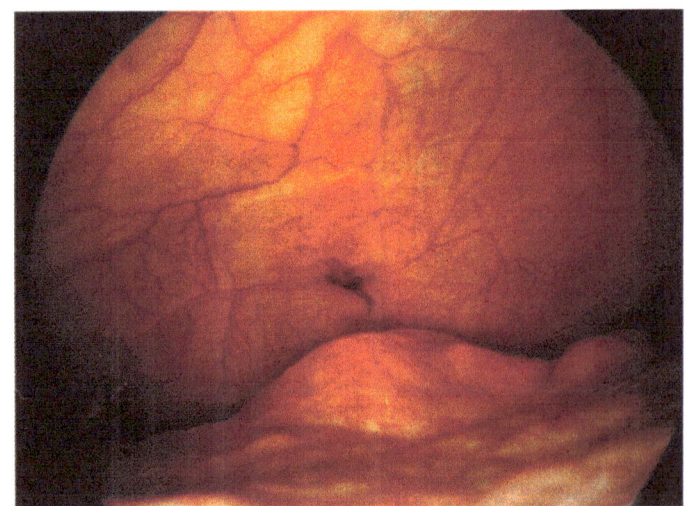

5

guided biopsy failed to clarify the diagnosis, laparoscopy was performed not so much to check the characteristics of the lesion, which was hidden behind the liver, but above all to search for any other nodules and to check the laparoscopic appearance of the organ surface, which echographically appeared as an extensive band with low echoes. Laparoscopy revealed cirrhosis and, protruding on the surface, two nodules; these were clearly neoplastic and localized at the hypoechogenic area. Biopsy confirmed carcinoma of the liver (Fig. 5.32).

When there are discrepancies between the findings, laparoscopy integrated with sonography allows for an echographic control after laparoscopy, and now we consider extensive hypoechogenic areas as possibly due to neoplastic infiltration. If the fibrin plug is inserted in the biopsy hole to mark the point from which the biopsy is taken (Fig. 5.33), it confirms that this echographic feature indicates hepatocarcinoma.

◄————————————————————

Fig. 5.27. Ultrasound axial scan of the left lobe of the liver. Roundish superficial hypoechogenic formation with a slight "hump," which is demarcated with respect to the surrounding parenchyma, which has hypoechogenic patches. Finding dubious

Fig. 5.28. Same case as in Fig. 5.27. An irregular, moderately vascularized formation with clear borders can be seen on the surface of the left lobe of the liver; it is difficult to interpret. Biopsy: *adenoma of the liver*

Fig. 5.29. Echography. Roundish "hypoechogenic" image with clear border on the parenchyma, which is slightly hyperechogenic and dyshomogeneous. *Metastasis to the liver*?

Fig. 5.30. Medium-sized nodules of the cirrhotic type. At the center is a pink, lard-like nodule. *Diffuse hepatocarcinoma of the liver with cirrhosis* suspected. Confirmation with biopsy

Fig. 5.31. Echographic oblique right subcostal scan with the patient in lateral left decubitus. A hyperechogenic, highly dishomogenous parenchyma with patches mainly on the deeper strata. The most superficial stratum has a reduced echogenicity, but it is equally dishomogeneous with small hypoechogenic areoles. In the deeper layers are roundish hypoechogenic areoles

Fig. 5.32. Same case as in Fig. 5.31. Left lobe of the liver; superficial nodulation from which protrudes a small pink mass, with a clear border. On the wall is the hole from the previous fine-needle biopsy. *Hepatocarcinoma* probable. Confirmation with biopsy

It is important here to point out that a primary liver neoplasm can give an echographic picture that is uncertain for malignant neoplasia even in the absence of associated cirrhosis (Fig. 5.34). Laparoscopy can give a clear picture of extensive but superficial areas of neoplastic tissue (Fig. 5.35). Probably the ultrasound picture is uncertain because the lesions are so thin.

Liver angioma may have, as mentioned above, a typical echographic picture, thus making the diagnosis easy, but it can give findings that are doubtful and that do not rule out a malignant form (Fig. 5.36). For some the diagnosis is always uncertain [70]. Thin-needle biopsy has also not improved the situation because it is considered risky and, above all, because its findings are often unreliable. If angioma is suspected, laparoscopy is definitely indicated. Some are of the opinion that laparoscopy should be performed prior to echoguided fine-needle biopsy because the latter is dangerous, particularly when lesions are superficial [70].

A laparoscopic diagnosis is almost always reliable (Fig. 5.37). Also when the angioma revealed echographically is deep and presumably hidden, laparoscopy is still indicated because it can reveal the presence of other smaller undetected angiomas that allow a diagnosis.

Finally, it is important to bear in mind that a diagnosis of *hemangiosarcoma* can be made only with the macroscopic examination and if necessary with a target biopsy from the solid tissue area that is under laparoscopic guidance.

The mean percentage of dubious cases requiring laparoscopy is not easy to establish reliably: the criteria for the indication are highly subjective. In Fornari's series [56], for example, out of 63 patients with focal lesions revealed echographically, the negative finding for neoplastic cells from fine-needle biopsy was held to be dubious in 23 cases. Laparoscopy was therefore performed where a false negative was suspected and it demonstrated that in ten cases there was a primary carcinoma. In 3 out of 47 cases, Salmi et al. [71] laparoscopically diagnosed focal nodular hyperplasia that echographically and biochemically had appeared dubious. In our series of 260 cases in which echography and echoguided biopsy failed to provide a satisfactory diagnosis, laparoscopy solved the diagnosis in 15 (5.7%): three hepatocarcinomas, four metastases, and eight benign forms. Here it is of crucial importance to stress that laparoscopy is definitely indicated

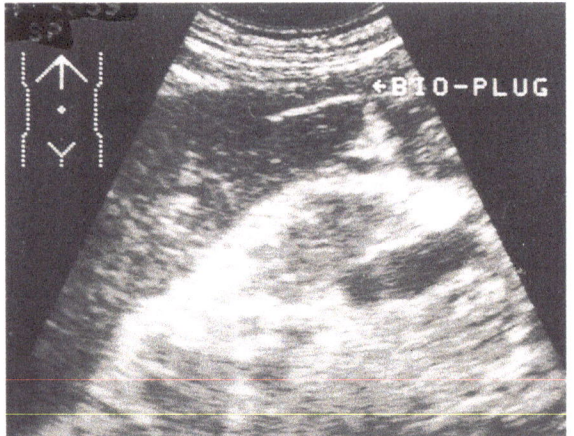

5.33

Fig. 5.33. Longitudinal echographic scan of the bord of the left lobe of the liver. In a hypoechogenic area n suspected of having a replacement lesion a laparoscop biopsy detected a *hepatocarcinoma*. The Bio-Plug i serted in the biopsy hole, which appears as a hype echogenic strip, indicates exactly the point where th tissue fragment was taken

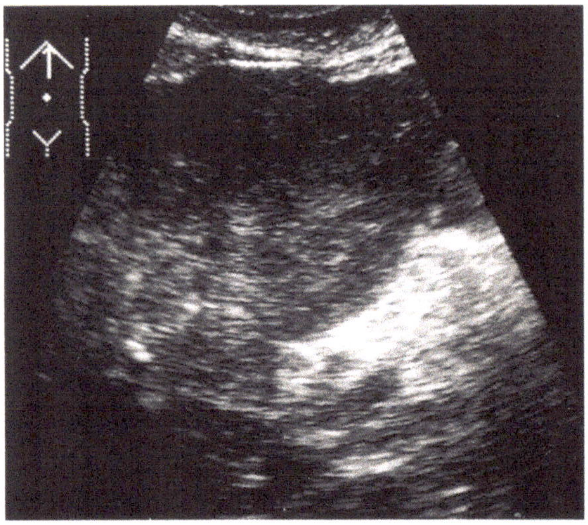

5.34

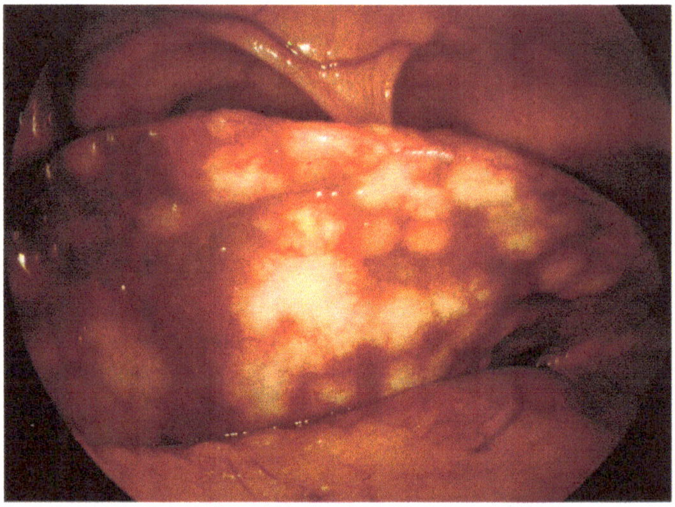

5.36

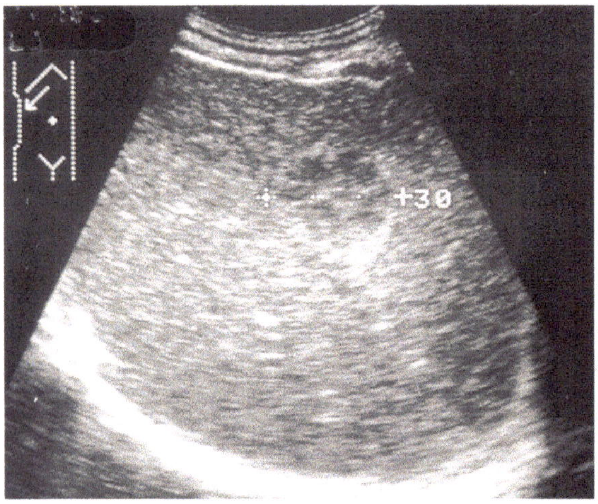

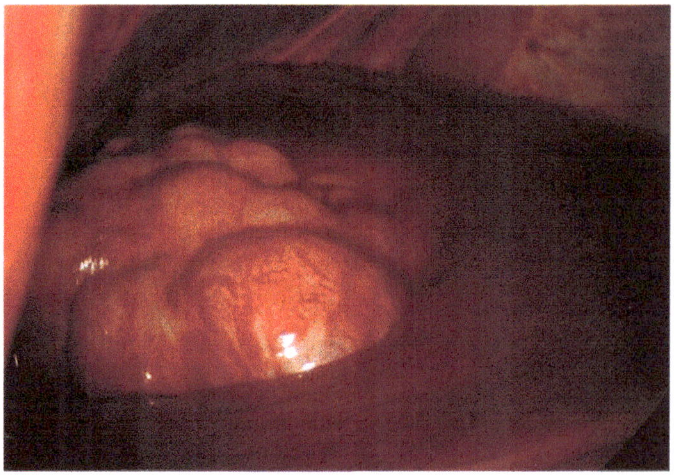

whenever the echography and fine-needle biopsy findings, considered in the light of the general clinical picture, are dubious; this is not rare and should always be borne in mind.

Although sonography is highly sensitive in the detection of focal liver lesions, some, particularly malignant neoplasms, do "escape" detection by this investigation. Echographically, the liver appears normal or presents slight echogenic alterations that appear insignificant. So some *negative sonographic findings* are "*false negatives*," and this occurs in a fairly high percentage of cases. We must therefore be cautious when considering the data in series from radiology institutes because the patient is unlikely to have a follow-up that can demonstrate whether the "negative" finding was false or not. The examination may therefore appear to be more sensitive than it really is. Tanaka et al., for example, submitted over 5000 subjects to echographic screening and detected 151 malignant tumors of the liver, 113 of which were found to be primary liver carcinomas. The sensitivity of echography was evaluated in 95% of the series. Subsequently, however, a further 24 cases of liver carcinoma were detected; these had escaped detection at the first echographic examination and had also been false negatives [72].

Fig. 5.34. Longitudinal scan of left lobe of the liver, which has an irregular margin (sinuous and nodular). Marked echostructural dyshomogeneity, prevalently hypoechogenous in the superficial half and hyperechogenous in the deeper areas. No features typical of focal lesion, except for the suspect picture of a "hump" at the upper margin

Fig. 5.35. Same case as in Fig. 5.34. Left lobe of the liver raised by an adhesion. Lower surface has numerous extensive yellow-white areas that are isolated or confluent, with irregular shapes and a hazy outline. Liver neoplasm: metastasis? Cholangiocarcinoma? Biopsy: *cholangiocarcinoma*

Fig. 5.36. Oblique subcostal echographic scan of the left lobe of the liver. Roundish area with a mixed structure and interrupted hyperechogenic halos; inside hyperechogenic bands in rays. Normal echostructure in the rest of the parenchyma. Malignant neoplasm? Angioma?

Fig. 5.37. Left lobe of the liver; large extensive plurilobular formations, highly vascular with clear margins. *Angioma of the liver*

In this respect the most reliable data are from comparative studies made with laparoscopy or with other techniques so as to check the echographic diagnosis. Chen et al. [73] compared echography, CT, arteriography, and laparoscopy in 13 cases of primary liver carcinoma measuring under 3 cm (small hepatocellular carcinomas). The sensitivity of CT was 88% while that of echography was 84%. The sensitivity of laparoscopy was only 19%. In their series of 30 small hepatocellular carcinomas, Cottone et al. [74] laparoscopically demonstrated 3 false sonographic negatives. In the series of Spinelli et al. [58], false sonographic negatives were found in 2 out of 27 primary tumors and in 6 out of 48 metastases.

Among our 260 cases of focal liver lesions, 47 were overlooked at preliminary echography, being diagnosed later with laparoscopy, which was performed because the negative sonographic finding was considered dubious. Twenty were liver carcinomas; in ten of these cases sonography had revealed a normal liver; it had revealed a slight parenchymal dyshomogeneity in the other ten; this was considered unimportant. In 27 there were metastases, which were not detected with echography.

The different laparoscopic findings then almost always provide, apart from the diagnosis, also a satisfactory explanation for the failure of sonography. There are various causes for this: some depend on the well-known shortcomings of echography while others are less obvious, being revealed through a systematic comparison between the results of the different techniques. The *tumor size* is of great importance.

It is generally held that a primary or metastatic neoplastic nodule with a diameter of under 2 cm is likely to escape sonographic detection. Sonography may fail to detect even larger neoplastic nodules if these have *particular loci* that are not well explored with ultrasound. False echographic negatives are most likely to be made at the ligament insertion and the round and falciform ligaments of the liver (Fig. 5.38).

Another tricky site is at the margin of the liver, where quite large hepatic neoplasms (Fig. 5.39) can be overlooked with ultrasound. A *diffuse infiltration* of the parenchyma is equally difficult to detect with echography. In these cases the differences in the echogenicity of the cirrhotic liver and the neoplastic tissue are clearly slight and the picture may therefore be negative or show alterations that are considered insignificant. This is not a rare occurrence. In our series of liver carcinomas we

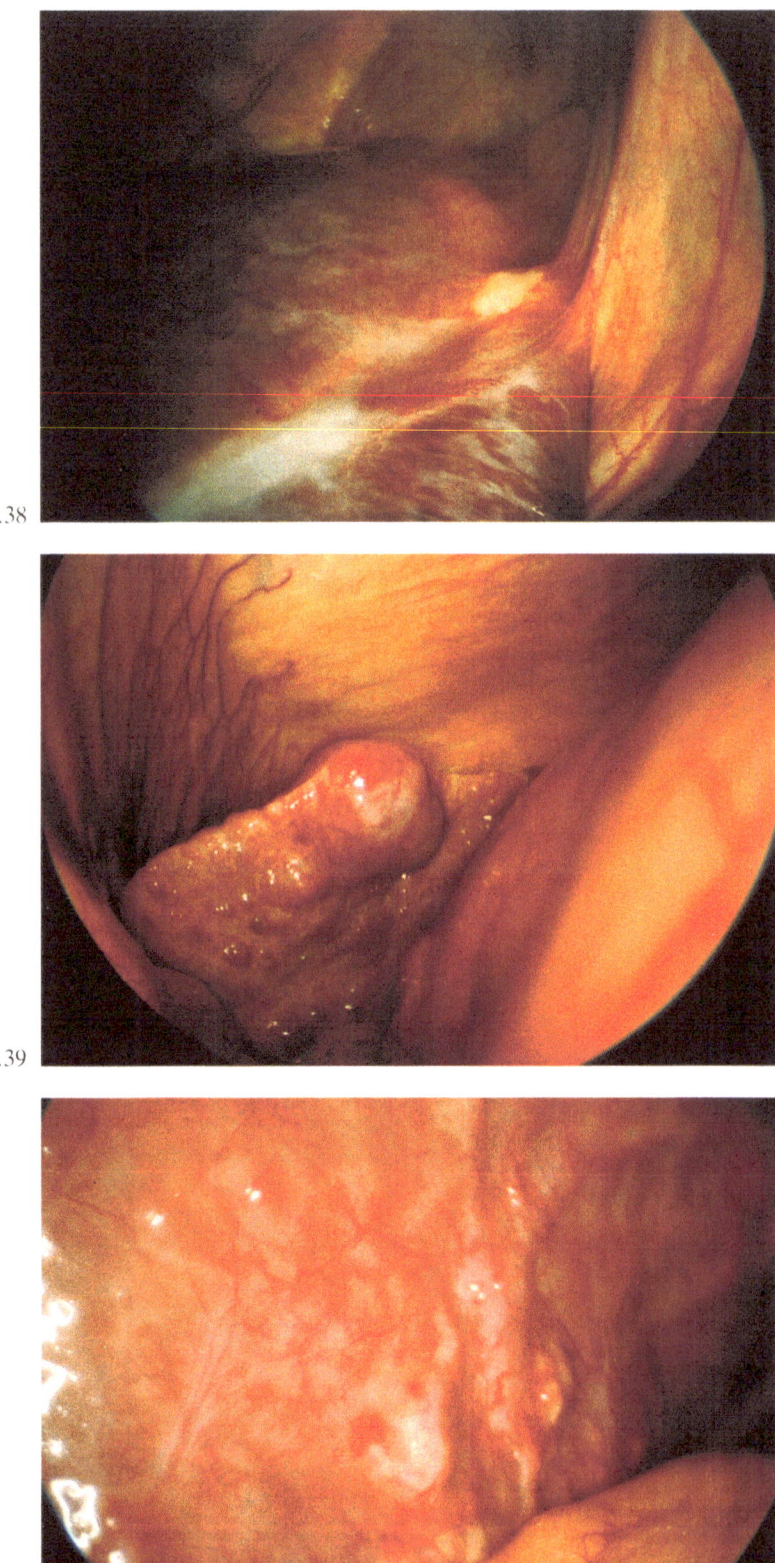

5.38

5.39

5.40

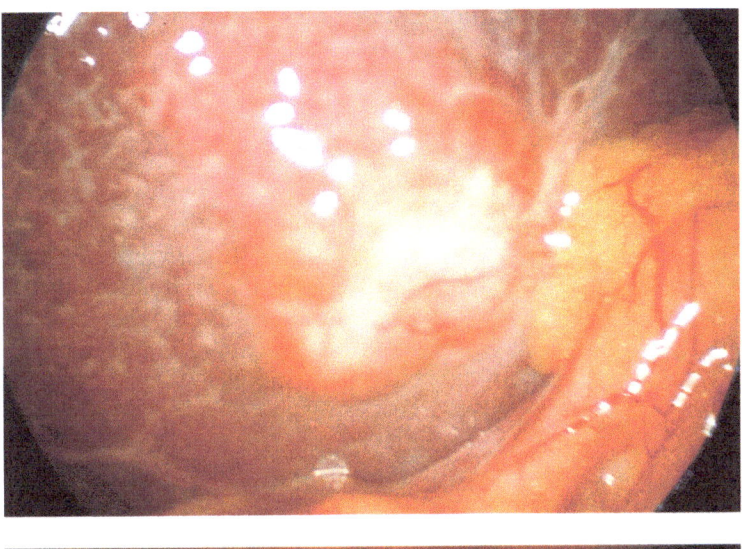

5.41

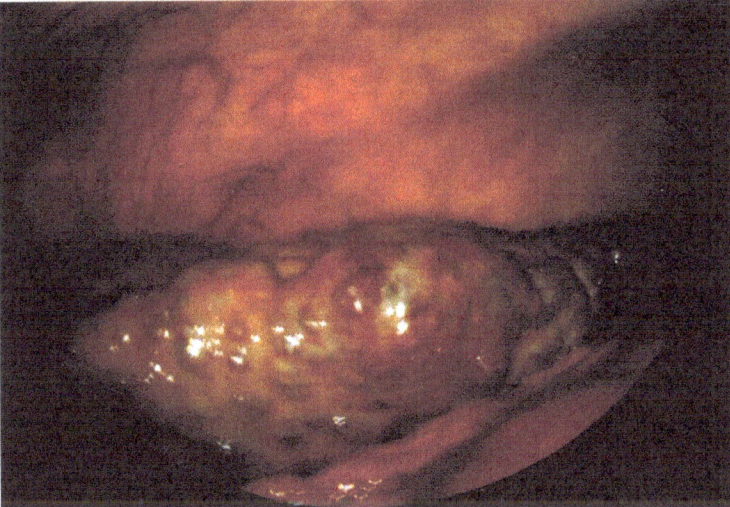

5.42

Fig. 5.38. Staging for carcinoma of the stomach. On the medial margin of the left lobe of the liver, at the base of the falciform ligament, is a yellowy-white plaque. Probably metastasis from epithelial neoplasia. Biopsy: *metastasis from adenocarcinoma*

Fig. 5.39. Left lobe of the liver stiff, raised with cirrhotic type of nodulation; a small protuberant neoformation at the margin. *Hepatocarcinoma with cirrhosis. Finding confirmed with biopsy*

Fig. 5.40. Surface of lower facies of the liver under high magnification: cirrhotic nodules are barely visible. Small nodules can be seen with vascular-type whitish branches. *Diffuse hepatocarcinoma* with involvement of the lymphatic network. Confirmation with biopsy

Fig. 5.41. Staging of carcinoma of the esophagus. Lower facies of the right lobe of the liver under high magnification. Cirrhotic nodulation: roundish protruding formation with whitish central crater. *Metastasis from epithelial neoplasia.* Confirmation with biopsy

Fig. 5.42. Lateral margin of the left lobe of the liver. Cirrhotic nodulation and intense cholestasis. A protuberant nodule with features suggesting neoplasia can be seen. Biopsy: *Hepatocarcinoma with cirrhosis*

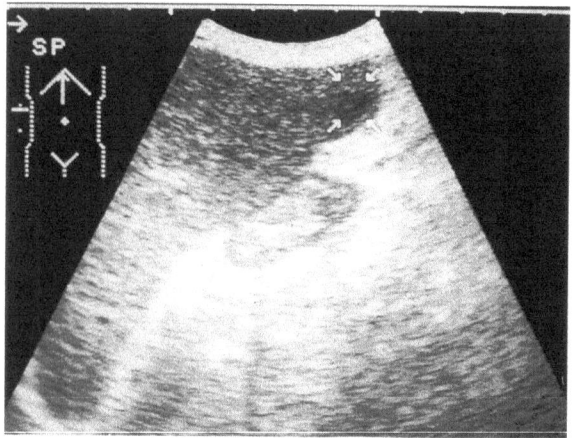

Fig. 5.43. Same case as in Fig. 5.42. After opportune changes in "gain," a small areola with a more marked echogenicity (→ *arrow*) is isolated at the site of the lesion indicated by laparoscopy on the margin of the left lobe

observed diffuse neoplastic infiltrations in 12 patients with negative ultrasound findings. Also with laparoscopy the diagnosis can be very difficult to make because at examination the neoplastic infiltration usually appears as a fine net sometimes with minute whitish nodules merging with the host tissue and therefore barely perceptible (Fig. 5.40).

Secondary tumors may also present as an infiltration of the entire parenchyma; laparoscopically the picture is difficult to interpret and can simulate a steatosis. In all these cases the diagnosis is made with biopsy.

It has been demonstrated that in the *presence of cirrhosis* the diagnostic sensitivity of echography is reduced. In our series, primary hepatocarcinomas that escaped detection at sonographic exploration were all associated with cirrhosis. Metastases occur more rarely on a cirrhotic liver but, when they are present, echography may fail to detect neoplastic nodules (Fig. 5.41), even ones that are large enough to be revealed in a normal liver. Figure 5.39 shows the main causes of failure with sonography: small dimensions, tumors on the liver margin, and association with cirrhosis.

All our cases in which laparoscopy demonstrated a primary or secondary tumor that had not previously been revealed were checked echographically at the end of the laparoscopic examination in a search for signs that might reveal a posteriori the presence of neoplasia. In only one case was

it possible to detect a carcinomatous nodule with a 2-cm diameter: a small, hazy, hypoechogenic area that escaped detection at the first examination (Figs. 5.42, 5.43). In some cases, echography demonstrated a superficial band of hypoechogenicity that was very hazy, without features typical for nodular lesions being observed. A fibrin cartridge, inserted at the biopsy hole, showed that the neoplastic tissue fragment had been taken directly from that area. The area itself showed no echographic alteration compatible with carcinomatous infiltration.

5.3.2 Conclusions

1. Sonography is an extraordinarily effective means for detecting and diagnosing focal lesions of the liver and for screening in normal subjects, above all in categories at risk of having a neoplasm.

2. With echoguided fine-needle biopsy the diagnosis can be clarified and the tumor type established. It is therefore the invasive technique of choice.

3. Echography with fine-needle biopsy and laparoscopy with target biopsy must be used in association and the decision to perform laparoscopy must be made on the basis of the results obtained with the previous examination using the following scheme.

a) If the echographic picture and the cytological and microhistological findings allow a certain and accurate diagnosis laparoscopy is superfluous. It is indicated only if a false echographic positive is considered possible and if further information that laparoscopy alone can provide is required (preoperative tumor staging, accurate evaluation of a hepatopathy, etc.)

b) If the echographic picture is doubtful and echoguided biopsy is unsuccessful or not significant, then laparoscopy is indicated because it can resolve the problem of a differential diagnosis above all for benign and malignant focal lesions of the liver.

c) If echography shows a normal liver but there is a clinical suspicion or the possibility of a primary or secondary tumor of the liver, then laparoscopy is indicated because it can demonstrate any "false echographic negative."

5.4 Portal Hypertension

Evidence of portal hypertension may be found by physical examination through: cutaneous collateral circulation in the usual sites, splenomegaly, and varices. Plain X-rays, arteriography, and, above all, esophagogastroscopy can be used to ascertain whether or not there are gastroesophageal varices and, if so, their severity. It therefore also shows whether there is a risk of hemorrhage. More recently sonography and CT have also been used to reveal accurately vein caliber in different areas [75–78]. Laparoscopy allows us to make a direct exploration of the abdominal cavity, and portal hypertension is visualized by inspecting the veins of the portocaval circulation. The laparoscopic study of portal hypertension integrates findings from other techniques.

5.4.1 Main Laparoscopic Findings

The main laparoscopic findings in portal hypertension are *collateral abdominal venous circulation* and *alterations of the spleen*. In portal hypertension endoscopic exploration reveals *abdominal vein alterations*. Collateral circulations should be searched for in the areas in which there could be anastomoses between the portal and caval systems.

However, laparoscopic findings at the large vessels are no longer of interest because imaging techniques now accurately reveal any alterations they may have. Normally vessels in the greater omentum are barely visible but in portal hypertension the omentum may appear grooved by tortuous, entwined veins of varying diameter that form a complex network. If large, these veins are revealed sonographically, but laparoscopic findings are useful when small veins are enlarged and turgid. Laparoscopy, however, is the only means to distinguish between a "collateral circulation" and venous turgidity due to "stagnation." Omental veins dilated by portal hypertension are bright red at laparoscopic inspection, showing an active blood flow, whereas in obstruction due, for example, to a tumor, the omental veins are equally distended but are dark red because they contain stagnant blood.

Mesenteric and gastric vein alterations are due to hypertension in the splenic vein, which is sometimes visible, and of the left gastroepiploic tributary of the portal vein through the splenic vein. It is also interesting to examine the lesser gastric

curvature veins, which sometimes appear altered in association with the dilation of the greater curvature veins, but also singly. This finding indicates an involvement of the right and left gastric veins in the collateral circulation and almost always indicates the presence of gastroesophageal varices.

Another valuable laparoscopic sign of portal hypertension is distention and turgor of the *paraumbilical veins*. These are part of the "portoaccessorial" system, which originates in the abdominal wall at the umbilicus, and they follow the falciform ligament near and immediately behind the round ligament, directly reaching the liver. Normally the blood from the umbilical regions runs in the right and left paraumbilical veins, and through these it reaches the left branch of the portal vein. When the portal circulation is obstructed below the entry of the paraumbilical veins, these veins are not affected. When the obstruction is upstream from their point of entry, the direction of flow in the paraumbilical veins is reversed, and a collateral circulation is formed that empties into the vena cava through anastomoses with the superior and inferior epigastric veins and the internal thoracic and subcutaneous abdominal veins.

At laparoscopy the paraumbilical veins thus appear distended and they hide the entire hepatic parenchyma at the anterior and the medial margins of the right lobe and follow the falciform ligament up to the umbilical region. In some cases, the paraumbilical veins are enlarged and emerge from both lobes and then reunite to form a single trunk. These collateral circulations show portal hypertension that is definitely caused by an intrahepatic obstruction. This finding is useful only if the alterations are an early, moderate, sign that could not be revealed sonographically.

Umbilical vein recanalization, which characterizes the so-called Cruveilhier-Baumgarten's syndrome, is easily revealed with simple ultrasound and so here laparoscopy is no longer of value. However, some consider this finding unreliable because it has also been obtained with ultrasound in patients without portal hypertension [79]. The round ligament becomes a large ectatic tortuous blue vein with a U-shaped curve, sometimes becoming enormous. Trocar introduction is therefore dangerous, but now laparoscopy is no longer required preliminary sonography is being used (see Sect. 2.2.1).

The finding of altered small peritoneal veins is particularly characteristic of the laparoscopic se-

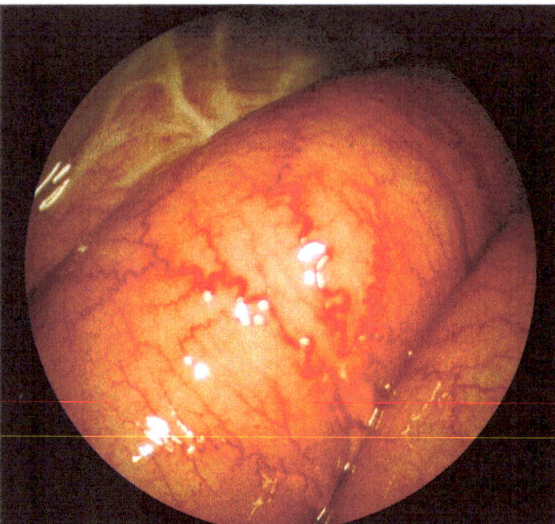

Fig. 5.44. *Collateral circulation from portal hypertension*; dilated and turgid small veins on the serosa of the small intestine

meiology for portal hypertension and is still of great interest, even today. These vessels are too small to be studied by sonography, CT or arteriography. Only with laparoscopy can these findings, which are of considerable practical importance, be obtained. Here laparoscopy is most important because it clarifies the morphological aspects and distribution of any small vessel alterations.

Normally the peritoneal vessels are thin and form a loose, barely visible network. In portal hypertension alterations in these vessels can be seen; they affect both the parietal and visceral surfaces. Raised, tortuous, dilated vessels are visible on the serosa of the intestinal loops, where they form a dense vascular network (Fig. 5.44). This is most evident at the parietal peritoneum – the veins are distended with blood, more numerous, and raised. There are many anastomoses, and in some cases true plexuses are observed.

It is opportune here to stress the characteristics of this "passive" congestion, in which the vessels appear distinct and well demarcated against the peritoneum, which retains its normal color; they must be distinguished from the characteristics of active congestion, in which the vessels are hazy and the peritoneum is reddened. These alterations are found where there are natural or newly formed communications between the portal and caval systems – the necessary conditions exist here for a collateral circulation.

Alterations of the small vessels of the *falciform ligament and the diaphragm* are due to the circulation forming on the system of the accessory portal veins of the "diaphragmatic group" and consist of a very distinct vascular network.

An accentuated venous pattern on the falciform ligament is often found in normal subjects; this may be particularly visible against the thin membrane of the ligament. This finding should, however, be considered significant only when the passive congestion is conspicuous and extends to the peritoneal vessels of the upper abdominal wall, which indicates communication with the systemic circulation.

The collateral circulation of the *biliary tree* is detected through the presence of congested veins on the serosa of the visible portions of the gallbladder. This circulation is due to increased pressure in the cystic accessory portal veins, and results in retrograde flow into the vena cava system (Fig. 5.45). These findings are infrequent, but they are highly indicative of portal hypertension.

The *Retzius system* veins are parallel and vertical, with frequent anastomoses in the lateral recesses of the abdominal cavity, along the line of the junction of the visceral and parietal peritoneum. These vessels represent the collateral circulation between the veins of the intestinal wall (portal vein tributaries) and the parietal veins (tributaries of the vena cava). At laparoscopy these alterations are hidden by the intestine so a careful search should be made with the patient in right and left lateral decubitus, so as to free these recesses and explore them completely.

The *larger omentum* at its more lateral part is attached to the abdominal wall directly beneath the spleen, in contact with its interior border, forming the *phrenocholic ligament*. This is best observed if the patient is put into a lateral right decubitus, with the trunk raised. Normally the ligament contains varying quantities of fat, has few blood vessels, and is taut between the upper wall and the abdominal organs, and only scantily vascularized. In portal hypertension, numerous veins of varying caliber originate from the visceral veins of the abdomen and run through the ligament, terminating on the upper wall near the ligament insertion.

In these cases, the visceral veins, tributaries of the portal system, use the phrenocolic ligament as a bridge to reach the wall and form an anastomosis with the caval veins.

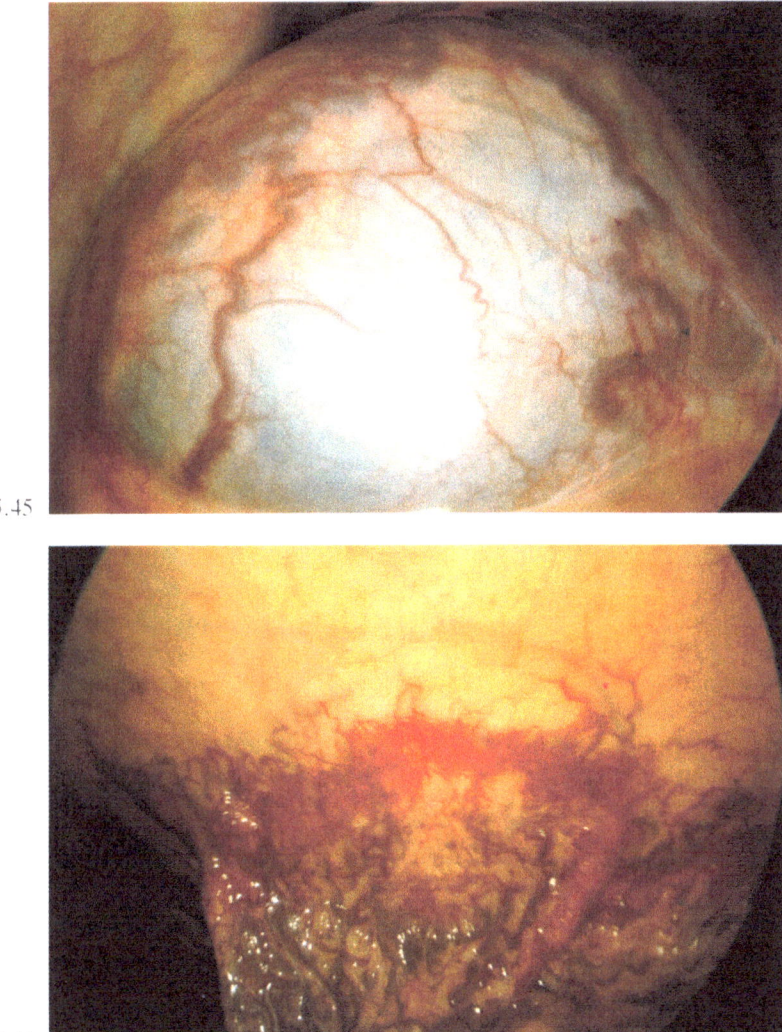

5.45

5.46

Fig. 5.45. *Collateral circulation from portal hypertension* formed by "cystic group" veins. Detail of the small veins on the serosa of the gallbladder wall; they appear dilated and tortuous

Fig. 5.46. *Collateral circulation from portal hypertension in adhesions.* Detail of the upper abdominal wall showing the insertion of a number of highly vascularized adhesions with multiple anastomoses with the parietal veins

If, either due to peritonitis or prior to surgery, *adhesions* are present between the organs and the wall, they may appear to have a rich venous network. This is a typical sign of portal hypertension, the adhesion serving as a newly formed bridge across which portal blood, under the influence of the increased portal pressure, drains into the systemic circulation (Fig. 5.46).

It is important to consider alterations of the spleen. In portal hypertension, the main finding is *splenomegaly*. This clinical sign can now be confirmed and well elucidated using imaging techniques, so now the advantages of laparoscopy are limited. If spleen enlargement is not severe, it cannot even be easily evaluated using endoscopy. Furthermore, in cirrhosis the spleen presents no particular or significant laparoscopic characteristics, the picture corresponding to that of the so-called fibrous or fibrocongestive splenomegalies, which may be due either to a primary splenopathy or which may be associated with or be secondary to liver cirrhosis. It is tricky establishing whether the splenomegaly is due to portal hypertension or another factor. There are no morphological visceral alterations to allow a reliable judgment to be made. The only criterion allowing a differentiation is that in some cases there are vein alterations revealing a collateral portacaval circulation, thus allowing us to link the splenomegaly with portal hypertension. But on these occasions portal hypertension may be severe enough to cause splenomegaly, but fail to cause any visible vein alterations, and because of this it cannot be detected laparoscopically. Nor can any link be found between the degree of spleen enlargement [80] seen laparoscopically and the portohepatic gradient, measured using suprahepatic vein catheterization [83]. It is therefore clear that splenomegaly cannot be considered a reliable sign of portal hypertension.

Biopsy is usually disappointing, generally revealing nonspecific alterations which are not conducive to making the diagnosis. Spleen biopsy is not indicated unless there are signs of splenopathy of a different nature.

Laparoscopic inspection of the spleen is therefore of little use for ascertaining portal hypertension in the cirrhotic patient.

In the presonographic era, laparoscopy was particularly important because it provided reliable signs of the state of the liver and therefore gave information as to whether hypertension was intra-, pre-, or posthepatic. Now it is fairly easy to distinguish between the different forms with sonography. Prehepatic portal hypertension in particular gives very clear sonographic pictures. Laparoscopy is therefore no longer used for this purpose. But it is still valuable, for it reveals collateral circulations consisting of small peritoneal vessels, vessels that imaging techniques fail to reveal. Laparoscopy enables us to detect: (a) the *early signs* of portal hypertension and (b) the *different "types"* of collateral circulation.

5.4.2 Present Indications for Laparoscopy

1. The initial alterations occur at the smaller veins, and laparoscopy enables us to discover the *early signs* of a collateral circulation. It is particularly important to explore areas of the peritoneum, such as the falciform and phrenocolic ligaments, the lateral peritoneal recesses, and adhesions, because here collateral circulations tend to form first, there being natural connexions between the two venous systems (see Fig. 5.1).

2. Laparoscopy is therefore the most sensitive means for ascertaining even moderate portal hypertension signs and it provides findings that enable us to distinguish between *different types of collateral circulation.*

Esophagogastroscopy, sonography, and CT demonstrate the presence of collateral circulations made up of large veins. Laparoscopy can also be used to study the circulations of the smaller veins. Although the larger veins are important for portal flow, the smaller veins are equally important from a functional viewpoint because they are very numerous. If the endoscopic and sonographic findings are combined, a complete chart for the large and small veins is obtained showing all the collateral circulations in each particular case.

The collateral circulations can have completely different characteristics. In some cases they involve the entire venous bed, on other occasions only a part of it. Although this is difficult to explain, we can say that the collateral circulation in portal hypertension can definitely be either *total* or *regional* [81]. And with the help of laparoscopy *three types of collateral circulation* can be found, each having a different clinical picture.

Type I is characterized laparoscopically by severe and extensive abdominal vessel involvement (Fig. 5.47); the gastric veins are spared, and varices are not present at gastroscopy. Of the 311 cases of portal hypertension in our series, 119 were type 1 (38.4%). Although gastroesophageal bleeding does not occur in this category, ascites is common [51 cases (42.9%)].

Type II is the opposite of type 1; the peritoneum is laparoscopically normal and the collateral circulation develops exclusively along the gastric veins (right, left, and short) (Fig. 5.48). Gastroesophageal varices are a significant finding at gastroscopy and arteriography, while the small peritoneal vessels are not involved. This group accounts for about 16% of all cases of portal hypertension. Gastrointestinal bleeding occurs at an early stage in more than 68% of cases, but ascites is rare [three cases (1.5%)].

In *type III* (45.6% of cases of portal hypertension) gastroesophageal varices are present and peritoneal veins are involved, the collateral circulations utilizing all or most of the available anastomotic connections (Fig. 5.49). The effect of the portal hypertension is evenly distributed throughout the intraabdominal venous system. The clinical picture is characterized by ascites [67 cases [47%)] and gastrointestinal bleeding [41 cases (29%)], which occurs in fewer cases (29%) and only at an advanced stage.

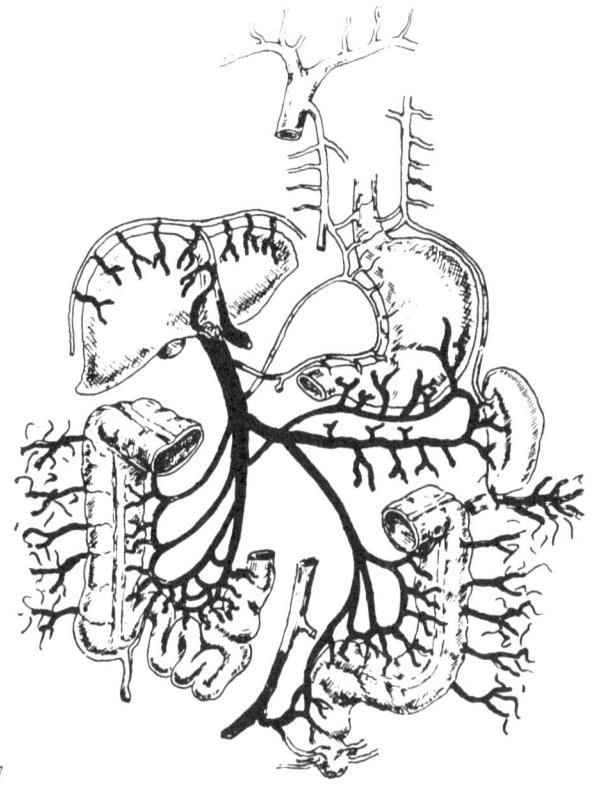

5.47

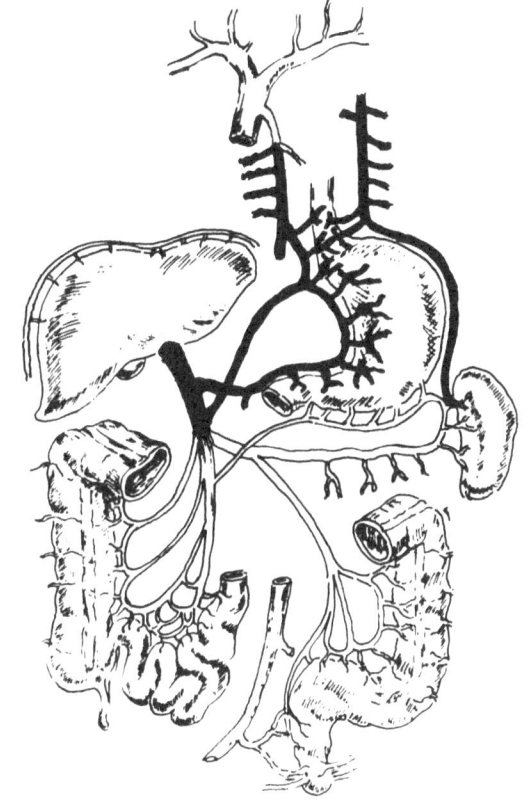

5.48

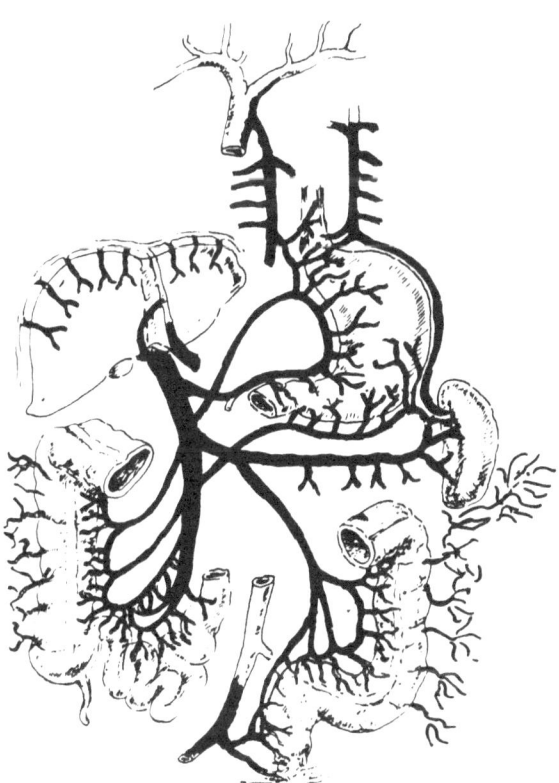

5.49

Fig. 5.47. *Dagnini's type I collateral circulation* [81]. The peritoneal venous system is involved: accessory venae portae, Retzius system, gastroepiploic vein and its branches; the umbilical vein may be recanalized. The right and left gastric veins and the venae gastricae breves are unaffected

Fig. 5.48. *Dagnini's type II collateral circulation* [81]. The peritoneal, gastroepiploic vein and its branches, etc. are unaffected (no laparoscopic signs of portal hypertension). The collateral circulation has developed exclusively at the expense of the right and left gastric veins and venae gastricae breves, which anastomose with the espophageal plexus

Fig. 5.49. *Dagnini's type III collateral circulation* [81]. All sections of the venous bed are involved. There are anastomoses at every level between the portal and caval systems

Our classification is most useful for predicting the likelihood of esophageal variceal bleeding and is therefore of particular value to the surgeon. A type II collateral circulation, associated with a high risk of bleeding, is the specific finding that indicates bleeding is almost inevitable in these patients. Surgical or endoscopic treatment is not indicated in type I patients, and is rarely indicated in type III patients.

The classification clearly indicates that patients with type II collateral circulation have the highest risk of hemorrhage because the gastroesophageal varices bear the entire pressure from portal hypertension, so hemorrhage is almost certain to occur. These patients therefore appear the most suitable candidates for prophylactic treatment especially now, with effective low-risk procedures, such as endoscopic sclerosis of varices.

Prophylaxis is undertaken but it is not yet certain whether the sclerosis is beneficial when performed in patients considered at risk endoscopically, but who have not yet had a hemorrhage. According to some, prophylaxis reduces the number of hemorrhages by two-thirds [82–84], while others [85–86] have misgivings.

The results depend greatly upon patient selection. When the predictive criteria used by the Japanese school [87] for the endoscopic findings of gastroesophageal varices were combined with those for laparoscopy (patients with type II collateral circulation according to our classification), then patients bound to have hemorrhages could be chosen and the results of prophylactic sclerosis improved upon.

5.4.3 Conclusions

1. Imaging techniques detect alterations in the larger veins, but laparoscopy is still of value because it identifies collateral circulations formed by small vessels that are too small to be detected with ultrasound.

2. By laparoscopically studying the small peritoneal vessels, we identify early collateral circulations and can then divide them into *three categories* of portal hypertension, thus identifying which patients are most likely to have hemorrhages from ruptured gastroesophageal varices.

References

1. Dagnini G, Bergamo S, Caldironi MW, Marin G, Patella N, Salmi A (1979) Validità e limiti delle prove diagnostiche in epatologia. Laparoscopia ed epatobiopsia. In: Attualità in diagnostica e terapia delle malattie del fegato e delle vie biliari. Il pensiero scientifico Editore, Roma
2. Vogel HM, Scherer K, Look D (1980) Comparative studies of laparoscopy, histology and gray-scale echotomography in diffuse diseases of the liver. Endoscopy 12:166–174
3. Mörl M (1987) Laparoscopy-present situation and prospects. Endoscopy 19:167–168
4. Buscarini L, Sbolli G, Civardi G, Di Stasi M, Fermi S, Buscarini E, Cavanna L, Fornari F (1987) La biopsie percutanée guidée sous échographie modifie-t-elle les indications de la laparoscopie en hépatologie? Acta Endoscopica 2:85–87
5. Savarino V, Magnolia MR, Scalabrini P, Piciotto A, Percario G, Bonello A, Zentilin P, Dodero M, Celle G (1987) Are sonography and radionuclide investigation alternative or complementary in diagnosing liver diseases? A comparison between these methods and laparobiopsy. Ital J Gastroenterol 19:5–9
6. Celle G, Savarino V, Picciotto A, Magnolia MR, Scalabrini P, Dodero M (1988) Is hepatic ultrasonography a valid alternative tool to liver biopsy? Report on 507 cases studied with both techniques. Dig Dis Sci 33(4):467–471
7. Lindner H (1973) Why laparoscopy? Acta Gastroenterol Belg 36:595–602
8. Henning H (1987) Hepatomegaly and inflammatory disease of the liver and gallbladder. In: Sivak MV (ed) Gastroenterologic endoscopy. Saunders, Philadelphia
9. Dagnini G (1980) Chronic persistent hepatitis. In: Clinical laparoscopy. Piccin Medical, Padua
10. Boyd WP (1982) Relative diagnostic accuracy of laparoscopy and liver scanning techniques. Gastrointest Endosc 28(2):104–106
11. Lewis E (1984) Screening for diffuse and focal liver disease: the case for hepatic sonography. J Clin Ultrasound 12:67–73
12. Sandford NL, Walsh P, Matis C, Baddeley H, Powel LW (1985) Is ultrasonography useful in the assessment of diffuse parenchymal disease? Gastroenterology 89:186–191
13. Dodero M, Celle G, Rovida S (1981) Ruolo attuale della laparoscopia in epatologia. Recenti Prog Med 4:400–408
14. Morèto M, Tertillano M, Zabella M, Suàrez M, Ibànez N (1988) Diagnostic yield and endoscopic patterns of laparoscopy in the diagnosis of granulomatous hepatitis. Endoscopy 20:294–297
15. Savarino V, Biggi E, Manzi C, Derchi L, Testa R, Cicio GR, Picciotto A (1980) Il valore dell'ecotomografia in rapporto alla laparobiopsia nella diagnosi delle epatiti diffuse. Minerva Dietol Gastroenterol 26:79–84
16. Buscarini L, Fornari F, Felice G (1985) La diagnosi delle epatopatie diffuse e a focolaio: ecografia e

laparoscopia a confronto. Sanità – Telex 106:58–67

17. Fukumoto Y, Okita K, Kodama T, Moda K, Nazida T, Pakimoto I (1980) Peritoneoscopic findings and liver function in chronic liver disease. Endoscopy 12:68–75

18. Anthony PP, Ishak KG, Nayak NC, Poulsen HE, Scheuer PJ, Sobin LH (1977) The morphology of cirrhosis: definiton, nomenclature and classification. Bull W H O 55(4):521–540

19. Ursin E, Spech HJ, Liehr H (1974) Laparoskopie and Lebersarkoidose. Med Klin 69:681–686

20. Le Verger JC, Gosselin M, Launois B, Gastard G (1977) Sarcoidose et hipertension portale. Présentation de 2 cas et revue de la littérature. Gastroenterol Clin Biol I:661–669

21. Castañeda Guillot C, Gragoso Arbelo T (1984) La laparoscopia en la enfermedad de Wilson. Rev Cubana Pediatr 56:221–226

22. Onji M, Yamashita Y, Kato T, Kondo H, Bandon H, Horiike N, Ohta Y (1987) Laparoscopic histopathological analysis of gentle undulation findings observed in patients with primary biliary cirrhosis. Endoscopy 19:17–19

23. Nord HJ (1982) Biopsy diagnosis of cirrhosis: blind percutaneous versus guided direct vision techniques. A review. Gastrointest Endosc 28(2):102–104

24. Coppo M, Paterlini P (1987) Aggiornamento di alcuni aspetti della cirrosi epatica. G Clin Med 2:69–85

25. Anonymous (1971) Clarity and confusion in active chronic hepatitis. Br Med J 4:126–127 (editorial)

26. Heit HA, Johnson LF, Rabin L (1978) Liver surface characteristics as observed during laparoscopy correlated with biopsy findings. Gastrointest Endosc 24:288–290

27. Pagliaro L, Rinaldi F, Craxi A, Di Plazza S, Filippazzo G, Gatto G, Ginova G, Magrin S, Maringhini A, Orsini S, Palazzo U, Spinello M, Vinci M (1983) Percutaneous blind biopsy versus laparoscopy with guided biopsy in diagnosis of cirrhosis. A prospective, randomized trial. Dig Dis Sci 28(1):39–43

28. Orlandi P (1979) Observer error in morphological diagnosis of chronic active hepatitis and cirrhosis. Ital J Gastroenterol 11:5–8

29. Zotti S, Papaleo E, Marin G, Patella M, Bergamo S, Caldironi MW, Cecchetto A, and Dagnini G (1981) Laparoscopy and liver biopsy in the morphological diagnosis of cirrhosis: concordance and diagnostic validity. Ital J Gastroenterol 13:14–17

30. Dagnini G, Zotti S, Marin G, Caldironi MW, Patella M, Cecchetto A (1986) Laparoscopy and guided biopsy in the diagnosis of cirrhosis. Ital J Gastroenterol 18:93–96

31. Galambos JT (1985) Classification of cirrhosis. Am J Gastroenterol 64(6):437–451

32. Harihara S, Monna T, Yamamoto S (1980) The prognostic value of peritoneoscopic findings in patients with liver cirrhosis. Gastroenterol J.P.N. 15(4):379–384

33. Scheuer PJ (1970) Liver biopsy in the diagnosis of cirrhosis. Gut 11:275–278

34. Orlando R, Lirussi F, Muraca M, Naccarato R, Okolicsanyi L (1988) Smooth liver surface may conceal cirrhosis. Evidence for the late development of nodular surface of the cirrhotic liver. Endoscopy 20:323–325

35. Pagliaro L, Simonetti R, Craxi A, Spanò C, Filippazzo M, Palazzo U, Patti S, Giannuoli G, Maraffa A, Colombo M, Tommasini M, Bellentani S, Villa E, Manenti F, Caporaso N, Coltorti M, Del Vecchio-Blanco C, Farsi P, Smedile A, Verme G (1981) Alcohol and HBV infection as risk factor for hepatocellular carcinoma in Italy: a multicentric, controlled study. Hepatogastroenterology 30:48–50

36. Buscarini L, Sbolli G, Cavanna L, Civardi G, Di Stasi M, Buscarini E, Fornari F (1987) Clinical and diagnostic features of 67 cases of hepatocellular carcinoma. Oncology 44(2):93–97

37. Dagnini G (1987) Laparoscopy in cirrhosis and portal hypertension. In: Sivak MV (ed) Gastroenterologic endoscopy Saunders, Philadelphia

38. Attali P, Prod'homme S, Pelletier G, Papoz L, Buffet C, Etienne J (1985) Carcinomes hépatocellulaires en France. Aspects cliniques, biologiques et virologiques chez 197 malades. Gastroenterol Clin Biol 9:396–402

39. Chlebowski R, Tong M, Weissman J, Block J, Ramming K, Weiner J, Bateman J, Chlebowski J (1984) Hepatocellular carcinoma: diagnostic and prognostic features in North American patients. Cancer 53:2701–2706

40. Luna G, Florence L, Johansen K (1985) Hepatocellular carcinoma: a 5 year institutional experience. Am J Surg 149:591–594

41. Nagasue N, Yukaya H, Hamada T, Hirose S, Kanashima R, Inokuchi K (1984) The natural history of hepatocellular carcinoma. A study of 100 untreated cases. Cancer 54:1461–1465

42. Nagasue N, Yukaya H, Ogawa Y, Sasaki Y, Akamizu H, Hamada T (1985) Hepatic resection in the treatment of hepatocellular carcinoma: report of 60 cases. Br J Surg 72:292–295

43. Dagnini G, Caldironi MW, Aldinio MT (1986) Tumori epatici primitivi: laparoscopia. Il fegato 32:121–124

44. Dagnini G, Zotti S, Caldironi MW, Piccigallo E (1984) La laparoscopia e la biopsia epatica nella diagnosi dei tumori del fegato. Ther Essenz Clin 12:641–643

45. Zaman S, Melia W, Johnson R, Portman B, Johnson P, Williams R (1985) Risk factors in development of hepatocellular carcinoma in cirrhosis: prospective study of 613 patients. Lancet I 8442, 1357–1359

46. Association for the Study of the Liver (AISF) (1984) Hepatitis B virus infection markers in chronic liver disease in Italy. The results of a multiregional investigation. Ital J Gastroenterol 16:195–200

47. Zotti S, Piccigallo E, Rampinelli L, Romagnoli GC, Tufano A, Dagnini G (1986) Primary and metastatic tumors of the liver associated with cirrhosis. A study based on laparoscopy and autopsy. Gastrointest Endosc 32(2):91–95

48. Dagnini G, Caldironi MW, Marin G, Buzzaccarini O, Tremolada C, Ruol A (1986) Laparoscopy in abdominal staging of esophageal carcinoma. Gastrointest Endoscopy 32(6):400–402

49. Buffet C, Pelletier G, Etienne JP (1983) Que reste-t-il de la laparoscopie en 1983? Gestroenterol Clin Biol 7:134–140

50. Le Carrer M, Poupon RY, Ballet F, Darnis F (1980) Les infection du liquide d'ascite chez le cirrhotique: étude clinique et biologique de 36 épisodes observés au cours d'une année. Gastroenterol Clin Biol 4:640–645

51. Ebara M, Ohto M, Shinagawa T, Sugiura N, Kimura K, Matsutani S, Morita M, Saisho H, Tsuchya Y, Okuda K (1986) Natural history of minute hepatocellular carcinoma smaller than three centimeters complicating cirrhosis. A study in 22 patients. Gastroenterology 90:289–298

52. Boyce WH, Jr, Nord HJ (1981) The hepatic nodule. Gastrointest Endosc 27(2):104–105

53. Boyd WP (1982) Relative diagnostic accuracy of laparoscopy and liver scanning techniques. Gastrointest Endosc 28(2):104–106

54. Lightdale C (1984) Screening for diffuse and focal liver disease: a gastroenterologist's viewpoint. J Clin Ultrasound 12:93–94

55. Spinelli P, Dal Fante M, Garbagnati F, Masciadri N, Pizzetti P (1984) Ultrasonography in the diagnosis of hepatic tumors. Ital Surg Sci 14(2):103–110

56. Fornari F, Rapaccini GL, Cavanna L, Civardi G, Fedeli G, Buscarini L (1988) Diagnostic of hepatic lesions: ultrasonically guided fine needle biopsy or laparoscopy? Gastrointest Endosc 34(3):231–234

57. Dubbins PA, O'Riordan D, Melia WM (1981) Ultrasound in hepatoma: can specific diagnosis be made? Br J Radiol 54:307–311

58. Fornari F, Cavanna L, Civardi G, Foroni R, Rossi S, Tansini P, Di Stasi M, Buscarini E, Buscarini L (1985) Ultrasonically guided fine-needle aspiration biopsy: first-stage invasive procedure in the diagnosis of focal lesions of the liver. Ital J. Gastroenterol 17:246–251

59. Lewis E (1984) Screening for diffuse and focal liver disease: the case for hepatic sonography. J Clin Ultrasound 12:67–73

60. Buscarini E, Fornari F, Cavanna L, Di Stasi M, Civardi G, Buscarini L (1985) Laparoscopia ed ecografia nella diagnosi di epatopatia cronica e di neoplasia. Ultrasuonodiagnostica 6:15–22

61. Sandler MA, Petrocelli RD, Marks DS, Lopez R (1980) Ultrasonic features and radionuclide correlation in liver cell adenoma and focal nodular hyperplasia. Radiology 135:393–397

62. Rogers JV, Mack LA, Freeny PC, Jonson ML, Sones PJ (1981) Hepatic focal nodular hyperplasia: angiography, CT, sonography and scintigraphy. AJR 137:983–990

63. Porcel A, Tubiana JM, Joffre F, Monnier JP, Bigor JN, Chermet J (1982) Adénome et hyperplasie nodulaire focal du foie; intérêt des examens radiologiques: a propos de quinze observations chez l'adulte. Ann Radiol (Paris) 25:175–183

64. Mirk P, Rubaltelli L, Bazzocchi M, Busilacchi P, Candiani P, Ferrari F, Giuseppetti G, Maresca G, Rizzato G, Volterrani L, Zappasodi F (1982) Ultrasonographic patterns in hepatic hemangiomas. J Clin Ultrasound 10:373–378

65. Itali Y, Ohomoto K, Araki T, Furui S, Ilio M, Atomi Y (1983) Computed tomography and sonography of cavernous hemangioma of the liver. AJR 141:315–320

66. Onodera H, Ohta K, Oikawa M, Abe M, Kanno T, Yoda B, Goto Y (1983) Correlation of the real-time ultrasonographic appearance of hepatic hemangiomas with angiography. J Clin Ultrasound 11:421–425

67. Koch H, Henning H, Friederich K, Lüders CJ (1984) Laparoskopische Beobachtungen zum gelben Fleck einer fokalen Leberverfettung. Z Gastroenterologie 5:250–254

68. Scott WW, Sanders RC, Siegelmann SS (1980) Irregular fatty infiltration of the liver: diagnostic dilemmas. AJR 135:67–71

69. Solis Herruzo JA, Duran A, Colina F, Santalla F, Garcia-Cabezudo J, Muñoz-Yauge MT, Morillas JD (1985) Laparoscopic and histological problems in the diagnosis of nodular regenerative hyperplasia of the liver. Endoscopy 17:105–108

70. Solbiati L, Livraghi T, Del Pra L, Jerace T, Masciadri N, Ravetto C (1985) Fine needle biopsy of hepatic hemangioma with sonographic guidance. AJR 144:471–474

71. Salmi A, Paterlini A, Buffoli F (1985) Carcinoma epatocellulare su cirrosi (C.E.C.): diagnosi ecografica laparoscopica. G Ital Endosc Dig 3:368–369

72. Tanaka S, Kitamura T, Ohshima A, Umeda K, Okuda S, Ohtani T, Tasuta M, Yamamoto K (1985) Diagnostic accuracy of ultrasonography for hepatocellular carcinoma. Cancer 56:660–666

73. Chen DS, Sheu JC, Sung JL, Lai MY, Lee CS, Su CT, Tsang YM, Wang SM, Yu JY, Yang TH, Wang CY, Hsu CY (1982) Small hepatocellular carcinoma – a clinico-pathological study in thirteen patients. Gastroenterology 83:1109–1119

74. Cottone M, Marcenò MP, Maringhini A, Rinaldi F, Russo G, Sciarrino E, Turri M, Pagliaro L (1983) Ultrasound in the diagnosis of hepatocellular carcinoma associated with cirrhosis. Radiology 147:517–519

75. Glazer GM, Laing FC, Brown TW, Gooding GAW (1980) Sonographic demonstration of portal hypertension: the patent umbilical vein. Radiology 136:161–163

76. Ishikawa T, Tsukune Y, Ohyama Y, Fujikawa M, Sakujama K, Fujii M (1980) Venous abnormalities in portal hypertension demonstrated by CT. AJR 134:271–276

77. Juttner HU, Jenney JM, Ralls PW, Goldstein LI, Reynolds TB (1982) Ultrasound demonstration of portosystemic collaterals in cirrhosis and portal hypertension. Radiology 142:459–463

78. Kane RA, Katz SG (1982) The spectrum of sonographic findings in portal hypertension: a subject review and new observation. Radiology 142:453–458

79. Salmi A, Paterlini A (1986) Sonographic patent umbilical vein: lack of specificity for portal hypertension. Am J Gastroenterol 8(7):556–558

80. Zuin R, Gatta A, Merkel C, Zotti S, Amodio P, Milani L, Dagnini G (1982) Evaluation of peritoneoscopic and oesophagoscopic findings as indexes of portal hypertension in patients with liver cirrhosis. Ital J Gastroenterol 14:214–219

81. Dagnini G (1975) L'importanza della laparoscopia nello studio dell'ipertensione portale. Minerva Med 66:432–442

82. Paquet KJ (1982) Prophylactic endoscopic sclerosing treatment of the esophageal wall in varices – a prospective controlled randomized trial. Endoscopy 14:4–5

83. Paquet KJ, Koussouris P (1986) Is there an indication for prophylactic endoscopic paravariceal injection sclerotherapy in patients with liver cirrhosis and portal hypertensions? Endoscopy 18:32–35

84. Bovero E, Farese A (1987) Scleroterapia profilattica delle varici esofagee: contributo clinico-manometrico. G Ital Endosc Dig 3:223–228

85. Koch H, Henning H, Grimm H, Soehendra N (1986) Prophylactic sclerosing of esophageal varices – results of prospective controlled study. Endoscopy 18:40–43

86. Terblanche J (1986) Sclerotherapy for prophylaxis of variceal bleeding. Lancet 26:961–963

87. Beppu K, Inokuchi K, Koyanagi N (1981) Prediction of variceal hemorrhage by esophageal endoscopy. Gastrointest Endosc 27:213–218

6 Laparoscopy in Oncology

Laparoscopy is indicated in the diagnosis and the study of abdominal tumors:

1. When the diagnosis suggests that an abdominal neoplasm is probable or likely but the situation is not clarified by the clinical, laboratory, and radiological findings.
2. In abdominal "staging" of a known malignant tumor.
3. For "follow-up" and "restaging" of a malignant tumor under therapy.

Noninvasive techniques and echoguided fine-needle biopsy have not replaced laparoscopy in the *diagnosis of tumors*, but they have certainly reduced its indications.

Laparoscopy is now, however, used increasingly often by oncologists to *stage malignant tumors*. So although the use of noninvasive techniques has increased in recent years, there has also been a steady increase in the number of "oncological" laparoscopies performed. In 1980 at the Padua center, 44% of the 1150 laparoscopies performed had been requested by oncologists, but in 1988 58% of the 1220 laparoscopies performed were required by oncologists. In fact, in spite of the contribution from non-invasive techniques, most oncologists still consider laparoscopy indispensable in the staging and the follow-up of certain tumors [1].

We have already discussed the present status of laparoscopy in the diagnosis of malignant abdominal neoplasms. We consider laparoscopy here in the *staging* and *follow-up* of malignant abdominal neoplasms.

6.1 Staging of Malignant Tumors

It is of prime importance to ascertain whether metastasis from a malignant tumor whose primary site is known has reached and involved the abdominal organs. First the clinical situation should be ascertained accurately in each patient so as to complete the diagnosis and to predict the course of the disease; it is of vital importance to establish whether the tumor has spread to the abdomen, in order to decide upon the most suitable therapeutic approach. Moreover, the need for definite and reliable data is felt on two fronts: (a) because therapy may be surgical and the procedures used for it have become more radical and (b) because while radiotherapy and drugs may be very effective and specific they are also highly toxic, and must therefore be used with precision and caution, and be based on highly selective criteria. The complex choice of the more suitable therapy and, in turn, its outcome, now depends greatly upon our knowledge of all the factors characterizing each particular picture. Abdominal exploration, made using all the available methods, is a crucial part of the study protocol for patients with a known malignant tumor that must be classified according to its particular "stage of evolution."

With malignant tumor *staging* the extent of diffusion from a known tumor is established with a view to:

1. Choosing the appropriate therapy.
2. Establishing a prognosis on the basis of reliable data.
3. Having a reliable reference point for follow-up, also in order to evaluate the efficacy of the particular therapy used – this is done for practical purposes or research.

There are two classical types of staging:

1. "*Clinical*," which is based upon information from the clinical history and the physical examination, laboratory data, and noninvasive investigations with protocols based on each patient's needs and the tumor characteristics.
2. "*Pathological*," which is based on all the available anatomical and histological data (marrow

biopsies, blind or target organ biopsies, puncturing for cytology, findings from laparoscopy or surgery). Pathological staging gives more reliable results, often demonstrating that the tumor spread is more extensive than that suggested by the outcome of clinical staging.

The need for a pathological staging led to the use even of laparotomy in malignant lymphomas.

Laparoscopy is simple and quick to perform, relatively inexpensive, and entails a low risk. Moreover, because it allows direct visualization of the abdominal organs, it enables us to take target biopsies which, in turn, provide invaluable findings. This technique has therefore become an extremely important tool for the pathological staging of tumors, although it does have shortcomings. Signs of a tumoral spread are less likely to escape detection at endoscopic exploration if the exploration is made thoroughly and meticulously and if each abdominal sector is explored, with the patient in all the possible decubitus positions. Above all, a search should be made for the sites of diffusion typical of each tumor in order to detect the smallest and earliest signs of metastasization. However, if the lesion is inaccessible to the laparoscope, all the precautions are useless and for this reason the possibility of false negatives for each tumor type should always be borne in mind. When laparoscopy is used for the pathological staging of a tumor it is of course governed by the same standards as those for the diagnosis of abdominal tumors.

The first invasive maneuver used to assess whether laparoscopy is indicated is transcutaneous fine-needle organ biopsy, which is either guided or blind if no sonographic "target" is indicated.

(a) If the biopsy is *positive* and clearly shows metastasis to the endoabdominal structures, laparoscopy is superfluous. This finding must, however, be definite as otherwise "false positives" may be obtained. (b) If the preliminary study is doubtful, laparoscopy is called for. (c) If no abdominal spread is found but the tumor characteristics suggest that metastasis is possible, then laparoscopy is indicated.

6.2 Follow-up and Restaging

During therapy for a malignant neoplasm, the oncologist must be able to use all the information necessary to make as safe an appraisal as possible because he can thus see the most rational possible therapeutic strategy. Laparoscopy gives "pathological" data that are more reliable than clinical, radiological, and laboratory findings and it also provides highly useful information for staging. The technique was therefore also used in the follow-up of patients with tumors during therapy.

Laparoscopy is simple to perform and well tolerated and it can therefore be repeated from time to time, providing insight into the anatomopathological and histological situation, thereby enabling us to make the most reliable possible appraisal. It provides concrete criteria that indicate whether therapy should be interrupted or whether it should be adjusted. We were among the first to propose laparoscopic *follow-up* [2] for certain types of tumor. There is no doubt that laparoscopy is useful for occasionally making a "pathological" check of the abdominal situation, apart from and as well as exploratory laparotomy, which is widely used for carcinoma of the ovary.

Of course each tumor type presents particular problems and so there is no standardized strategy for follow-up. We used the following methodological scheme [3]:

1. If the *first laparoscopy* or laparotomy shows that the neoplasm has spread to the abdomen (spleen, liver, lymph nodes, and/or peritoneum, etc.) the aim of the second laparoscopy is to make a macroscopic and histological study to detect any changes due to therapy. The most opportune time to perform the laparoscopic control is decided upon in each individual case when a therapeutic cycle is completed – the oncologist decides this (type of tumor, variety, staging, etc.) and also establishes when the remission appears clinically complete.

Laparoscopy can be performed at different intervals, from a minimum of 3 to a maximum of 10 months and then later on it can be repeated several times.

In cases in which neoplastic lesions were evident at the first laparoscopy it is very important to make a morphological study and to compare the second laparoscopic findings with the descriptions and the photographs made at the first (Fig. 6.1). Multiple biopsies are, however, of crucial importance and should be taken from the areas with recognizable signs (such as residual scar tissue) of the neoplastic lesions (Fig. 6.2). Of course biopsies must be taken at all points in which traces of the tumor may be seen or suspected.

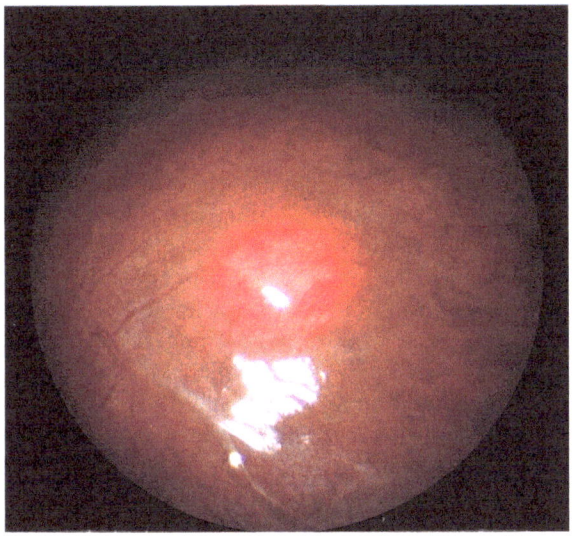
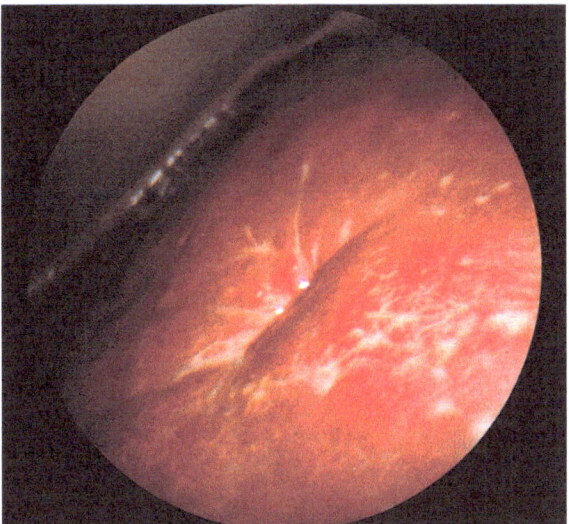

6.1

6.2

Fig. 6.1. Laparoscopic staging of a Hodgkin's disease lymphoma. Small roundish nodule that is raised slightly by the right lobe of the liver. Biopsy: *Hodgkin's disease lymphoma*

Fig. 6.2. Same case as in Fig. 6.2. Laparoscopic follow-up for Hodgkin's disease lymphoma performed 15 months later. Clinical remission achieved with polychemotherapy. Finding of scar tissue from the liver nodule. No traces of neoplastic tissue. Target biopsy: *negative*

2. Where the pathological staging did not demonstrate an abdominal spread, with a second look any prior negative finding can be checked. This is done mainly if, during therapy, any general or local clinical signs are observed (fever, weight loss, liver or spleen enlargement, lymphnode tumefaction) or if changes in the laboratory or radiological findings are found indicating that the tumor may have spread to the abdomen. Laparoscopy is performed to ascertain whether the various signs are related to the tumor or whether they have another cause or causes.

Finally, in the absence of new signs 24–36 months after suspension of therapy, control laparoscopy can be performed. In patients with a clinical recovery it can be performed to ascertain whether there is also a corresponding anatomical remission. I prefer to call this examination "*restaging*" as here we are dealing with an appraisal made at a distance, and to reserve the term "follow-up" for the controls which are made during therapy.

Laparoscopy is of definite value for follow-up and restaging and it is unlikely to be replaced by noninvasive methods, even those accompanied by fine-needle biopsy. These techniques are not reliable enough for staging because they carry a risk of false negatives. Nor can they be used for a distance control because here it is extremely difficult to rule out a false negative for malignancy. Even with laparoscopy it is difficult to work out whether or not previously detected lesions have now been sterilized, and it is practically impossible to take a biopsy from all the neoplastic focuses, even when using the most meticulous possible technique. In some of our cases four out of five biopsies failed to evidence tumor traces and in only one sample were neoplastic cells found [4]. Although we cannot specify the percentage of false negatives, we can say that recovery from previously demonstrated hepatic or splenic metastases is not evaluated reliably by laparobiopsy and so any impression of recovery may be false. In patients with a previous diagnosis of cancer of the ovary, for example, laparobiopsy may give a negative finding after therapy. A second surgical operation is, however, required for it should guarantee that any neoplastic residue overlooked at laparoscopy will be found.

However, the advantages of endoscopic abdominal exploration should never be underestimated for, among other reasons, this technique obviates laparotomy. So, although it has shortcomings and although noninvasive techniques are now available, laparoscopy is indicated for the follow-up and the restaging of patients with malignant tumors.

At present laparoscopy is part of a study protocol for the staging and follow-up of some malignant tumors that can be classified as:

1. Systemic tumors
2. Tumors with a primary extraabdominal localization
3. Tumors with a primary endoabdominal localization

In malignant neoplasms, laparoscopy enables us to choose the most suitable therapy – radiotherapy, chemotherapy, or surgery, or a combination. Where therapy is mainly surgical, laparoscopy can show whether it should be radical or palliative.

6.3 Systemic Tumors: Malignant Lymphomas

In order to have an idea of the present role of laparoscopy in the study of malignant lymphomas, a brief outline of its history is required.

Therapy for lymphomas was the first to give important results in the treatment of malignant tumors and different therapeutic alternatives became available (radiotherapy and different types of chemotherapy with drugs used alone or combined). Therefore, because different types of therapy were available, it became important to be able to distinguish between the different stages of lymphoma evolution in order to choose the most appropriate therapy.

In 1971, at the Ann Arbor Conference a classification was put forward, and this is still used today. The four stages are as follows:

Stage I: involvement of a single lymph node region (I), a single organ, or a nonlymph node site (IE).

Stage II: involvement of two, or more, lymph node regions on the same side of the diaphragm (II), or involvement circumscribed by a non-lymph-node organ or site and of one region, or more, on the same side of the diaphragm (IIE).

Stage III: involvement of the lymph node regions above and below the diaphragm (III), which may be accompanied by a circumscribed involvement of a non-lymph-node organ or site (IIIE), or of the spleen (IIIS) or of both (IIISE).

Stage IV: diffuse involvement of one organ, or more, or of non-lymph-node tissue, sometimes with lymph node tumefaction.

The stages are then qualified with an A or B depending on whether or not there are general symptoms, such as weight loss, fever, night sweats, and/or an increased erythrocyte sedimentation rate.

The goal of therapy and the way in which it is administered vary depending on the stage specified for each patient. Although some variations have been made in recent years, the classical schemes are still valid, surgery being limited to the stage IA localized forms. Stage I and II patients also undergo radiation only while polychemotherapy is indicated for stage III and IV patients. It is important to ascertain lymphoma spread to the abdomen because this finding changes both the therapeutic strategy and the prognosis.

In 1968 at the Stanford Center Gladstein et al. proposed exploratory laparotomy with diagnostic splenectomy using a rigorously standardized "oncological" technique that comprises several lymph node biopsies and serialized spleen examinations in order to guarantee that staging would be more reliable. This is still the most valid method available. Laparoscopy was first introduced for lymphoma staging in 1971 by De Vita et al. [5], at a time when laparosplenectomy was widely used and was considered extremely successful because it had demonstrated that "pathological" staging was much better than "clinical" staging. Laparotomy with splenectomy and multiple biopsies did in fact show that in about 30% of cases the disease was anatomically more advanced than suggested by the "clinical" study [6].

Laparoscopy appeared able to guarantee a good "pathological" staging, although it was less accurate and this technique was considered a second choice in the staging protocol for malignant lymphomas. It was at first used only in patients who could not undergo laparosplenectomy. Later on, laparoscopy was also used where the tumor spread to the liver and spleen was clinically highly suspicious and laparotomy considered superfluous. Gradually the oncological endoscopic technique was improved, so laparoscopy became a more effective means for staging; about 10 years ago laparoscopic results were comparable with subsequent laparotomic results in the study of the liver, but in the study of the spleen laparotomic results were highly superior. Laparoscopy and splenic biopsy revealed only 70%–75% of splenic lesions successively demonstrated with laparosplenectomy.

When systematic laparosplenectomy had been used for a few years, its shortcomings emerged: its mortality rate was negligible, but it had a high morbidity rate (up to 37%), with different types of immediate postoperative complications: pleural leakage, abscesses, intestinal canalization disturbances, and thromboembolic phenomena due to thrombocytosis associated with a high piastrinic adhesivity. These sequelae were not particularly serious but they led to a delay in initiating therapy. Above all, the most serious late complication, which occurred after radio- and polychemotherapy, was sepsis; this potentially fatal sequela was the most worrying aspect of laparosplenectomy. Observed in up to 21% of cases, if almost exclusively affected splenectomized patients and was a consequence of immune deficiency [7]. Moreover, these observations were later confirmed. Healthy individuals who undergo splenectomy for trauma are also at a higher risk of developing bacterial infections, above all from pneumococcus or from type B *Haemophilus influenzae*. Among a total of 459 patients with lymphomas, 88 underwent splenectomy and subsequent polychemotherapy; 28% of these developed severe sepsis. Of the 371 patients who received chem. therapy alone without splenectomy, only 15.2% developed sepsis [8]. It was therefore opportune to ask whether the advantages of highly accurate staging compensated for the possible immediate complications of laparosplencetomy, particularly in view of their severity at a distance. Because of these reservations, fewer laparosplenectomies were performed, while there was a corresponding increase in the number of laparobiopsies; this technique was less accurate, but it was practically devoid of immediate or late complications and also was less costly.

In the early 1980s the procedure for the "pathological" staging of malignant lymphomas could be summarized as follows [3, 9]:

In *Hodgkin's disease lymphoma*, radiotherapy alone was used for stages I, IIA, and IIIA, while polychemotherapy was used for the other stages. The choice of therapy depended greatly upon staging, which therefore had to be accurate. The first invasive investigation consisted of laparoscopically guided splenic and hepatic biopsy; if the tumor was found to have spread to the spleen and liver, then these findings provided enough information for an appropriate therapy to be chosen. False laparoscopic negatives were made in about 25% of cases, so, if laparobiopsy findings were negative, then laparosplenectomy was always performed so as to avoid making false negatives and to initiate appropriate therapy. When these schemes were used, the number of surgical operations performed in Hodgkin's disease lymphoma was slightly reduced, with definite advantages, important ones being that therapy could be started immediately and hospital stay reduced.

In *non-Hodgkin's disease lymphoma*, on the other hand, laparotomy with splenectomy was almost completely abandoned, being replaced by laparoscopy. This tumor has an early and rapid diffusion and radiotherapy alone appeared inadequate, even in the early stages. A perfect laparotomic staging, with its disadvantages and risks, was considered superfluous because polychemotherapy was always used.

Nowadays a reliable appraisal for lymphoma staging must take into account two aspects that have substantially modified the situation: noninvasive techniques and technical and methodological progress by laparoscopy in oncology.

6.3.1 Imaging Techniques

In malignant lymphoma *noninvasive imaging techniques* do not give findings that are particularly conducive to discovering the signs of an abdominal diffusion. Liver and spleen involvement can give rise to different sonographic findings, depending on their type of diffusion. Moreover, focal lesions, which are quite infrequent, give rise to a hazy picture, which can be either hyper- or hypoechogenic. However, lesions under 1 cm in diameter cannot be detected. If the lymphomatous tissue diffusely infiltrates the spleen or the liver, and this commonly occurs, there may be a slightly generalized irregularity, with a prevalent increase or decrease in echoes, and this is difficult to interpret. In the vast majority of cases, however, the sonographic finding appears completely normal. In patients with lymphomatous infiltration the findings for the liver are frequently negative. Sonography sufficiently accurately indicates whether there is spleen or liver enlargement, but this datum is not very important because these organs can have normal dimensions even when the lymphoma has spread to them. They may, on the other hand, be enlarged but not contain the tumor. Overall, sonography does not reliably indicate diffuse lymphomas of the liver and spleen.

Our experience with sonography in lymphoma staging has been disappointing. In only 20% of cases of malignant Hodgkin's disease (41) and non-Hodgkin's disease (54) lymphoma were nodules echographically revealed in the spleen; in the remaining cases the picture was normal, or with slight, apparently insignificant modifications.

Only rarely are there liver nodules large enough for sonographic detection, so findings are positive in less than 5% of cases and this is in agreement with Bolondi et al., who found a sensitivity of 5.2% [10].

Computed tomographic scan is highly sensitive in the search for lymph nodes, but it does not satisfactorily reveal whether or not the abdominal organs are affected. In his staging for Hodgkin's disease patients, Castellino found that CT scan had a sensitivity of 64% for spleen tumors and 25% for liver tumors. He considered the efficacy of the different noninvasive or slightly invasive techniques in the staging or Hodgkin's disease lymphoma, and confirmed that angiography with lymphography is still the best available imaging technique in the evaluation of the aortic, caval, and iliac lymph nodes, stating that: (a) CT scanning more precisely defines the extent of bulky lymph node disease and also evaluates the higher paraaortic lymph nodes, which are not usually opacified with lymphography, but is not effective in the assessment of splenic or hepatic involvement in Hodgkin's disease, although its performance in these areas is as good as that of other imaging techniques; (b) ultrasound scanning provides information similar to that from CT although rigorous studies evaluating its accuracy have not been performed to provide information for decision making [11].

Magnetic resonance appears to be highly sensitive for liver lymphomas, but it is not so specific [12]. At present few series have been reported on this aspect, and not many appear to be in favor of this technique [13].

Fine-needle biopsy is simple to perform and highly effective; it has certainly enhanced the diagnostic potential of sonography and CT scan. It is very suitable for the puncturing of enlarged lymph nodes, in particular of the splenic or mesenteric hilum, of abdominal masses and, of course, the liver and spleen. Biopsy can be guided by echographic images or made blind if no focal lesions are demonstrated. As fine-needle biopsy, frequently used with brilliant results for the diagnosis of abdominal organ tumors, has not yet been widely applied in lymphoma staging, it is impossible to evaluate accurately its diagnostic potential in this branch.

Lymph node puncturing appears worthwhile because in about two-thirds of cases it allows us to diagnose lymphomatous infiltration and to make a satisfactory histological typification of the lymphoma. It is certainly more difficult than epithelial metastasis to diagnose, but it is fairly easy to recognize histiocytic and Hodgkin's disease lymphomas [14]. Liver and spleen puncturing give different results depending on whether focal lesions are detected with ultrasound and therefore a target biopsy is made, or biopsy is blind because no target can be found. Jansson et al. [15] obtained positive findings in Hodgkin's disease lymphoma with blind liver biopsy in only 1 case among 59 – in another 4 positivity was suspected. This failure is explained by the fact that Hodgkin's disease lymphoma often spreads in the form of small nodules that are unlikely to be reached by puncturing (Fig. 6.3). However, with non-Hodgkin's disease lymphomas the results are better: among 79 biopsies both in the liver and the spleen there were 9 positive and 9 suspect findings. Yet a "suspected" diagnosis does not allow staging, and so in these cases invasive techniques must be used.

The authors also point out that with a cytoaspirate it is often difficult to distinguish between normal and diseased lymphocytes, so some of the negative findings are presumably false. Here I feel it opportune to add that, for the same reasons, normal lymphocytes may be considered neoplastic, thus giving rise to false positives. Cavanna et al. [16] point out that simple CT and echographic images can provide important information, although this is valid only for clinical staging. Echoguided fine-needle biopsy used in non-Hodgkin's disease lymphoma patients with ultrasound-detected focal lesions gave the following results: in 13 out of 14 cases the diagnosis was confirmed: 11 true positives and 2 true negatives (checked laparoscopically), a success rate of 92%. This is a very high percentage but it is not absolute. It can only refer to cases with lymphomatous sites in the liver and spleen, nodules large enough for ultrasound detection and target biopsy. These conditions are ideal for the diagnosis, but they are quite rare. If all lymphomas are taken into consideration, then in the large majority of cases the liver and spleen have a "normal" ultrasound appearance, and it is possible to make a diagnosis with fine-needle biopsy in a far lower percentage of cases.

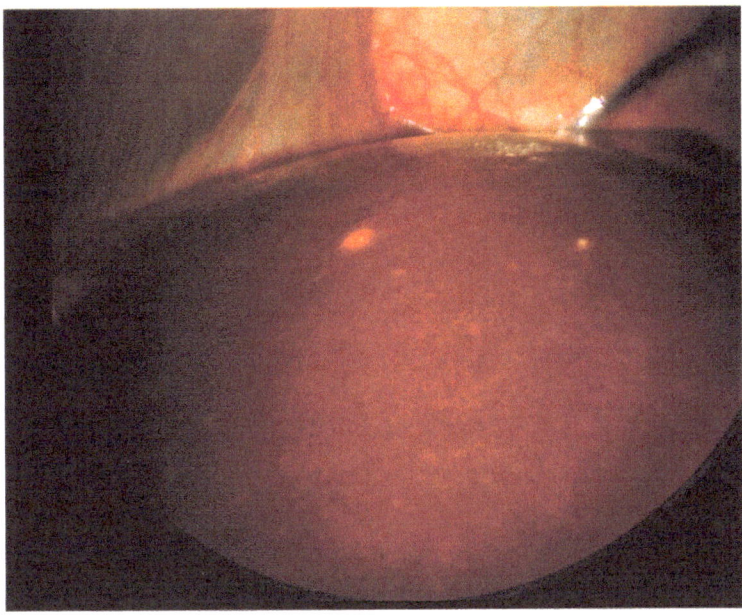

Fig. 6.3. Staging. View of the entire surface of the left lobe of the liver. Two tiny yellowy-white patches can be seen; there are others that are barely visible. Target biopsy: *Hodgkin's disease lymphoma*

These techniques are still very important and they are bound to improve. Therefore "ultrasonically guided fine-needle biopsy" can be considered a new, useful procedure in the management of patients with lymphoma. It can aid staging, restaging, and follow-up of such patients and, when it gives positive findings, it obviates more aggressive diagnostic procedures such as laparoscopy and exploratory laparotomy [17–20].

6.3.2 Progress in Oncological Laparoscopy

The *technique for oncological laparoscopy* is basically the same as it was several years ago, although progress has been made in hepatic and splenic biopsy (cutting needles, Bio-Plug, etc.) and they have greatly enhanced the results.

The method for oncological laparoscopy has greatly improved. A particularly thorough examination is made of all the explorable abdominal areas, with the patient in all types of decubitus position, while a probe is used to raise and shift the liver, spleen, omentum, etc. We can thus observe the largest possible organ surface area, discover any lesions, and search for enlarged lymph nodes (Fig. 6.4), peritoneal spread, etc. (Fig. 6.5). In lymphoma, in particular in its initial stages, the findings can be very few and far between and difficult to detect. *Spleen involvement*, which is the first step in subdiaphragmatic lymphoma diffusion, can appear as simple plaques or yellowish-white nodules that are isolated or confluent. In the earlier stages, when the spleen size is normal or there is only slight enlargement, it is difficult to see gross lesions. Small nodules, spots, or slight protuberances predominate. Very often the spleen, even if infiltrated by lymphomatous tissue, appears normal or has a slight alteration, such as a color variation or it has a surface scabrosity that is of uncertain significance. In the *liver* the lesions have analogous characteristics. Here too, in the early stages, gross conglomerates are rare: small nodules or spots against a normal liver are frequently observed (Fig. 6.3). Very often the liver has alterations that are not significant, with an accentuated lobular pattern and a yellowish hue that suggests local or diffuse steatosis (Fig. 6.6), or may be variegated and have bluishred spots. Very often the organ appears entirely normal. Considerable difficulty can be encountered in making a laparoscopic appraisal of the spread of a lymphoma to the abdominal organs. When the liver or spleen lesions are large (patches, nodular forms, etc.), then interpretation is easy. But if they are small and their number is limited they may be overlooked, so a careful search must be made in

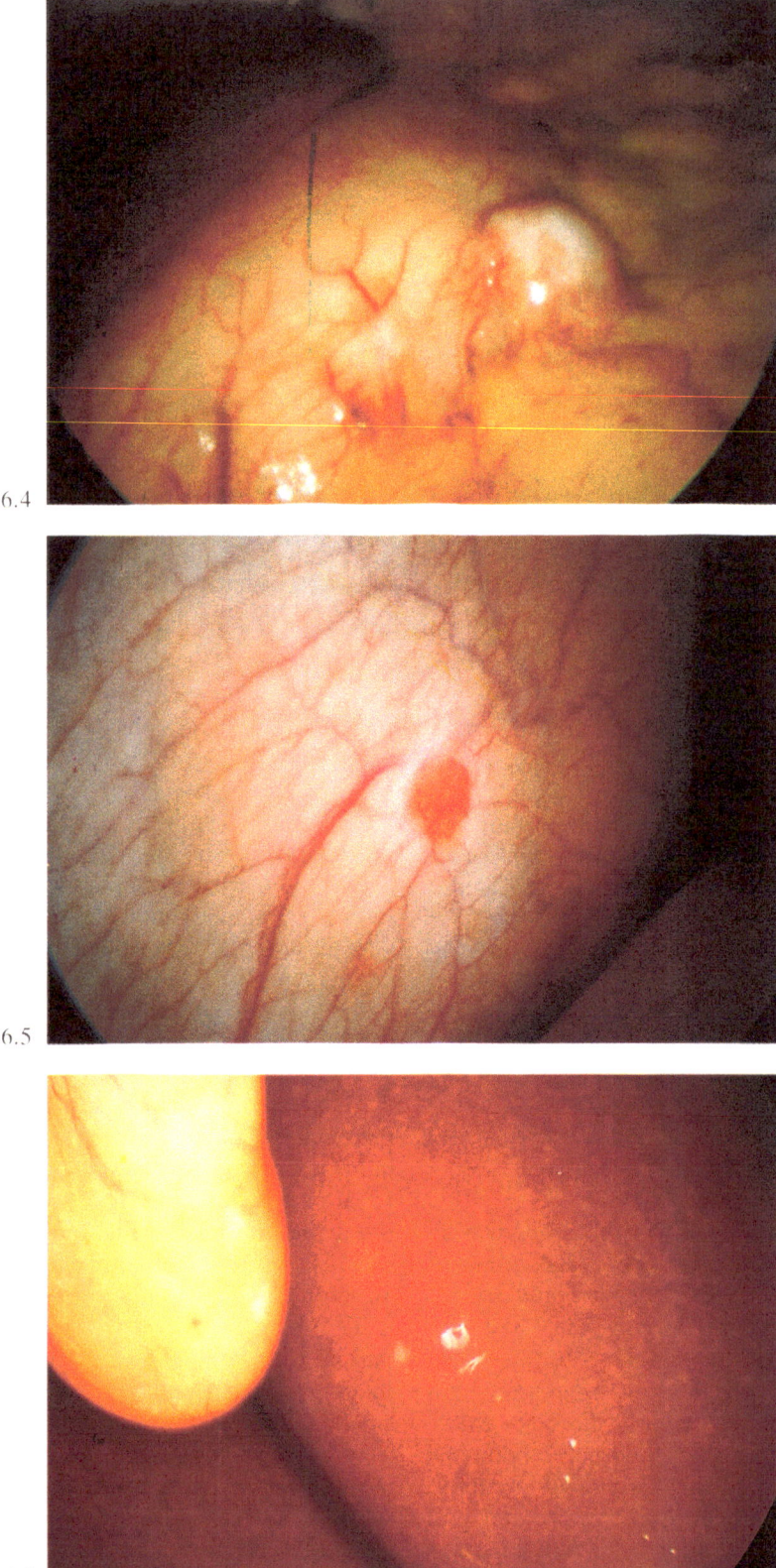

6.4

6.5

6.6

all areas of the organ. Where there is diffuse infiltration without apparent signs of lesions, the diagnosis is only bioptic. This technique has been greatly improved and the results now obtained can be highly satisfactory. As mentioned above, splenic biopsy has greatly improved the results of laparoscopy in the staging of malignant lymphomas. The validity of laparoscopy in this field cannot be considered if spleen biopsy is not routinely complementary to the technique, as for liver biopsy.

Of course the laparoscopic biopsy sample is taken from the lesion and this is the ideal condition for obtaining reliable and accurate data (Fig. 6.7). But it should be stressed that, above all in the absence of visible lesions when target puncturing cannot be performed, multiple biopsy is of great value. Of course the likelihood of collecting neoplastic tissue depends upon the size and number of samples taken. This applies in particular to staging of lymphomas (Fig. 6.8).

This was supported both for the liver and spleen [9, 21] and has also been recently reemphasized [22]. Monconduit et al. [23] studied patients with lymphoma without macroscopic liver lesions and found that in 4% of cases the histological finding was positive if a biopsy was taken from only one lobe, but it was positive in 17% if the biopsy was taken from both.

Multiple biopsies are even more important in the study of the diffusion of lymphomas to the spleen. In our series of 171 patients who underwent laparoscopy for staging Hodgkin's disease lymphomas and who were at clinical stages I and II, 21 patients had negative macroscopic splenic and liver findings. Biopsy was decisive because it demonstrated that the tumor had spread to these organs. Biopsy was taken from the liver in seven patients, four samples being taken from each: in

six cases neoplastic tissue was present in all the samples while in the remaining patient two samples were positive and two negative. Biopsies of the spleen were taken from 14 patients and in 8 the histological finding was positive in all the tissue samples obtained: in the remaining six, some samples were positive while others were negative. This indicates that with a single biopsy there would have been a considerable likelihood of making false negatives. In order to reduce further the number of false negatives, especially the splenic ones, we felt it opportune to set out some rules for performing biopsy on the basis of the single macroscopic findings as well as to explore the abdominal cavity in all its sectors, by searching in particular for the sites of any lymphoma propagation.

1. When both the spleen and liver appear laparoscopically normal, the following multiple biopsies must be obtained: three from different parts of the spleen and four from the liver – two from the right and two from the left lobe. If the spleen is not involved then neither is the liver [24]; in only one case has a lymphoma in the liver only been reported [25]. However, if at examination the spleen appears normal, we cannot rule out a lymphoma diffusion and so biopsies must also be taken from the liver.

2. When lesions suggest a lymphoma diffusion, target biopsies must be obtained. If only the spleen is affected, then four biopsies must be taken from the liver, even if it appears normal because it may be involved. If only the liver alone appears to be involved and the macroscopic finding is definite, then target organ biopsy is sufficient; it would be superfluous to take a biopsy from the spleen because, above all in non-Hodgkin's disease lymphoma, spread to the liver is unlikely without spleen involvement.

Since we started using this scheme, laparoscopy has become a far more effective method for malignant lymphoma staging.

The percentage of errors has considerably diminished and, although the problem of false negatives has always been negligible for the liver, we can now safely claim, in agreement with others [21, 20], that laparoscopic results are as valid as those of exploratory laparoscopy. The greatest progress has, however, been made in the study of the spleen, for here false laparoscopic negatives were made in a fairly high percentage of cases. In the last series of 244 Hodgkin's disease lymphomas

---

◄————————————————

Fig. 6.4. Staging. On the gastric serosa of the great curvature of the stomach can be seen nodular, whitish, raised formations. Biopsy: *non-Hodgkin's disease lymphoma*

Fig. 6.5. Staging. Normal parietal peritoneum. Flat pink plaque, with distinct border that is difficult to interpret. Biopsy: *peritoneal diffusion of Hodgkin's disease lymphoma*

Fig. 6.6. Staging. Detail of the surface of the liver which can simulate an accentuation in the lobular pattern from steatosis. Lymphomatous infiltration suspected. Biopsy: *non-Hodgkin's disease lymphoma*

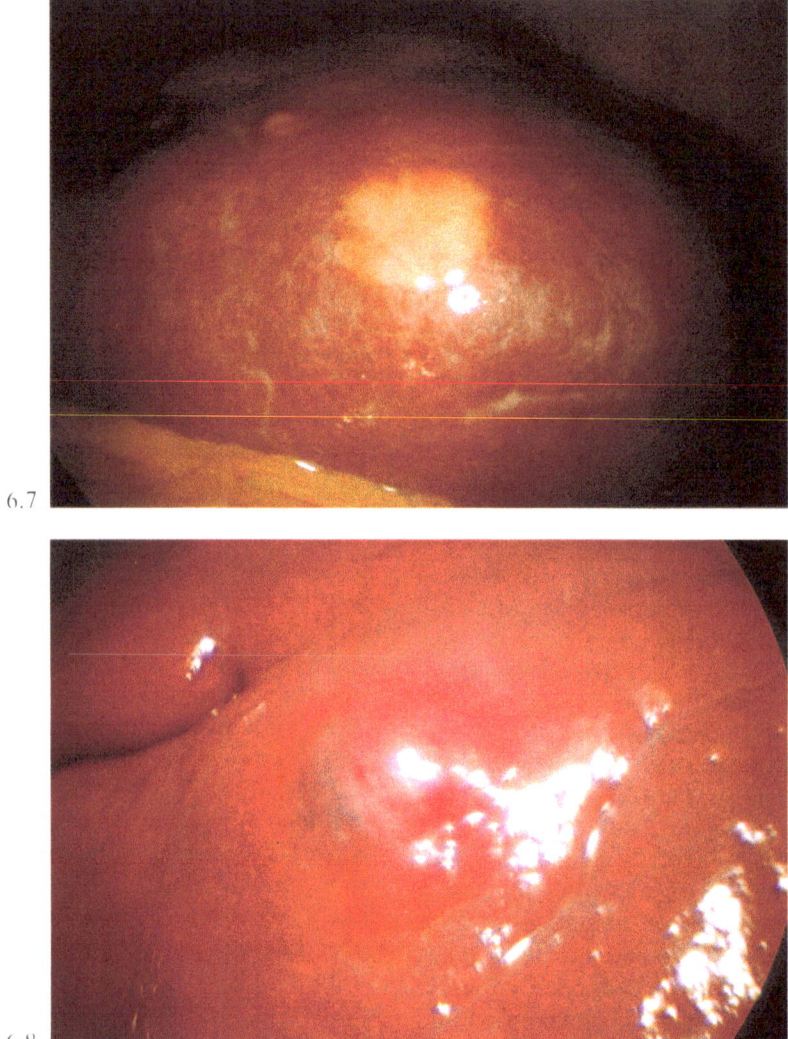

6.7

6.8

Fig. 6.7. Staging. Detail of the spleen surface on which can be seen a whitish plaque probably due to lymphomatous diffusion. Target biopsy: *non-Hodgkin's disease lymphoma*

Fig. 6.8. Staging. Surface of the spleen under high magnification has a normal appearance with a few insignificant irregularities. Multiple biopsies: *infiltration from Hodgkin's disease lymphoma*

we studied for staging, laparoscopically guided biopsy findings, made using the above-mentioned method, were negative for 80 patients; they subsequently had laparotomy with splenectomy to check the negative findings. In only eight cases had a neoplastic infiltration escaped laparoscopic detection; in six this affected only the spleen and in the remaining two it also involved the liver [26]. The percentages of false laparoscopic negatives in Hodgkin's disease lymphoma have therefore dropped in recent years – from 20%–25% down to 10%.

An overall consideration of the results of staging for malignant lymphomas attests to the progress made. In 171 of our Hodgkin's disease lymphoma stage I and II patients, laparoscopy showed a lymphoma infiltration to the spleen in 11% and to the liver in 7.6%. In about 30% of cases both the liver and spleen laparoscopically appeared normal, the neoplastic infiltration being detected only through biopsy.

In this series the laparoscopic findings resulted in an upstaging of categories with respect to the

Table 6.1. Laparoscopic and histological findings in 171 cases of Hodgkin's disease lymphoma, clinical stages I–II

Positive biopsy	Macroscopically negative
Spleen 19 (11%)	6
Liver 13 (7.6%)	4
Stage advancement after laparoscopy: 18.6%	

Table 6.2. Laparoscopic and histological findings in 147 cases of non-Hodgkin's disease lymphoma, clinical stages I–II

Biopsy positive	Macroscopically negative
Spleen 29 (20%)	14
Liver 22 (15%)	13
Stage advancement after laparoscopy: 35%	

clinical classification; in 18.6% of cases the percentages were very close to those obtained with laparosplenectomy (Table 6.1).

A non-Hodgkin's disease lymphoma is highly aggressive and has a greater tendency to spread rapidly to the liver and spleen without there being any nodular lesions, so the results of laparoscopic staging are even more indicative. Laparoscopy showed spleen involvement in 20% and liver involvement in 15% of 147 patients at clinical stages I and II. Forty-eight percent of the spleen tumors and 59% of the liver tumors could not be detected laparoscopically, but only histologically. Overall, on the basis of laparoscopic findings in 35% of cases stages I and II were upstaged to stages III and IV (Table 6.2).

Finally, it should be stressed that no accidents occurred in 244 Hodgkin's disease lymphomas and in 271 non-Hodgkin's disease lymphomas studied with laparoscopy and liver and spleen multiple biopsies.

6.3.3 Present Indications for Laparoscopy

Thanks to improvements in technique and method, laparoscopy is now almost on par with laparosplenectomy in the staging of lymphomas. At present laparoscopy has many advantages over surgery, its only disadvantage being that it is more likely to give rise to false negatives, although this occurs in only 10% of cases. The individual oncologist must therefore decide which of the following to use in each situation: (a) surgery for an accurate initial appraisal, in spite of its disadvantages, hinderances, sequelae, risks, and expense, or (b) laparoscopy, which gives a slightly less accurate staging but has no sequelae, risks, or high costs and therapy can be started immediately. Another disadvantage of laparotomy for staging is that it is almost always followed by adhesion formation, which hinders or precludes any later laparoscopies for follow-up, thus denying the oncologist data that would be very useful in deciding the therapeutic strategies.

At present laparotomy with splenectomy is performed less often than previously, only being used when strictly necessary. The larger oncology centers at Milan and Padua have a clear strategy for the study of malignant lymphomas in order to work out the most appropriate therapeutic program for each case and to decide upon the most rational possible therapeutic means. In *non-Hodgkin's disease lymphoma* laparoscopy alone is always performed. The main reason for this is not to have strict staging, because only small percentages of cases (no more than 20%) are stages I and II, and in any case polychemotherapy is always performed regardless of the stage, but rather to establish a clear anatomohistological reference point for subsequent evaluation of the outcome of therapy. The follow-up must therefore be based upon a specification of the prognosis.

In *Hodgkin's disease lymphoma* staging must be very rigorous in cases in which roentgen therapy is the only therapeutic program and in which it must be certain that patients are stage I and IIA. False negatives cannot be made. The use of laparosplenectomy is usually linked to the type of therapy used. In Stanford's group, and in general in the United States, where roentgen therapy is used for stage I, II, and IIIA patients, laparosplenectomy is still widely used. Laparoscopy is reserved for patients at a more advanced stage. Now, in the Italian centers the first invasive investigation to be used is laparoscopy with multiple biopsies. Laparosplenectomy is not only used when the laparobioptic findings are negative for abdominal diffusion, but also and mainly in cases in which there are elements, such as spleen enlargement or lymph node enlargement, that suggest that the lymphoma has spread to the abdomen. In the oncological center of Padua, this criterion is used:

from 1985 to 1987 among patients who underwent preliminary laparoscopy only five underwent laparosplenectomy – three of these were positive.

Furthermore, the protocols for therapy in recent years have been modified because polychemotherapy has given such favorable results that there is a tendency to use it also in association with roentgen therapy for stage II patients. Consequently, if a stage IIS or stage III patient is laparoscopically classified as stage II, the error is not serious because the same therapeutic protocol can be used for all these stages. This also explains why laparosplenectomy is now used less often in the staging of Hodgkin's disease lymphomas, in spite of the fact that it is more accurate than laparoscopy.

Needless to say if echography and fine-needle biopsy demonstrate that there is a definite spread to both the spleen and liver, then laparoscopy is redundant. However, if the spleen is positive and the liver is negative, laparoscopy must be performed in view of the high percentage of false negatives from liver fine-needle biopsy in Hodgkin's disease lymphoma. The appraisal of liver involvement with any change in stage is important because, if there is a change, then therapy must be adjusted accordingly. *Laparoscopic follow-up and restaging* are particularly useful in lymphomas: therapy is particularly effective against lymphomas and its effect is often rapid. Moreover, in order to evaluate the results so as to regulate the therapeutic approach on their basis, it is of prime importance to add an examination providing pathological data to the routine clinical and laboratory controls.

However, considerable difficulty is met in the laparoscopic follow-up. The lesions detected at the "first look" either are static or have regressed. These findings are certainly useful when the patient is under therapy because they allow us in each case to adjust the therapeutic program or keep it as it is. Any impression of a remission or a cure from a lymphoma is, however, much less reliable. In fact, the neoplastic tissue may no longer be recognizable to the naked eye; one may only see traces of the lesion, which may appear as thin plaques or in the form of scars with different shapes and sizes – the latter may be retracted and deep or superficial. However, a laparoscopic impression of a recovery is not too reliable. The laparoscopic examination may be useful because it can guide the biopsy-taking from all the visible focuses. But the diagnosis is only reliable if one or more samples demonstrate the presence of neoplastic tissue.

If the biopsy is negative, then this is an indicative finding, but it cannot guarantee that the tumor has become sterile. These cases must therefore be carefully checked and, if necessary, submitted to a new control laparoscopy at a later date. The uncertainties arising as to whether there has been a histological "recovery" from a malignant lymphoma show that in the follow-up noninvasive techniques accompanied by transcutaneous biopsy cannot be proposed. The shortcomings of these techniques are well known for staging, but their shortcomings are even greater in follow-up and restaging.

6.4 Primary Extraabdominal Tumors

Laparoscopy has the advantage of enabling us to extend systematic "pathological" staging to tumors for which exploratory laparotomy has been rarely performed.

Abdominal endoscopic exploration was found to be of particular value for the pathological staging of tumors of the breast, esophagus, and lungs as well as for melanoblastomas. The clinical and laboratory pictures often suggested that the tumor stage was lower than the true stage the tumor had actually reached. These tumors have similar characteristics: an epithelial matrix, a marked tendency to metastasize to the abdomen, in particular the liver. Furthermore, elective radical therapy for them consists of the surgical excision of the tumor. Of course, this is feasible if a local tumor is excisable and also if there is an adequate guarantee that the tumor has no distant metastases.

Before deciding to perform radical surgery it is of crucial importance to know whether the abdomen is tumor free. This applies in particular to primary tumors with an extraabdominal localization, because in such cases the abdomen is not incised and no abdominal metastases can be searched for.

For a certain period, laparoscopy was systematically indicated for the staging for these tumors, but now the situation has changed.

6.4.1 Breast Cancer

Because breast carcinoma has a marked tendency to metastasize to the liver, laparoscopy is indicated in the protocol for its staging. To demonstrate the usefulness of this investigation in establishing whether the tumor is localized in its site of origin, and consequently whether radical surgical excision could be performed, we cite our results obtained in the presonographic era. In 22 out of 147 breast carcinomas with no clinical, laboratory, or radiological signs of spread to the abdomen, laparoscopy demonstrated metastases to the liver (15%). In another 100 cases with some signs that could lead to a suspicion of distant spread, liver metastases were found in 37. On the basis of these data in a large number of cases the type of operation used was modified, as was the prognosis.

The procedures now used for staging have changed. Breast cancer metastasizes to the liver usually in the form of fairly large multiple nodules which take root in the usually normal liver tissue. In a really high percentage of cases imaging techniques can detect these lesions. Moreover, the peritoneum, which is difficult to study reliably with noninvasive examinations, is more rarely involved, any involvement occurring at a late stage. As there are ideal conditions for a satisfactory echographic staging, laparoscopy is no longer necessary.

Furthermore, in cancer of the breast, the primary cancer can be studied preliminarily and patients unlikely to have metastases can be distinguished from those that are more likely to have distant metastases. The distinction is made by analyzing the mammary sites using the TNM scheme, three basic elements of the disease being evaluated: (a) primary tumor (T), (b) lymph nodes (N), and (c) distant metastases (M). In the T1, NO, N phases distant metastases are exceptionally rare and so abdominal staging is useful, starting with the cases classified as T2 and, in particular, T2b, those with adhesions to the fascia or to the pectoral muscle or T3b, N2, and, of course, MO, M1a, and M1b.

There is thus little likelihood of false abdominal negatives being made and now sonographic staging is systematically used. Laparoscopy is no longer part of the study protocol. However, in the odd case in which ultrasound findings are doubtful, then laparoscopy must be performed: in breast cancer staging, any images that might be interpreted as metastases or liver angiomas call for clarification with laparoscopy.

6.4.2 Esophageal Carcinoma

Radical surgery for esophageal cancer has been greatly improved in recent years and so the need for accurate staging has been felt even more strongly.

Radical surgery, sometimes associated with radiotherapy, is the therapy of choice. Yet this type of surgery is complex and prolonged and carries high intraoperative and anesthesiological risks. Moreover, it is usually performed on aged subjects whose general health may already be poor [27–30]. Radical surgery therefore may be reserved for patients without metastasis, and this can be ascertained only with a systematic and reliable staging protocol. Cancer of the esophagus frequently gives rise to abdominal metastasis. With a view to obtaining an accurate subdiaphragmatic appraisal, laparoscopy has for the past few years been included in the clinical study program. This technique is very useful in the detection of abdominal metastases that escape clinical staging; it is accurate in the selection of patients for radical surgery, and has almost totally replaced exploratory surgery alone. We were among the first systematically to use laparoscopy in esophageal carcinoma staging [3, 31]. Our experience has above all confirmed that abdominal metastases are almost absent in tumors localized at the upper third, but their frequency progressively increases from the middle third to the cardiac forms. Second, we must stress that laparoscopy very frequently reveals metastases in cases in which the abdomen appears uninvolved at clinical staging.

In our series of 369 patients with carcinoma of the esophagus abdominal spread was found in 14% (Table 6.3) [32].

In the light of the above considerations for breast cancer staging one might assume that imaging techniques can also provide accurate staging for tumors of the esophagus. The latter, after all, have analogous characteristics; they have the same epithelial matrix as well as the same tendency to metastasize to the liver; the metastases are almost always multiple, nodular, and large enough to be detected sonographically.

Yet the situation for cases of esophageal cancer is different. Esophageal carcinoma metastasizes not only to the liver but, in a high proportion of cases, to other abdominal organs. Table 6.3 shows that a recurrence to the liver occurs in 10% of cases but the peritoneum, omentum, lymph nodes, and stomach considered together have a higher

Table 6.3. Number and site of abdominal metastases as related to location of esophageal or cardia cancer

Abdominal metastases (52 cases:14%)

Location	No. of cases	Liver	Peritoneum	Omentum	Gastric wall	Lymph node
Upper third	28	–	–	–	–	–
Middle third	96	4	2	–	1	1
Lower third	156	15	5	3	4	3
Cardia	89	15	11	3	13	7
Total	369	37(10%)	18 (4.9%)	6(1.6%)	18(4.9%)	11(3%)

proportion of secondaries, which are found in 14.4% of cases. Invasive techniques fail to detect tumors at the parietal and visceral peritoneum or at the omentum unless the masses are large (Fig. 6.9). Laparoscopy can on the other hand discover plaques and small single or isolated nodules on the serosa (Fig. 6.10).

Spread to the external stomach wall should never be underestimated; often it cannot be revealed with esophago-gastroscopy, but can be suspected and detected with endoscopic echography, the finding being easily obtained with laparoscopy, with also allows a bioptic sample to be taken. Finally, worthy of mention are regional lymph nodes which, when small, may not be detected with sonography. If they are detected, it cannot be established whether their enlargement is due to neoplastic infiltration or to an unimportant reaction.

Therefore, as in all abdominal tumors, laparoscopy is superfluous when sonography and any echoguided fine-needle biopsy unequivocally reveal that the tumor has spread to the abdomen. Otherwise, in cancer of the esophagus imaging techniques do not guarantee a reliable staging. This concept is confirmed by making a comparison between echography and laparoscopy [33] or using the two techniques in combination. We used the latter to stage 86 patients. Preliminary echography showed that four definitely had metastases to the liver and echoguided fine-needle biopsy confirmed the diagnosis. These patients were not submitted to a radical surgery program and no further investigatory examinations were made. In another three cases echography failed to resolve the problem, calling attention to suspect liver images: in one case laparoscopy revealed liver metastasis, in another a neoplastic diffusion, not, as suggested by echography, to the liver – but to the omentum. In the remaining patient the endoscopic examina-

tion was negative. In five cases, the sonographic finding suggested a neoplastic infiltration to the lymph nodes, which were enlarged but not enlarged enough to allow fine-needle target biopsy. Laparoscopy with biopsy showed a neoplastic infiltration in two cases and simple aspecific adenitis in a further two. In the remaining case a neoplastic tumor was found; it was peritoneal, not lymph nodal. The echographic finding was negative for metastasis in the remaining 56 cases. Laparoscopy did, however, demonstrate that the tumor had spread in four: in one to a cirrhotic liver in the form of an apparently single nodule with a diameter of a few millimeters (Fig. 6.11); to the spleen in another as a small isolated nodule (Fig. 6.12), to a perigastric node (one case), and to the gastrohepatic ligament (one case). Laparoscopy can therefore confirm or rectify the echographic diagnosis in suspicious cases, and may obviate any false positives. Above all, it reveals any false echographic negatives. The latter cannot be considered negligible in the liver, where sonography failed to detect metastases in 1.5% of cases, but more so for other sites, where errors were made in 4.5% of cases.

––––––––––––––––––––––––––––––––––––➤

Fig. 6.9. Staging. Detail under high magnification: in the adipose tissue of the greater omentum is a small fleshy formation. *Omental metastasis from carcinoma*

Fig. 6.10. Staging. Detail under high magnification: small whitish plaque, only just visible on the parietal peritoneum of the diaphragm. *Peritoneal metastasis from carcinoma*

Fig. 6.11. Staging. Surface of the left lobe of the liver with nodules of the cirrhotic type. In the center can be seen a small whitish nodule. *Metastasis to the liver from carcinoma on medionodular cirrhosis*

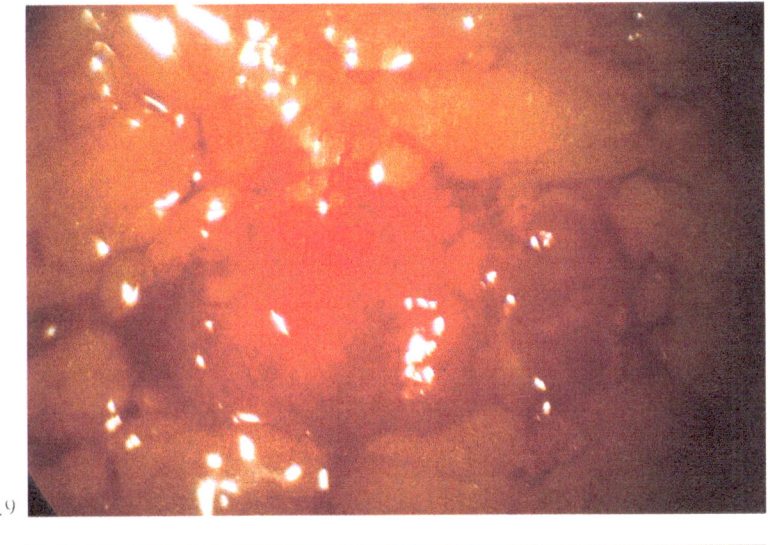

6.9

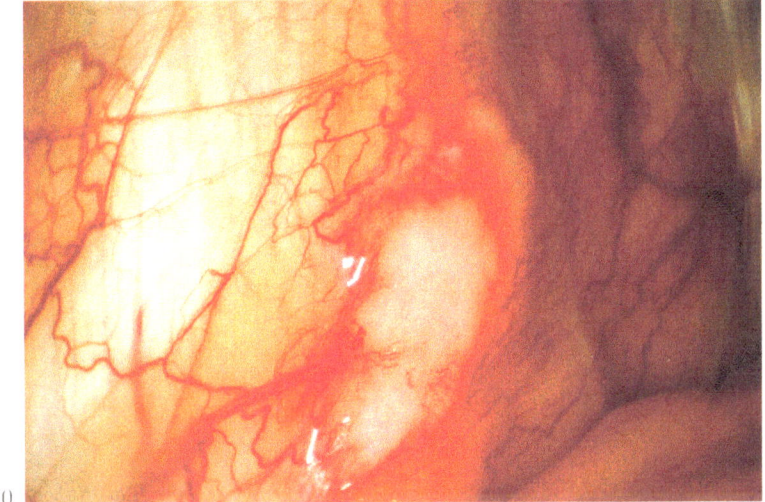

6.10

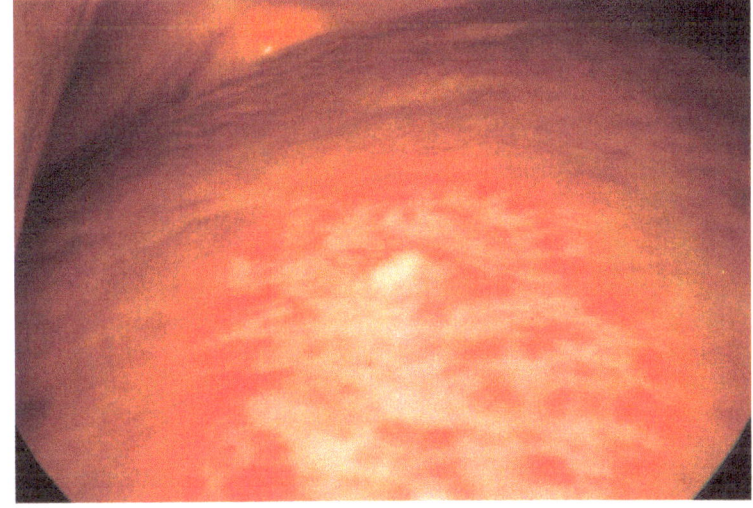

6.11

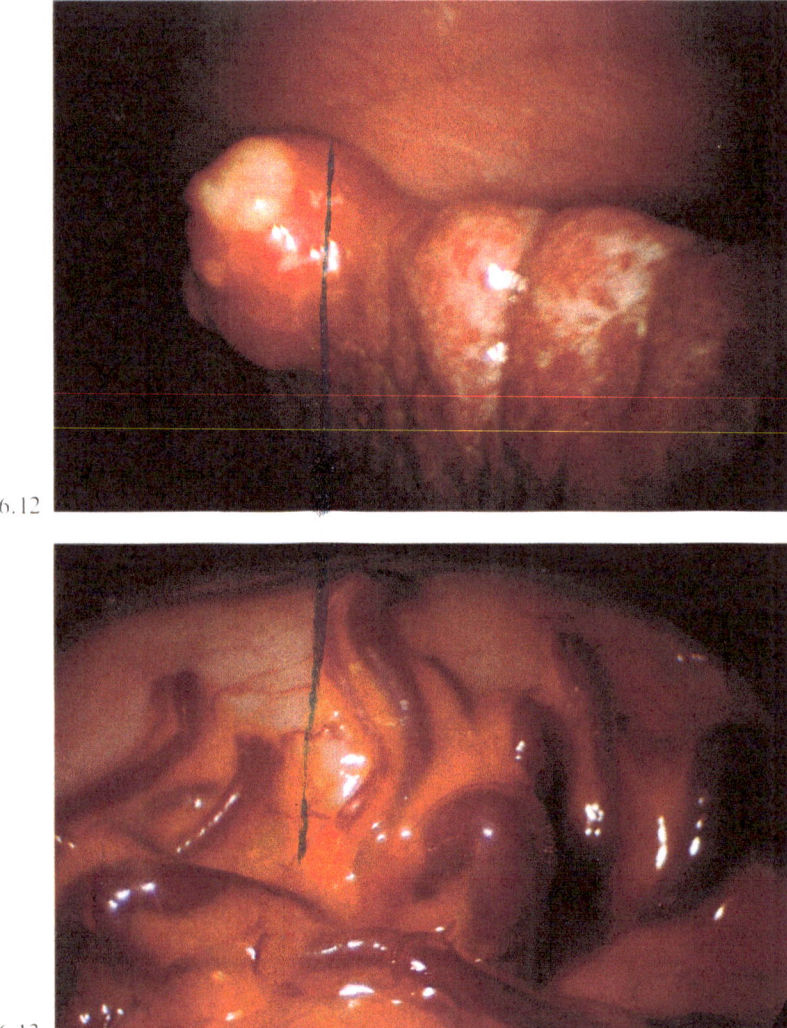

6.12

6.13

Fig. 6.12. Staging. Small unevenly spherical nodule protrudes on the spleen margin, partly covered by splenic tissue, with a central whitish area. *Metastasis to the spleen from carcinoma*

Fig. 6.13. Staging. Dilated and turgid veins of the greater gastric curvature. *Marked collateral circulation from portal hypertension*

Laparoscopy is therefore very useful in the staging of esophageal cancer, and echographolaparoscopic integration is still the most effective diagnostic instrument available. Of course it is a prerequisite for radical surgery to rule out abdominal metastases. Laparoscopy effectively provides this information.

In esophageal cancer, however, laparoscopy can provide other important data about the liver,

thereby indicating whether or not surgery is indicated. As is known, esophageal tumors are frequently associated with chronic alcoholism and therefore a high number of patients have alcoholic hepatitis.

Laparoscopy with biopsy is the ideal method for diagnosing, classifying, and evaluating a liver disease and its severity as well as for collecting all the anatomo-histological findings that, when pooled with the clinical and laboratory data, allow a more accurate functional appraisal to be made; and this is of crucial importance in deciding whether or not the patient can undergo surgery. The importance of this aspect of the laparoscopic staging of esophageal cancer was confirmed in our series of 369 patients [32], in 56% of which associated chronic alcoholism was found; 14% of these had frank cirrhosis and another 14% had noncirrhotic hepatopathy.

Another important finding is made only with laparoscopy: collateral circulations due to portal hypertension in esophageal cancer with cirrhosis. Because these can develop in the abdominal cavity at the expense of the small vessels, they are difficult to detect sonographically. They can give rise to dramatic pictures (Fig. 6.13): hyperplasia, dilation, and turgor of veins, and the formation of true plexuses. When collateral circulations are large, forming above all on the phrenocholic ligament or on any adhesions at the expense of the Retzius system, they seriously hamper or even preclude a radical esophageal operation. Here therefore laparoscopy is indispensable for it gives the surgeon information about any alterations to the abdominal venous circulation, which may mean that radical surgery is contraindicated. In about 6% of cases in our experience, the surgeon decided to perform palliative surgery because there was severe cirrhosis and a laparoscopic finding of marked collateral circulations from portal hypertension.

Finally, it should be mentioned that cirrhosis hinders the sonographic detection of liver metastasis because there is only a slight difference between the echogenicity of neoplastic tissue and that of liver tissue. Moreover (three cases in our experience) a sonographically revealed nodule considered metastatic turned out to be primary hepatocarcinoma when laparoscopic and target biopsy findings were obtained. Therefore, in the staging of esophageal cancer, laparoscopy is an examination of fundamental importance. It may be avoided only if echography and echoguided biopsy guarantee that there is abdominal metastasis.

6.4.3 Lung Tumors

In view of the frequency with which lung tumors give metastases to the liver, for several years a subdiaphragmatic appraisal has been made before making any surgical excision. A clinical and radiological study was required, but a pathological staging made with surgical exploration was also considered necessary; more recently this has been replaced by laparoscopy.

The latter has proved very useful; it detected abdominal tumor spread that had escaped detection at the previous examination, and there was a consequent upstaging. Often diagnostic errors,

above all "false positives," can be corrected. Laparoscopy confirms the known tendency of lung cancer to metastasize to the liver and other organs even in the early stages. In 14% of cases of lung tumors clinically localized to the thorax, Oliviero et al. [34] found abdominal metastasis. Thanks to combined laparoscopy and marrow biopsy, Tancini et al. [35] upstaged patients with a "clinically localized" form in 15.3% of cases. Moreover, thanks to this technique they discovered that 7 out of 38 patients considered inoperable because of a finding of distant spread were in fact operable because it demonstrated that there were no abdominal lesions. In 1980, in our series laparoscopy demonstrated that 7% of 86 lung tumors without clinical signs of distant spread were found to have metastasis. Even then it was reasonable to conclude that laparoscopy should be used in the pretherapeutic appraisal of bronchial carcinomas and that it was indispensable in anaplasic and small cell tumors [36].

It is necessary here to make a clear distinction between *bronchogenic carcinomas* (epidermoid carcinoma, adenocarcinoma, large cell cancer) and *small cell tumors*.

For *bronchogenic carcinomas* the observations made for breast cancer are applicable. Any metastases occur almost exclusively in the liver; they are nodular, almost always multiple, and therefore make up fairly large elements adhering to a usually normal parenchyma. They therefore have enough features for sonographic detection and they give images that indicate the suitable sites for fineneedle target biopsies. These tumors can be satisfactorily staged for surgery, which is the principal form of therapy, on the basis of a simple clinical, laboratory, and sonographic study and, where necessary, a slightly invasive procedure such as transcutaneous puncture. For these reasons laparoscopy no longer has a role in this protocol. It can, however, be performed in some cases if the findings are dubious.

The above points do not apply to *small cell lung carcinoma*, which has a marked tendency for early diffusion. Like other types of malignant lymphoma [37], it spreads extremely rapidly. This explains why this tumor is so sensitive to radio- and chemotherapy, which have definitely improved its prognosis [38]. Where possible therapy also includes surgical ablation. There is disagreement as to whether it is opportune to perform surgery in these cases. In any case, surgery must be performed on patients selected on the basis of strict criteria: it must be established whether a particular T1- and T2-stage primary tumor is resectable. In other words, the following must be ruled out: spread to distant or mediastinic lymphatics, metastasis to the brain, thorax, liver and suprarenals. But also for those who believe in polychemotherapy alone, it is important to discover whether there is diffusion to the liver because the prognosis also depends on this, as does the therapeutic program. The latter varies depending on the form found and whether this form is extensive or localized. Moreover, if the extent of tumor spread is accurately established, then a reference point is also established so that during therapy the results obtained can be assessed. This is particularly important in small cell tumors, for which therapy programs have not been altogether standardized. Comparisons made recently between noninvasive techniques and laparoscopy indicate that the former do not always give reliable results.

In 1987 Hansen et al. compared the efficacy of sonography with echoguided biopsy with that of laparoscopy with target biopsy in the staging of these tumors. In 25% of 131 patients the liver was involved: the metastases were sonographically detected in 86% and laparoscopically detected in 76% of cases. Sonography with biopsy therefore appears to be more effective in the detection of liver metastases in patients with small cell lung cancer. Laparoscopy, however, detected liver involvement in another five patients with negative ultrasound findings [39].

In our latest series of 86 patients studied with "echography for laparoscopy" we had similar percentages: 24.5% of cases with ultrasound – detected liver involvement, without laparoscopy being performed, and 4.6% with neoplastic abdominal diffusion diagnosed laparoscopically after a negative echographic finding had been obtained. The relatively high number of failures with sonography can be explained by analyzing the different ways in which small cell tumor metastasizes to the abdomen, above all by the fact that, like lymphoma, this tumor often gives rise to *atypical hepatic and extra-hepatic metastases* [40].

In a series of ours consisting of 138 small cell carcinomas without clinical signs suggesting abdominal diffusion, liver metastases were found in 35 cases (25%). In 19 cases (54%) the metastases had macroscopic morphological characteristics that were typical of metastases from epithelial tumor: multiple, small, and large pinkish white nodules with a central umbilication. In another 15 cases,

on the other hand, the lesions to the liver gave atypical pictures: (a) scattered micronodules that were hardly revealed at all; these were whitish, semitransparent, and without central craters (eight cases) (Fig. 6.14); (b) small, flat superficial whitish plaques with hazy margins (five cases) (Fig. 6.15); and, finally, (c) no macroscopic signs of neoplastic tumors (two cases) [41].

Echography can reliably detect metastatic nodules of a certain size and thickness, but it is far less effective when lesions are small and flat. It is impossible to make an echographic diagnosis in cases in which lesions are not endoscopically visible and tumor infiltration can only be detected histologically. Moreover, small cell lung tumor can give extrahepatic metastases that, in our series, accounted for 18%. These different localizations should be laparoscopically searched for with great care. We have found isolated nodular metastases on the parietal peritoneum (Fig. 6.16) and in the spleen. Splenic metastases appear as small translucent whitish nodules (Fig. 6.17). This feature, already pointed out for the liver, can be an indicative, if not pathognomonic, macroscopic sign of a secondary small cell cancer. The diagnosis must always, however, be confirmed with biopsy. These particular forms and localizations are likely to escape detection with noninvasive techniques, and here laparoscopy is therefore preferable to them.

It is necessary to explore carefully all the sites in which a metastasis might occur. As well as the sites already specified, the pelvis must be carefully examined, for here there may be metastases to the ovary.

Finally, as the tumor can involve the liver without giving rise to macroscopically recognizable alterations, at least two bioptic samples should be taken from each lobe, even if the liver appears normal. So the rules for lymphoma should be followed. Because of the similarities with malignant lymphomas, when staging this tumor, we always took three splenic biopsies from an apparently normal spleen. After finding that about 100 cases checked were all negative, we abandoned this practice, taking spleen biopsy only when visible lesions were present.

Finally, small cell tumor can metastasize to the lymph nodes, but usually these metastases can be detected echographically; fine-needle biopsy should be taken to ascertain whether they are neoplastic because the ultrasound image does not allow us to establish this. In fact it is not rare for

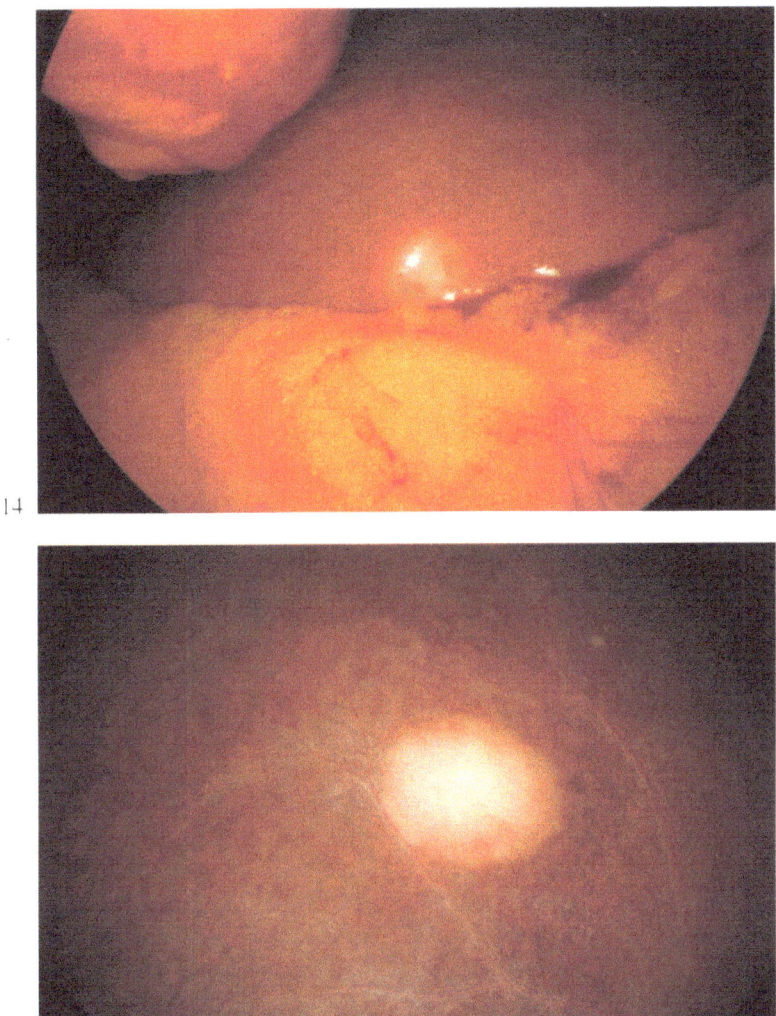

6.14

6.15

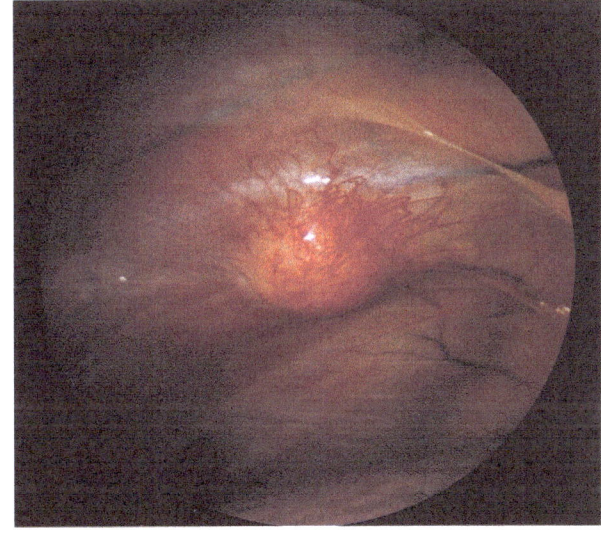

Fig. 6.14. Staging. Margin of the left lobe of the liver with a roundish, grayish-red plaque that has a gelatinous appearance. *Metastasis to the liver from pulmonary microcytoma*

Fig. 6.15. Staging. Small roundish, flat whitish plaque. *Metastasis to the liver from pulmonary microcytoma*

Fig. 6.16. Staging. Isolated nodule with marked passive ▶ congestion on the parietal peritoneum of the upper wall of the abdomen. *Metastasis to the peritoneum from pulmonary microcytoma*

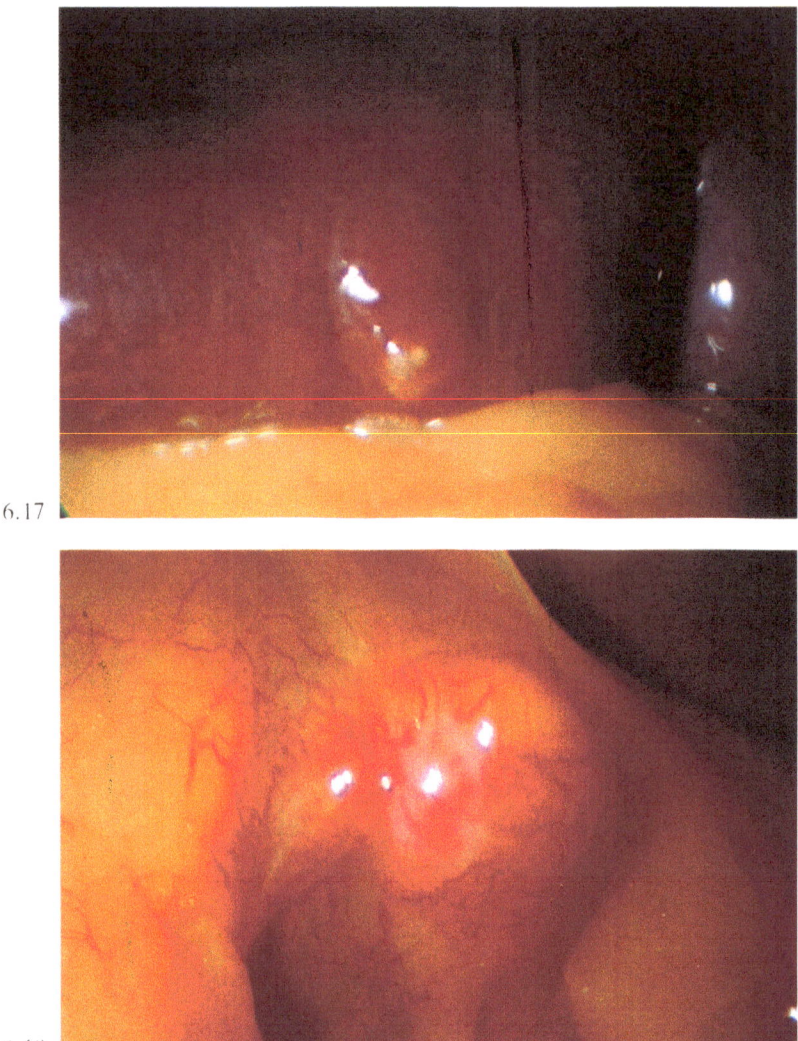

6.17

6.18

Fig. 6.17. Staging. Small nodule of the spleen, slightly protruding. *Metastasis to the spleen from pulmonary microcytoma*

Fig. 6.18. Staging. Nodule in the omental adipose tissue. *Lymphatic metastasis from microcytoma?* Confirmation with biopsy

aspecific adenopathy to become so large that it simulates neoplastic diffusion. Where a finding is negative or dubious, laparoscopy should be performed (Fig. 6.18).

Sonography with echoguided biopsy is still the first technique used in the staging of small cell lung tumors. But it is valid only in cases in which there is definitely an abdominal diffusion. If the finding

is negative, laparoscopy is indicated, just as it is for malignant lymphomas [39, 40].

Finally, laparoscopy can be indicated to study the effect of therapy. If the initial echography demonstrated metastases, then echography can be repeated many times over and is irreplaceable – for it gives constant information on any modifications during therapy. But to investigate any remission after therapy has been completed, echography and cytology or microhistology are inadequate. Even with laparoscopy there are numerous pitfalls in establishing whether the disease has become "negative" although laparoscopy is more likely to detect any remaining neoplastic tissue (Fig. 6.19, 6.20). This can often be detected macroscopically; failing this, then it is detected with multiple biopsies. The follow-up must be made with laparos-

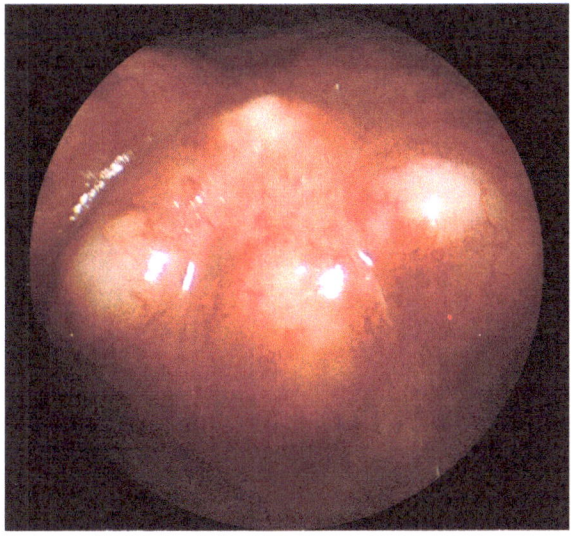

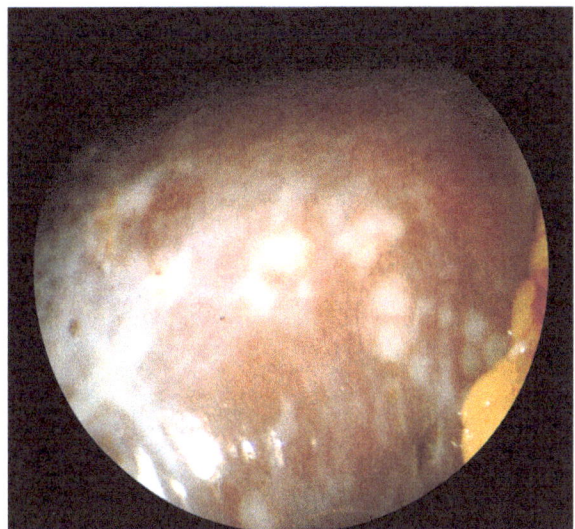

6.19

6.20

Fig. 6.19. Staging. Metastasis with multiple nodules from *pulmonary microcytoma* on the left lobe of the liver

Fig. 6.20. Same case as in Fig. 6.19. Follow-up after 4 months' treatment: clinical remission. The nodules have disappeared but there are still plaques with thickened Glisson's capsule. Macroscopic finding of persistent neoplastic tissue. Confirmation with biopsy

copy in cases that were considered negative at the echographic staging.

6.4.4 Melanoblastoma

Skin melanoblastoma grows rapidly and tends to have both a local and a distant spread via the blood, which passes through the lymphatic stations. The prognosis and likelihood of any cure depend mainly on the *local conditions of the primary tumors*, which are divided into five categories on the basis of (a) their degree of penetration following Clark's scheme and (b) their stage of evolution. The most widely used classification is that proposed by the WHO Melanoma Group; it is very simple and specifies three stages: I, melanoma with neither regional nor distant metastases; II, melanoma with regional metastasis, but without distant metastasis; and, III, melanoma with distant metastasis.

An exact staging was considered of prime importance in the choice of therapy and protocol for the clinical, laboratory, and radiological study, which of course has now been greatly enriched

by CT and sonography. However, the characteristics of melanoblastoma preclude a sufficiently reliable staging, and for this reason in the late 1970s laparoscopy appeared a suitable method to compensate for any inadequacies of clinical staging. Bleiberg [42] found abdominal metastases in 23%. We had much lower percentages [6%] in our first series of 115 patients who had been more rigorously selected, and classified as the first (Clark IV–V) or second stage.

Imaging techniques have greatly reduced the requests for laparoscopy in the staging of melanoblastomas. The present study protocols in fact included only sonography or CT scan [43, 44]. Yet these programs are highly inaccurate. In a series of 297 laparoscopies performed in patients with a negative ultrasound finding for abdominal metastases to stage melanoblastoma, we found that sonography has several pitfalls. Abdominal metastases were discovered in almost 15% of cases; 67.5% were hepatic, 27.9% peritoneal, and 4.6% splenic.

Liver metastases are therefore the most frequent form, but only half of the lesions found laparoscopically were large enough to be detected echographically, having diameters of over 2 cm. The others were smaller – 24% were between 1 and 2 cm (Fig. 6.21) and 27.5% were 1 cm or less and therefore too small for ultrasound detection (Fig. 6.22). Peritoneal tumors then account for almost 28% of the abdominal metastases; with echography it is always extremely difficult to detect peritoneal lesions, but melanoblastoma metastases in particular can be simple spots that are so small and thin that they are only detected

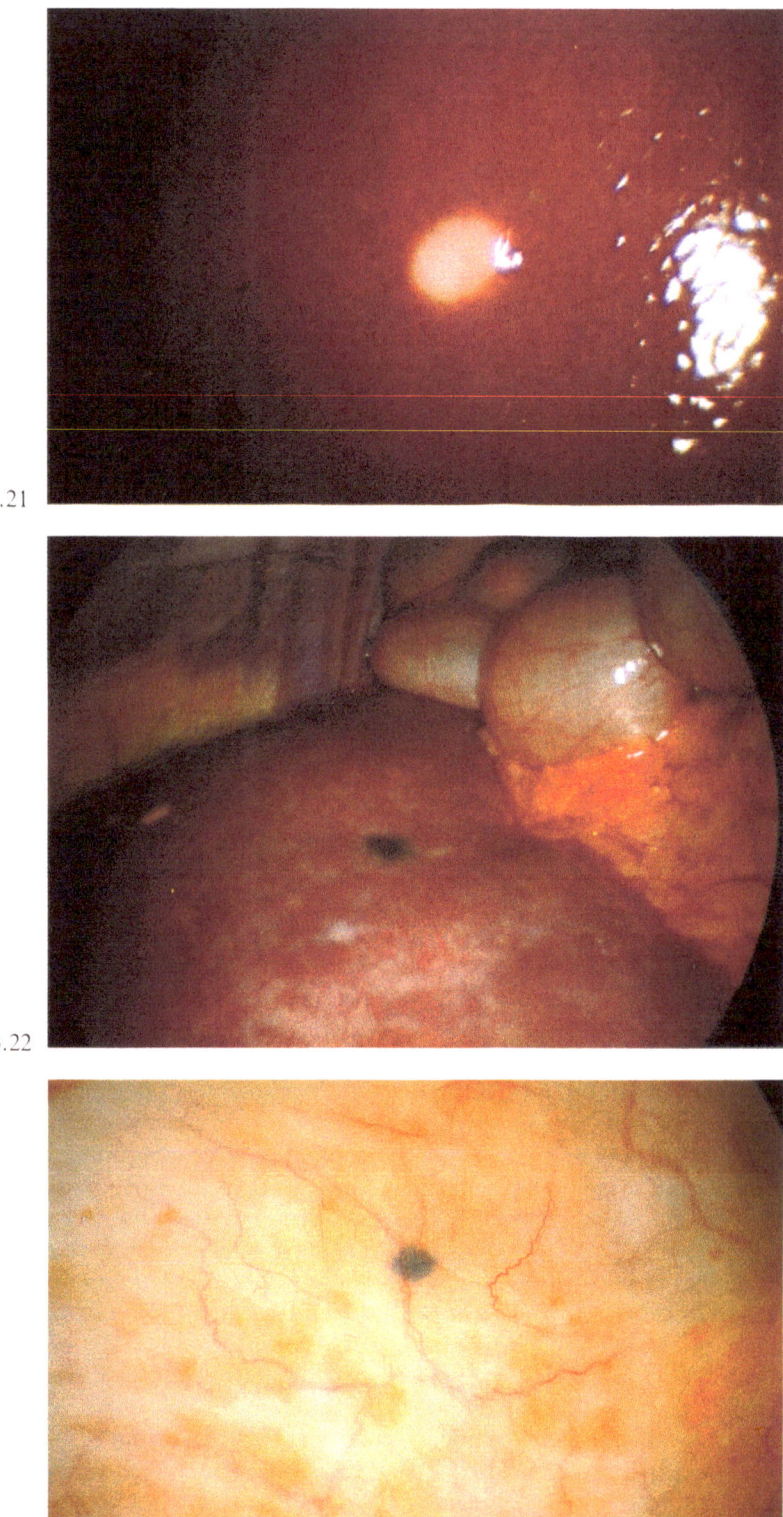

6.21

6.22

6.23

with endoscopy, and this is possible only because they are black (Fig. 6.23). We studied a series of 35 patients with sonography and fine-needle laparoscopically guided biopsy and our findings confirmed that sonography is inadequate in the detection of abdominal metastases from melanoblastoma: in four cases (11.5%) false ultrasound negatives were found.

So laparoscopy is far superior to imaging techniques in the staging of melanoblastoma. Yet nowadays it is hardly ever used. This is perhaps due to the fact that, even if it is only approximate, clinical staging provides an adequate guide for therapy. Treatment consists of surgery, the primary tumor being excised as widely as possible together with any regional lymph nodes involved. Adjuvant therapy (radiopolychemotherapy or immunotherapy used singly or in combination) have as yet not given appreciable results. Therefore the accurate staging that laparoscopy can guarantee and that in other tumors is indispensable for choosing the most suitable therapeutic strategy has not yet proved particularly useful in melanoblastoma because it does not modify or change the therapeutic protocol. Therefore, until the different types of therapy are changed, laparoscopy will continue to be considered superfluous in the staging of melanoblastoma, in spite of the fact that it is highly effective.

6.5 Primary Endoabdominal Tumors

The type of search made for metastases from tumors with a primary endoabdominal site varies depending on the following. If the primary tumor is situated in an organ within the abdominal cavity and elective therapy is surgical, then laparotomy is above all exploratory. When performing it the surgeon can collect all the information necessary

for staging and can decide whether a radical excision of the neoplasm can be made or palliative surgery performed; he or she may decide to do nothing at all. However, accurate preoperative staging can obviate many useless laparotomies, only curative surgery being performed.

Clinical staging has been greatly improved by imaging techniques, which allow us to detect most of the metastases to the liver, which is the most frequent site for tumors from the digestive tract. Therefore laparoscopy is used much less often in such cases. But, in particular situations, it is still found to be useful, and it is sometimes indicated in the preoperative staging of *carcinoma* of the *stomach*, *intestine*, *pancreas*, and *liver*. Of the endoabdominal tumors, cancer of the ovary is considered elsewhere.

6.5.1 Stomach Carcinoma

As already stated for the other *epithelial* tumors, sonography and echoguided biopsy can demonstrate a more advanced diffusion of the tumor in the abdomen than can traditional clinical staging, and it can change the therapy plan or program. Yet it must be borne in mind that sonography can give false negatives for small localized liver metastases with particular sites and it is unlikely to evidence peritoneal lesions. Cancer of the stomach has a strong tendency to spread to the nearby structures, to the greater and lesser omentum, in particular. If the neoplastic infiltration is massive, there is considerable thickening of and marked modification in the adipose tissue, most of which is replaced and this is detected with sonography. But often in its initial stages, this phenomenon is slight and can only be diagnosed, or even only just suspected, with direct visualization. In fact, the omentum has small rose-colored or whitish plaques with a hazy outline, which are harder than the surrounding fat (Fig. 6.24). Sometimes the infiltration is not even visible: the adipose tissue still has its normal characteristics, being only slightly harder and more rigid. Of course the diagnosis must be confirmed by biopsy. Laparoscopy can provide useful information on the state of the stomach wall, that is on the P parameter, which is added to the other TNM system parameters and that is usually established intraoperatively. P1, P2, P3, and P4 are used to indicate respectively the involvement of the mucosa, submucosa, muscularis, and serosa. With laparoscopy we can detect a P4

Fig. 6.21. Staging. Small roundish plaque on the liver, which has a normal appearance. *Apigmented melanoblastoma*

Fig. 6.22. Staging. Lateral posterior extremity of the left lobe of the liver: tiny roundish plaques, one of which is black and two whitish-pink. *Pigmented and apigmented metastasis from melanoblastoma*

Fig. 6.23. Staging. Parietal peritoneum. Tiny black spot. *Peritoneal metastasis from melanoblastoma*

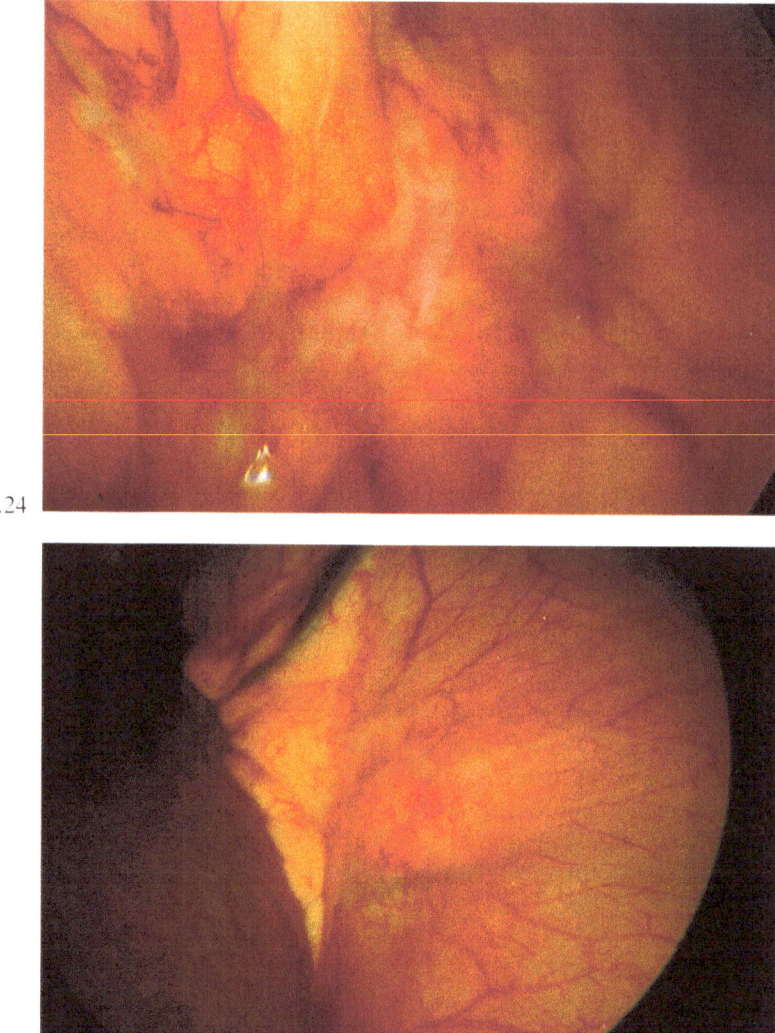

6.24

6.25

Fig. 6.24. Staging. Detail of adipose tissue of the omentum, the center of which appears to be replaced by whitish-red plaques with hazy outlines. *Omental infiltration from gastric carcinoma*

Fig. 6.25. Staging. Detail of the lesser gastric curvature; *on the left*, the fat of the lesser omentum and the border of the left lobe of the liver. *In the center* can be seen a subserous plaque that is slightly raised and devoid of vessels. *Subserous diffusion of gastric carcinoma*

(Fig. 6.25), which is generally inaccessible to other types of exploration, fiberscopy in particular.

Finally, it should be stressed that regional lymph node enlargement is very common in cases of gastric carcinoma. Enlargement does not always depend on neoplastic infiltration and, even if the

lymph nodes are detected echographically, transcutaneous fine-needle puncture is difficult to perform. Laparoscopy allows the direct visualization of perigastric omental and mesocolon lymph nodes, etc., and it also enables us to take useful biopsy samples, using forceps.

We therefore believe that when radical surgery is being planned for patients with negative ultrasound findings then laparoscopy can be extremely useful.

6.5.2 Intestinal Tumors

In theory the problems connected with laparoscopy in intestinal tumors are very similar to those encountered in cancer of the stomach. In practice,

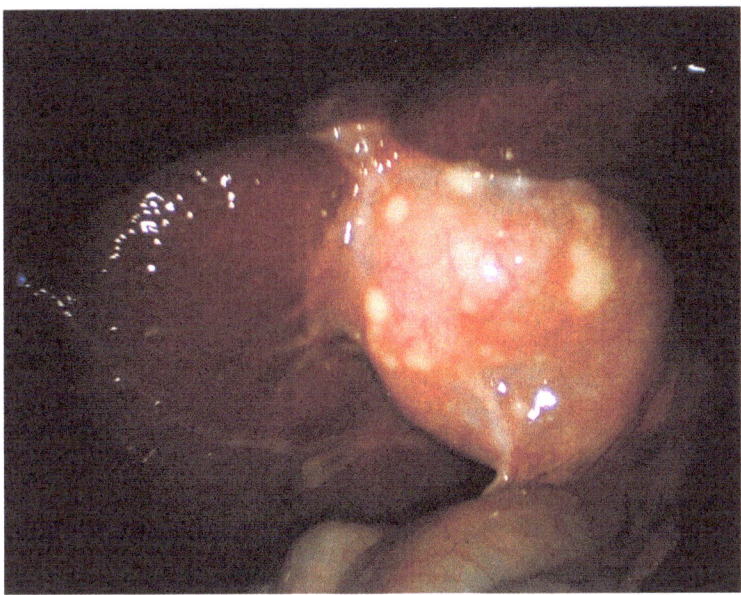

Fig. 6.26. Staging. Lower surface of the right lobe of the liver and the gallbladder, on the serosa of which can be seen some small whitish plaques of different shapes and sizes which are slightly raised. *Metastasis to the visceral peritoneum of the gallbladder from epithelial neoplasm*

however, laparoscopy does not have the same indications: patients with cancer of the large intestine must undergo surgery even if they already have metastasis, above all because there is a risk of occlusion, so the tumor must be exicised before this occurs, also because primary tumor excision appears to cause regression of secondaries, and finally because encouraging results can be obtained by, where possible, resecting the liver metastases.

6.5.3 Pancreatic Tumors

Numerous investigation techniques are used in association with diagnosing carcinoma of the pancreas. Transhepatic cholangiography, endoscopic retrograde cholangiopancreatography, CT, ultrasound, visceral angiography, and perhaps nuclear magnetic resonance imaging have all contributed in various ways to evaluating tumor site, size, and spread.

It is possible to make a laparoscopic diagnosis of carcinoma of the pancreas, but it is not convenient. On the other hand, preoperative laparoscopic

staging can still be valid, even in the era of noninvasive techniques. We support this concept, and have already discussed it for mechanical jaundice. There are many alternatives in the therapy for pancreatic cancer; they include curative resection, palliative surgery, nonsurgical internal biliary stents, intraoperative radiotherapy, or no treatment at all. In order to choose, we must use an accurate pathological staging and laparoscopy is still the most reliable method for doing this. Recent findings have confirmed this. Using laparoscopy, Weiss et al. (1985) found peritoneal metastases in 25% of 32 cases of carcinoma of the pancreas for which echographic findings had been negative for metastases [45]. Warshaw et al. (1986) made a noninvasive preliminary study of patients with known pancreatic cancer who were candidates for curative resection or intraoperative radiotherapy; when findings were negative they performed laparoscopy. In 40 cases, they found that laparoscopy detected metastases that had escaped sonographic detection; the laparoscopic findings were confirmed by biopsy: small nodules of the liver (six cases), plaques of the parietal peritoneum (seven cases), and infiltration of the omentum (one case). Among the 26 negative cases that according to laparoscopy were also negative, in three, metastases were found with subsequent laparotomy, in two because the liver exploration had been incomplete, and in one because the metastasis was deep sited and therefore hidden. The overall accuracy of noninvasive techniques combined with laparoscopy was found to be 93%. The laparoscopic findings can decisively change the therapeutic strategy, and did so in 35% of the patients in this study [46].

We also use the same scheme as the surgeon, weighing up all the information in order to choose the most appropriate therapy. We perform laparoscopy whenever sonography does not reveal a tumoral diffusion. In our experience the most frequent cause of false sonographic negatives is peritoneal metastases (Fig. 6.26). The sensitivity and diagnostic accuracy of associated sonography and laparoscopy are extraordinarily high.

6.5.4 Liver Carcinoma

In recent years surgery for liver tumors has made considerable progress. Because surgical resection is always serious and, in the great majority of cases, the tumor is associated with cirrhosis, which further increases the risks, the operability of each patient must be assessed meticulously.

We have already stated (Sect. 5.3) that laparoscopy can often provide important data about the tumor, data that are not obtained with the preliminary investigations. It is worthwhile repeating here that laparoscopy enables us to: (a) see whether the size and extent of the hepatocarcinoma really do correspond to the sonographic finding and (b) ascertain whether there is a single nodule or whether there are multiple lesions and, if so, whether they involve one lobe or both (Fig. 5.26). These findings can modify the therapeutic program. Laparoscopy is therefore always indicated to complete the staging in candidates for radical liver resection.

Liver transplant for tumors calls for meticulous preparation if accidents are to be avoided. When waiting for the transplant, patients are systematically submitted to a complete staging that also includes exploratory laparotomy. Laparoscopy is never performed for this reason, but because the main aim of the investigation is to rule out peritoneal metastases, and here surgery can be less accurate than laparoscopy. In the future therefore laparoscopy should be used in staging for liver transplant candidates.

Finally, in recent years, in some liver carcinomas measuring under 4 cm, above all in subjects for whom surgery is contraindicated because of a severe coexisting cirrhosis, percutaneous echo-guided ethyl alcohol injections have been proposed [47]. Results have certainly been encouraging. Lap-

aroscopy has been used successfully to ascertain whether preconditions for the treatment exist and, above all, whether the node is single [48].

6.5.5 Ovarian Carcinoma

Considerable progress has been made in recent years in the treatment of primary carcinoma of the ovary. This has almost certainly depended upon improvements made in oncological surgery – a more satisfactory search is now being made for neoplastic tissue and its excision is more complete; the omentum and all the structures to which the tumor can metastasize can be excised. Progress also depends on the use of increasingly effective antiblastic drugs.

An overall improvement in the general approach for therapy has been obtained thanks to staging and follow-up, which enable us to choose the most appropriate combined protocols for each particular case.

Laparotomy, of course, is performed to excise the tumor and it is the first step in staging.

Laparoscopy was introduced for the staging of ovarian carcinoma in the early 1970s [49–56] because this tumor tends to have an early diffusion, both to contiguous structures, above all the peritoneum; it also has a strong tendency to spread to the diaphragmatic arches. Results with laparoscopy were found to be highly satisfactory because this technique is extraordinarily effective in the study of the peritoneal serosa. In particular it allows us to explore the more important areas, i.e., the diaphragmatic parts that are distended by pneumoperitoneum (Fig. 6.27). Moreover, with laparoscopy we can make a thorough examination of the peritoneal surface: thanks to the improved accuracy of optics and magnification, by moving the laparoscope nearer to the wall, we can detect the tiniest lesions, even the pin-head-sized ones. Ovarian cancer often spreads to the peritoneum in this way, with many tiny tumors forming.

Comparative studies made between laparoscopy and surgery demonstrate that laparoscopic staging of the upper quadrants is more satisfactory than surgical staging [49, 51], above all if a traditional subumbilical incision is used. On the other hand, also when an extended vertical incision is made above the umbilicus, diaphragmatic metastases are difficult to demonstrate if a laparoscope is not used during laparotomy [53].

Our experience, reported in 1978, fully confirms these results. In our first series of 51 cases of

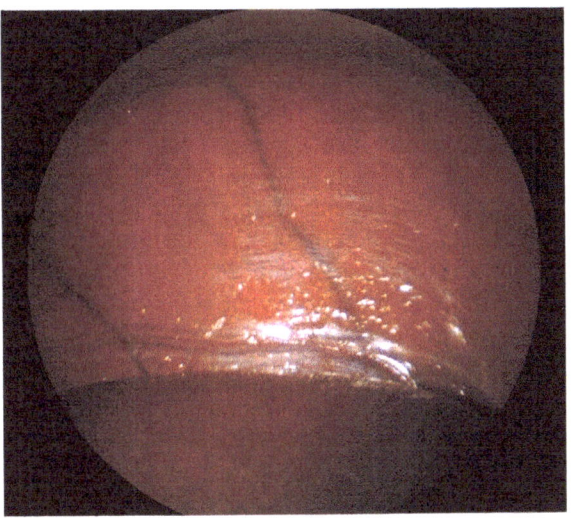

Fig. 6.27. Staging. Left hemidiaphragm is distended by pneumoperitoneum; on the parietal peritoneum are numerous small granules that are illuminated by the flash. *Multiple metastases from ovarian carcinoma to the parietal peritoneum of the diaphragm*

ovarian carcinoma [57], the peritoneal metastases found had a diameter of less than 3 mm in 38% of cases. Sometimes they were the size of a pinprick and could only be detected under high magnification with incident light (Fig. 6.28). Laparoscopy performed on a group of patients who had previously undergone surgery to excise the tumor and to make a staging was found to be of value. In 32 out of 38 patients surgically classified as stages I and II, laparoscopy confirmed the negative finding

for diffusion to the peritoneum. In the other six, however, it revealed that there were metastases to the peritoneum: in one case to the pelvic peritoneum and in the other five to the subdiaphragmatic serosa. Laparoscopy thus modified the stage in 16% of cases.

The results obtained with laparoscopy therefore suggest that this technique be used in the protocol for staging and a second step in staging, as a complement to surgery.

Laparotomy is thus made to: (a) confirm the clinical diagnosis, (b) excise the tumor, and (c) make an initial staging. Then, subsequently, with laparoscopy the exploration is completed and, in particular, the upper abdominal sectors are explored.

We are of the opinion that laparoscopy should also precede surgery. We always aim for this, as it appears to be ideal. Unfortunately, however, it cannot always be put into practice because often patients are sent to specialized centers after already undergoing surgery. Laparoscopy prior to surgery can be extremely useful because it enables us to: (a) confirm the diagnosis and establish the tumor type using reliable macroscopic and bioptic findings, (b) make a thorough peritoneal exploration of sectors most at risk, and (c) indicate to

Fig. 6.28. Staging. At high magnification on the parietal peritoneum can be seen some tiny granules, visible only under incident light. *Peritoneal metastasis from ovarian carcinoma*

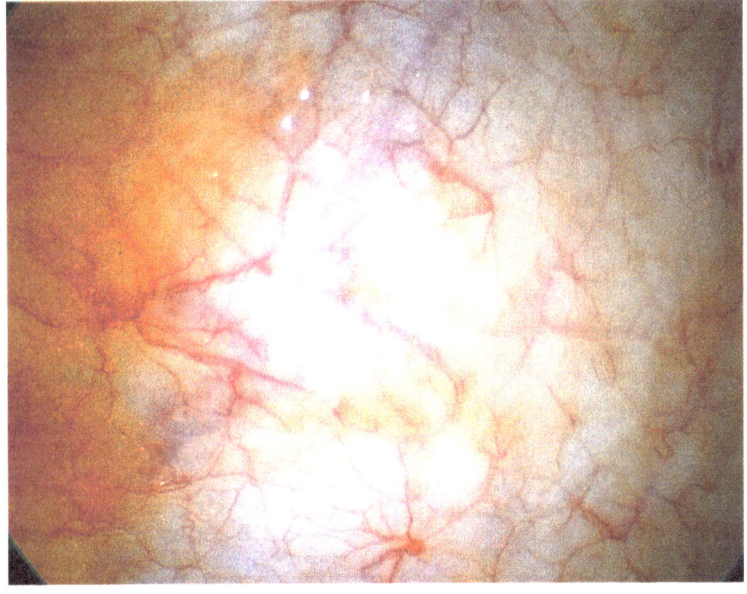

the surgeon the subsequent surgical procedure required for tumor excision and completion of the staging for the pelvis and retroperitoneum, where, as is well known, surgery is much more effective.

6.5.5.1 Imaging Techniques

Unlike for other tumors, the staging for ovarian carcinoma has not changed. This is because the tumor has a prevalent and early diffusion to the peritoneum and the omentum, where metastases are unlikely to be detected by ultrasound or CT scan. The latter techniques can diagnose metastases only when they are very advanced, that is if there are masses from an omental and mesenteric infiltration or if involvement from the parietal peritoneum is severe enough to cause a thickening of the wall, thus giving rise to a significant finding. At this stage, however, the disease is unlikely to have clinical signs (ascites, abdominal masses, etc.) that are sufficient evidence for a diagnosis of peritoneal diffusion.

Moreover, the main prerogative of imaging techniques, i.e., their ability to show liver metastases, is of little use in ovarian cancer because liver meatastases from this tumor are rare and are highly unlikely to appear as an early symptom. In all our series of laparoscopies for staging of ovarian tumors that are clinically or surgically classified as stage I or II, the abdominal diffusion involved the peritoneum and omentum only; we have never found a metastasis to the liver parenchyma. In the literature only in exceptional cases have metastases to the liver from ovarian carcinoma been found at this stage of the disease [56]. We found liver metastases in four patients with ovarian tumors but laparoscopy was performed not for staging of a known tumor, but to investigate important abdominal symptoms (ascites, hepatomegaly, masses, etc.) that had not been diagnosed clinically. In these patients laparoscopy demonstrated total and advanced ovarian carcinoma that had completely involved the abdominal organs.

Second, liver metastases from ovarian tumors are not always characterized by small or large multiple nodules with central craters, which usually are a typical sign of epithelial secondaries. They may instead appear small, soft, and gelatinous, resembling a vesicle. Their size and anatomical characteristics make these lesions, which can be revealed with laparoscopy, highly unlikely to be detected with sonography or other noninvasive techniques.

We are therefore of the opinion that imaging techniques, which are in any case included in the protocol for "clinical staging," are not of use in staging for ovarian carcinoma at its early stages, except for the rare occasions when they have images that are clearly metastatic, this being then confirmed by echoguided thin-needle biopsy.

This is also the opinion of the group at the "Tumor Institute" of Milan, who found that in 40% of cases laparoscopy showed abdominal localizations of ovarian cancer that was overlooked with imaging techniques [21].

6.5.5.2 Cytology

The main route of diffusion for carcinoma of the ovary is transcelomatic: the tumor cells detach from the neoplasm and enter the peritoneal fluid; variations in endoabdominal pressure due to respiration cause the peritoneal fluid to circulate continuously from the pelvis up to the lower diaphragmatic surface, above all through the right paracolic sulcus, the main communication between the supra-and submesocolic compartment. The peritoneal fluid is thus the main vehicle for transmission of cells from one part of the abdominal cavity to another.

Abdominal cytology therefore plays a very important role in the staging of these tumors [51–56]; the technique for obtaining material to study cells is an integral part of laparoscopy, which is completed by its findings.

During laparoscopy we can obtain a sample of physiological fluid from the cavity or, if no spontaneous liquid is found, a peritoneal lavage can be made. This is always done if no peritoneal lesions are found with a thorough exploration of the peritoneal surface. Although such cases appear to be negative, tumor cells may be found and a physio-

→

Fig. 6.29. Laparoscopic follow-up in patient with prior surgery for carcinoma of the ovary. Small fleshy nodule on the parietal peritoneum. Metastasis? Biopsy: *Metastasis from carcinoma of the ovary*

Fig. 6.30. Laparoscopic follow-up in patient who had prior surgery for ovarian carcinoma. On the parietal peritoneum of the pelvis can be seen a fleshy pink bilobular nodule. *Metastasis?*

Fig. 6.31. Same case as in Fig. 6.30. When biopsy was taken with forceps, residual suture material was found. Probably *granuloma from foreign body*. Histological confirmation

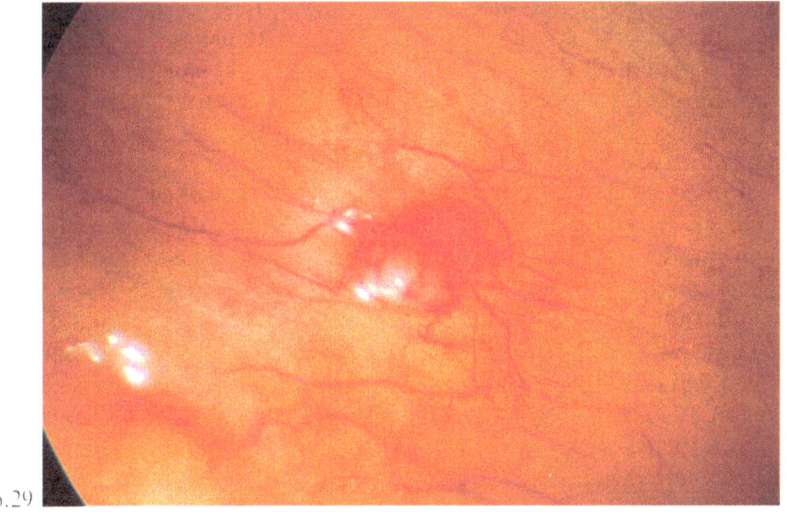

6.29

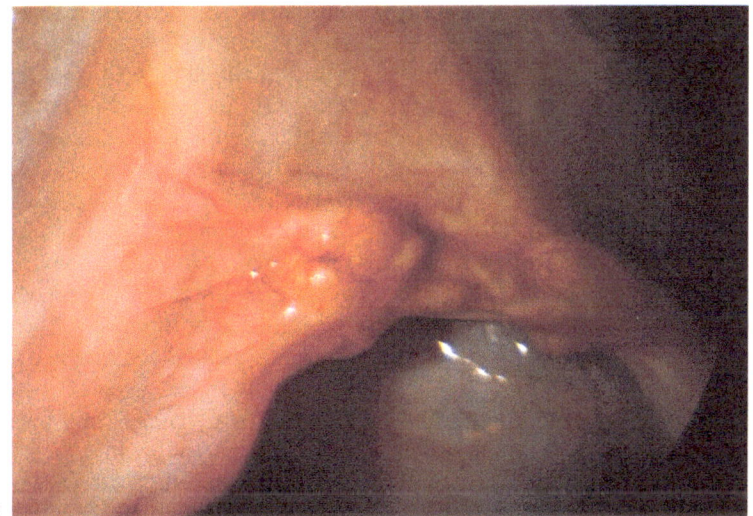

6.30

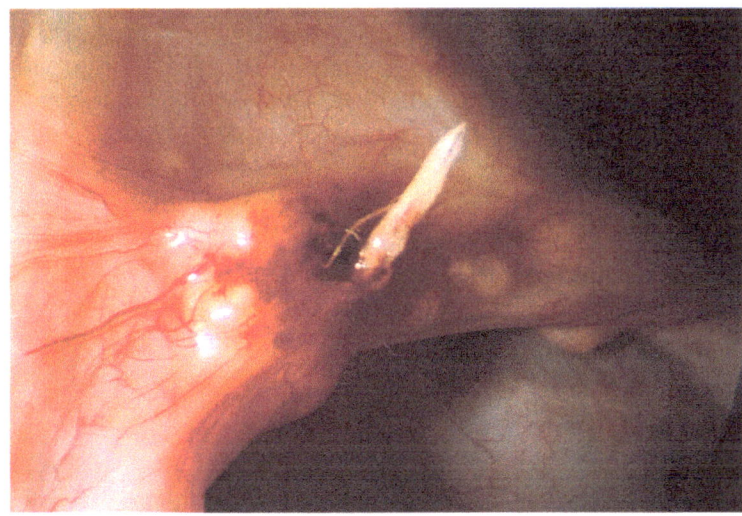

6.31

logical solution (500 ml at 37°C) is therefore injected into the cavity through the operating laparoscopic channel. The patient is then put into different decubitus positions for about 10 min so that the liquid comes into contact with all the surfaces of the peritoneal serosa. The liquid is then searched for with the naked eye in the different sites where, depending on the patient's position, it has collected, being aspirated using a long needle passed through the laparoscope. We usually manage to recover 300–350 ml of the 500 ml liquid originally injected. The aspirated material must be sent immediately to the laboratory. Systematic cytological examination of either spontaneous or lavage fluid enables us to detect neoplastic cells in the abdomen in 6%–8% of cases that are macroscopically negative at laparoscopy [54, 56]. In our series we found similar percentages (7.36%), with a corresponding upstaging [57].

6.5.5.3 Follow-up and Restaging

Surgery has long been entrusted with checking results during, and at the termination of, therapy. The so-called "second look" and, where necessary, "further looks" were made both to have a restaging, and to excise any remaining neoplastic tissue resistant to radio- or polychemotherapy. For the above-specified reasons for staging and because it is easy to repeat and causes minimal trauma, laparoscopy is now used systematically in the follow-up and restaging of ovarian carcinoma [56–61].

The series reported in the literature are highly heterogeneous and an accurate evaluation of the results is therefore difficult. We can, however, say that if laparoscopy is performed during a clinical remission in patients with a previously detected abdominal metastasis, in 25%–35% of cases it can show that these have persisted; in our latest series laparoscopic findings were positive for metastases in 33% of patients who had apparently been cured [61].

The difficulty involved in making laparoscopic "searches" with this technique does have its limitations. After completion of therapy any neoplastic remains may be minimal and can be overlooked, even during an extremely thorough search.

Moreover, in patients who have undergone one laparotomy or more, especially if recent, small nodules, spots, or thickenings of an uncertain nature are often found in the abdomen. In these cases it is essential to take bioptic specimens of

suspected lesions that could be metastases (Fig. 6.29), inflammatory reactions, or granulomas. It is not unusual to find foreign body granulomas, residues of suture material, or inflammatory reactions adjacent to malignant lesions (Figs. 6.30, 6.31).

Finally, the adhesions consequent to prior surgery can limit the exploration, thus making the laparoscopic finding less reliable. The pitfalls should always be false negatives. Of course as in staging, spontaneous liquid or physiological solution injected must be submitted to cytological examination as, in the absence of visible lesions, this can evidence whether the tumor has persisted.

In subjects submitted to therapy, however, cytological findings must be used with great caution. We found that in 13 out of 38 cases in which neoplastic lesions were present and confirmed by biopsy, cytology was negative. This is due to the fact that the isolated tumor cells are less resistant and consequently any negative cytological findings are not completely reliable.

There are therefore many pitfalls and laparoscopy cannot replace surgery for a reliable appraisal at the completion of therapy for carcinoma of the ovary. Yet it is an extremely valuable supportive technique, particularly when dealing with the delicate problem of choosing, on the basis of concrete, objective evidence, the most opportune moment for a "second" or "further" surgical "look." Now laparoscopy and surgery are used in combination following a procedure that is universally considered valid [57–62]. When a therapeutic cycle considered adequate for a complete sterilization of the neoplastic tissue has been completed, an anatomical check must be made in order to evaluate the outcome of therapy and to decide how to continue with therapy. Laparoscopy is now used to do this, not laparotomy. The most appropriate therapy is therefore chosen in a rational way, on the basis of laparoscopy using the following scheme.

1. Laparoscopy shows that there is still neoplastic tissue in the form of small peritoneal omental lesions, etc., that are confirmed bioptically, or the macroscopic examination is negative but the cytological finding, from spontaneous liquid or lavage, indicates that neoplastic cells are present. In this case, because clinical remission has no corresponding anatomical sterilization, therapy must be continued, and any necessary modifications made to it. In such cases, it provides important indications for the continuation of therapy,

and obviates superfluous surgery. It does this, as already stated, in about one-third of patients.

2. Laparoscopy not only demonstrates that residual neoplastic tissue is present, but also reveals remaining, quite large, formations at the omentum, small pelvis, etc., that were refractive to therapy and that require exeresis. In these cases, endoscopy indicates that surgery must be performed to excise the neoplastic tissue. Laparotomy is therefore performed because of an exact indication and for therapeutic purposes.

3. Laparoscopy does not detect neoplastic lesions and cytology is negative. Anatomically the disease appears to be in remission. Unfortunately, however, as the negative laparoscopic finding is not reliable, a surgical "look" is required to check whether there has been a complete sterilization of the process or not. As already stated for staging, surgical exploration in the small pelvis provides a greater guarantee.

Combined laparoscopy and surgery, used as an alternative on the basis of these criteria, is the most effective and rational means available in the management of ovarian tumors.

6.6 Conclusions

1. The integration between echography and laparoscopy can give highly satisfactory results in the study of abdominal neoplasms by reducing the number of unnecessary laparoscopies and by giving an overall increase in the diagnostic potential.

The scheme we employed for a combined echographic and laparoscopic study of abdominal tumors is as follows: (a) clinical suspicion of abdominal neoplasm and (b) staging, follow-up, and restaging of malignant neoplasm.

2. For the *diagnosis of abdominal tumors*, laparoscopy, as has already been stated, is not indicated as often as it was, its indications being inversely proportional to the ability of non-invasive techniques and fine-needle biopsy to diagnose the different types of tumor in each organ.

3. On the other hand, in recent years laparoscopy has made great steps forward, the progress being made both in technique and in "oncological" methodology. This has considerably increased its diagnostic potential in this field.

Laparoscopy is therefore still valid in *staging*, *follow-up*, and *restaging*, above all for tumors with characteristics that make them difficult to detect with imaging techniques. In particular some fundamental points must be stressed [62]:

1. Laparoscopy is used systematically in the study of malignant lymphomas. It has practically replaced laparosplenectomy in non-Hodgkin's lymphomas. In Hodgkin's disease laparosplenectomy is used when laparoscopy with multiple biopsy reveals no evidence of disease in order to avoid false negatives. Laparoscopy is also used in follow-up examinations to facilitate rational therapeutic decisions.

2. Small-cell lung cancers are now managed with "pathological" staging thanks to laparoscopy. This modality was not previously used. Laparoscopic staging gives a fairly high percentage of "upstagings" as compared with clinical staging. Laparoscopy is also used regularly in the follow-up of these tumors.

3. Laparoscopy has introduced systematic staging in the management of esophageal carcinomas where previously the possibility of pathological staging was completely ignored. Information on tumor diffusion and possible alcoholic liver disease is crucial in the choice of correct therapy.

Ultrasound Findings

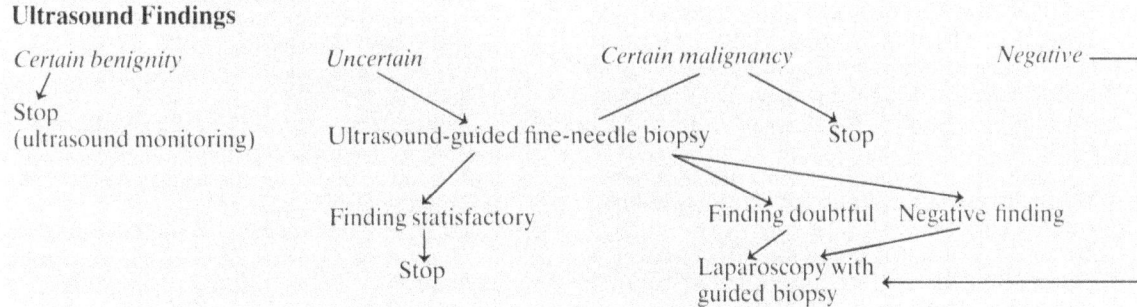

4. Laparoscopy has an important role in the management of ovarian cancer today, where it is associated with surgery for both staging and follow-up. Exploration of the diaphragmatic peritoneum with biopsies allows detection of metastatic disease often not revealed by laparotomy.

References

1. Spinelli P, Pizzetti P, Dal Frate M (1985) La laparoscopia in oncologia. Med Paziente 1:40–45
2. Dagnini G, Bergamo S, Caldironi MW, De Stavola G (1977) Esempi e proposte di follow-up laparoscopico di neoplasie maligne. In: Abstracts of the 7th Congress Soc Ital End Digest Palermo
3. Dagnini G (1980) Attuali vedute sullo staging e sul follow-up laparoscopico nei tumori maligni. G Ital Gastroenterol Endosc 3:1–8
4. Dagnini G (1982) Considérations à propos de la surveillance laparoscopique des localisations abdominales des tumeurs malignes sous traitement. Acta Endoscopica 12(1):91–96
5. De Vita VT Jr, Bagley CM Jr, Goodell B, O'Kieffe DA, Truyllo NP (1971) Peritoneoscopy in the staging of Hodgkin's disease. Cancer Res 31:1746–1750
6. Aisenberg AC (1978) The staging and treatment of Hodgkin's disease. N Engl J Med 299(22):1228–1232
7. Weitzman S, Aisenberg AC (1977) Fulminant sepsis after the successful treatment of Hodgkin's disease. Ann J Med 62:47–50
8. Dionigi R, Monico R (1984) Le infezioni in chirurgia oncologica. Proc 8th Nat Congr Sico. Monduzzi, Bologna
9. Spinelli P (1980) La laparoscopia nello staging dei linfomi maligni. In: Veronesi U, Emanueli H. et al. (eds) Progressi diagnostici in oncologia. Ambrosiana, Milano
10. Bolondi L, Gandolfi L, Labò G (1984) Diagnostic ultrasound in gastroenterology. Piccin Butterworths, Padova
11. Castellino RA (1982) Imaging techniques for staging abdominal Hodgkin's disease. Cancer Treat Rep 4:697–700
12. Richards MA, Webb JAW, Reznek RH, Davies G, Jewell SE, Shand WS, Wrigley PFM, Lister TA (1987) Riconoscimento della diffusione di un linfoma maligno al fegato per mezzo della risonanza magnetica a bassa forza di campo. Br Med. J 6:250–256
13. Weinreb JC, Brateman L, Maravilla KR (1984) Magnetic resonance imaging of hepatic lymphoma. Am J Radiol 143:1211–1214
14. Zornosa J, Cabanillas FF, Altoff TM, Ordonez N, Cohen MA (1981) Percutaneous needle biopsy in abdominal lymphoma. A J R 136:97–103
15. Jansson SE, Bondestam S, Heinonen E, Gröhn P, Vuopio P (1983) Value of liver and spleen aspiration biopsy in malignant disease when these organs show no signs of involvement in sonography. Acta Med Scand 213:279–281
16. Cavanna L, Fornari F, Buscarini E, Foroni R, Rossi S, Buscarini L (1985) Ultrasonically guided biopsy in pathological staging of non-Hodgkin's lymphomas. Haematologica 2:132–135
17. Pontifex AH, Keimo P (1984) Application of aspiration biopsy cytology. Cancer 53:553–556
18. Buscarini L, Cavanna L, Fornari F, Rossi S, Buscarini E (1985) Ultrasonically guided fine-needle biopsy: a new useful technique in pathological staging of malignant lymphoma. Acta Haematol. 73(3):150–152
19. Suzuki T, Shibuya H, Hoshimatsu S, Suzuki S (1987) Ultrasonically guided staging splenic tissue core biopsy in patients with non-Hodgkin's lymphoma. Cancer 60:879–882
20. Reguzzoni G, Limido E, Lesinigo E, Montalbetti L, Airaghi ML, Rocca F (1988) La laparoscopia nello staging dei linfomi. Recenti Prog Med. 79(5):206–209
21. Spinelli P, Pizzetti P (1987) La laparoscopia nel carcinoma ovarico: possibilità e limiti. Atti giornate di radiologia diagnostica oncologica. Monduzzi, Bologna
22. Jaffe ES (1987) Malignant lymphomas: pathology of hepatic involvement. Semin Liver Dis 7(3):257–268
23. Monconduit M, Paillot B, Piguet H (1980) Apport de la laparoscopie au diagnostic de l'atteinte hépatique des hématosarcomes. A propos de cent examens. Sem Hop Paris, 56, 439–444
24. Colby TV, Hopper RT, Warnke RA (1982) Hodgkin's disease: a clinicopathologic study of 659 cases. Cancer 49: 1848–1858
25. Gordon CD, Sidawy MK, Talarico L, Kondi E (1984) Hodgkin's disease in the liver without splenic involvement. Arch Intern Med 144:2277–2278
26. Miola E, Marin G, Nitti D, Salvagno L (1985) Attualità in tema di staging laparoscopico del linfoma di Hodgkin. G Ital Endosc Dig 3:378
27. Earlam R, Cunha-Melo JR (1980) Oesophageal squamous cell carcinoma. A critical review of surgery. Br J Surg 67:381–390
28. Akiyama H, Tsurumaru M, Kawamura T, Ono Y (1981) Principles of surgical treatment for carcinoma of the esophagus. I. Analysis of lymph-node involvement. Am Surg 194:438–446
29. Wong J (1981) Management of carcinoma of oesophagus. JR Coll Surg Edinb 26:138–148
30. Skinner DB, Dowlatshahi KD, Demeester TR (1982) Potentially curable cancer of the esophagus. Cancer 50:2571–2575
31. Caldironi MW, Marin G, Buzzaccarini O, Tremolada C, Ruol A, Dagnini G (1984) Lo staging laparoscopico delle neoplasie esofago-cardiali. G Ital Endosc Dig 7(1):17–23
32. Dagnini G, Caldironi MW, Marin G, Buzzaccarini O, Tremolada C, Ruol A (1986) Laparoscopy in abdominal staging of esophageal carcinoma. Gastrointest Endosc 32(6):400–402

33. Shandall A, Johnson C (1985) Laparoscopy or scanning in oesophageal and gastric carcinoma? Br J Surg 72:449–451

34. Oliviero G, Constans P, Solvignon F (1980) La laparoscopie pour recherche des métastases hépatiques au cours des cancers bronchopulmonaires (115 laparoscopies). Rev Fr Mal Respir 8:163

35. Tancini G, Marchini S, Volonterio A, Barni S, Spinelli P (1982) Impiego combinato della laparoscopia e della biopsia ossea nella determinazione dello studio del carcinoma a piccole cellule del polmone. Valutazione di 116 casi consecutivi. Tumori 68:81–84

36. Dagnini G (1980) Clinical laparoscopy. Piccin Medical, Padua

37. Livinston R (1980) Small-cell carcinoma of the lung. Blood 4:575–584

38. Oldham RK, Greco FA (1980) Small-cell lung cancer. A curable disease. Cancer Chemother. Pharmacol. 4:173–177

39. Hansen SW, Jensen F, Pedersen NT, Pedersen AG, Hansen HH (1987) Detection of liver metastases in small-cell lung cancer: a comparison of peritoneoscopy with liver biopsy and ultrasonography with fine-needle aspiration. J Clin Oncol 5(2):255–259

40. Dagnini G (1987) Laparoscopy in small cell lung cancer. In: Abstracts of the international conference on small cell lung cancer. Ravenna, pp 53–55

41. Patella M, Bergamo S, Tufano A, Miola E, Dagnini G (1984) Lo staging ed il follow-up laparoscopico del microcitoma del polmone. G Ital Endosc Dig 7(1):25–30

42. Bleiberg H, La Meir E, Lejeune F (1980) Laparoscopy in the diagnosis of liver metastases in 80 cases of malignant melanoma. Endoscopy 12:215–218

43. Doiron M, Bernardino M (1981) A comparison of non-invasive imaging modalities in the melanoma patients. Cancer 47:2581–2584

44. Silverman P, Heaston D, Korobkin M, Seigler H (1984) Computed tomography in the abdominal metastases from malignant melanoma. Invest. Radiol. 19:309–312

45. Weiss SM, Skibber JM, Mohinddin M, Rosato FE (1985) Rapid intraabdominal spread of pancreatic cancer. Arch Surg 120:415–416

46. Warshaw AL, Tepper JE, Shipley WV (1986) Laparoscopy in the staging and planning of therapy for pancreatic cancer. Am J Surg 151:76–79

47. Ohoto M, Sugiura N, Ebara M (1986) Treatment of hepatocellular carcinoma by alcohol injection into tumor and irradiation. Jpn J Cancer Chemioter 13(part II):1625–1634

48. Salmi A (1988) Iniezione percutanea ecoguidata di alcool: terapia palliativa del carcinoma epatico primitivo associato a cirrosi. Risultati preliminari. Recenti Prog Med 79:449–451

49. Bagley CM Jr, Young RC, Schein PS, Chabner BA, De Vita VT (1973) Ovarian carcinoma to the diaphragm frequently undiagnosed at laparotomy. A preliminary report. Am J Obstet Gynecol 116:397–400

50. Rosenoff SH, De Vita VT, Hubbard S, Young RC (1975) Peritoneoscopy in the staging and follow-up of ovarian cancer. Semin Oncol 2:223–228

51. Piver MS, Lopez RG, Xynos F, Barlow JJ (1977) The value of pre-therapy peritoneoscopy in localized ovarian cancer. Am J Obstet Gynecol 127:288–290

52. Lacey CG, Morrow PC, Di Saia PJ, Lucas WE (1978) Laparoscopy in the evaluation of gynecologic cancer. Obstet Gynecol 52:708–712

53. Mangioni C, Bolis G, Molteni P, Belloni C (1979) Indications, advantages and limits of laparoscopy in ovarian cancer. Gynecol Oncol 7:47–55

54. Spinelli P, Pilotti S, Luini A, Spatti G, Pizzetti P, de Palo G (1979) Laparoscopy combined with peritoneal cytology in staging and restaging ovarian carcinoma. Tumori 65:601–610

55. Tolino A, Mastrantonio P, Di Serio C, Berruto Caracciolo G (1981) Laparoscopic staging of ovarian carcinoma. Eur J Gynecol Oncol 2:113–118

56. Ozols RF, Fisher RI, Anderson T, Makuch R, Young RC (1981) Peritoneoscopy in the management of ovarian cancer. Am J Ostet Gynecol 140:611–619

57. Marin G, Caldironi MW, Piccigallo E, Bandini F, Nicoletto O, Dagnini G (1984) Lo staging ed il follow-up laparoscopico del tumore ovarico. G Ital Endosc Dig 1(7):31–38

58. Piver MS, Shashikant BL, Barlow JJ, Gamarra M (1980) Second-look laparoscopy prior to proposed second-look laparotomy. Obstet Gynecol 55:571–573

59. Giardina G, Sismondi P, Prelato L, Zola P (1980) Utilità della seconda laparotomia e della laparoscopia nel follow-up delle pazienti in trattamento per tumori ovarici. Minerva Ginecol 32:699–701

60. Jing Q, Ai-da, Li-chuan L (1984) Laparoscopy in the diagnosis and management of ovarian cancer. J Reprod Med 29(7):483–488

61. Dagnini G, Marin G, Caldironi MW, Piccigallo E, Miola E (1987) Laparoscopy in staging, follow-up and restaging of ovarian carcinoma. Gastrointest Endosc 33:80–83

62. Dagnini G, Marin G (1986) Laparoscopy in staging and follow-up of tumours: is its role of secondary or essential importance? In: Dobrilla G (ed) Problems and controversies in gastroenterology. Cortina International, Verona

7 Emergency Laparoscopy

Only since the 1960s has laparoscopy been used for abdominal emergencies. Until then laparoscopy had been considered contraindicated in acute abdomen because the premedication required, pneumoperitoneum, was considered too risky. It was also thought that trauma from the examination might cause a further deterioration in the patient's condition. Yet the first attempts at laparoscopy in patients with acute abdomen proved that the risks were minimal and, moreover, information and invaluable data were obtained in situations in which an accurate diagnosis had to be made quickly [1, 2].

The now widespread use of emergency laparoscopy depends on the successful results obtained when the first attempts were made. Llanio was a true pioneer in this area, making an extraordinary contribution to the use of emergency laparoscopy. In Cuba in 1965 he founded an important center to provide constant day and night emergency laparoscopic examinations. Emergency laparoscopy is usually performed to: (a) Clarify an uncertain diagnosis in cases of *acute non-traumatic abdomen* (suspicion of acute hepatobiliary diseases, appendicitis, peritonitis, acute pancreatitis, acute abdominal vascular diseases, etc.) or (b) recognize and clarify the site, type, and severity of any lesions in *blunt abdominal traumas* and in *multiple traumas.*

Laparoscopy achieved these aims in a highly effective way: as early as 1973 in a series of 1265 observations, Llanio reported that this examination resolved the diagnosis in 97% of cases and failed in only 0.12% [3]. Endoscopic findings allowed a useless laparotomy to be obviated, or it allowed any necessary surgery to be performed without incurring any additional risks.

In short, emergency laparoscopy was found to be:

1. Simple to perform (technically the same as a routine laparoscopy), well tolerated, and not particularly dangerous
2. Capable of detecting and clarifying in a high number of cases spontaneous or traumatic lesions causing acute abdomen
3. Almost always capable of establishing whether an immediate laparotomy is required or whether it would be useless
4. Finally, by revealing the site, nature, and features of the lesion, it "guides" any necessary surgical procedure and enables us to decide preoperatively upon the surgical approach.

Laparoscopy was therefore the ideal means for resolving problems from acute abdomen. In the early 1970s it was in fact believed that the diagnostic value of emergency laparoscopy was above dispute and that its use should be more widespread. Gastroenterologists, internists, and, above all, surgeons should therefore be persuaded to consider emergency laparoscopy a routine procedure, using it just as one uses a plain ray in acute abdomen or gastroduodenoscopy in upper gastrointestinal tract hemorrhages [4].

In spite of this, however, the use of emergency laparoscopy did not increase as it might have. Except for Llanio's series, which in 1977 already consisted of 6400 cases [5] and recently over 40000 (Llanio 1986, personal communication), in the different centers throughout the world only a small number of laparoscopies have been performed, amounting to no more than 2%–3% of all laparoscopies. In 1980, in Padua, where collaboration with surgeons has always been close, out of 1050 laparoscopies, 180 (18.5%) were requested for surgeons, but only 7% for emergencies. In view of the frequency of emergency abdomen, this figure is very small. It may depend on the fact that in theory emergency laparoscopy has numerous indications but that in practice they are few and far between, because the surgeon may often consider it unnecessary.

When presented with a clinical picture that shows that emergency surgery is necessary, the surgeon is of the opinion that an accurate diagnosis is not necessary. If, however, there are not enough clues as to whether emergency surgery is required, then laparoscopy can be decisive. On the one hand it demonstrates whether laparotomy is unnecessary and on the other it shows whether emergency surgery is required, thus obviating the dangers of tardy surgery. So laparoscopy has "potential" and "real" indications; in our view the latter are all the cases characterized by the need for emergency surgery rather than an uncertain dignosis [6]. So laparoscopy is almost always superfluous in cases in which the symptoms are clear but is, on the other hand, indicated more where there is an incomplete, insidious picture that gives rise to doubt, thus suggesting to the surgeon that he or she should wait. Of course the "area of doubt" is not clearly demarked and a request for laparoscopy is made on the basis of a subjective impression. For example, a series of 176 children were operated on for acute appendicitis; in 141 of these acute appendicitis, or another disease that justified the operation, was found. But in 20 cases no lesions were found; 14 patients underwent preliminary laparoscopy and in 6 cases this examination showed that surgery was not required [7]. Other authors are in favor of laparoscopy for cases in which appendicitis is suspected, for it allows the diagnosis to be changed and a useless laparotomy to be obviated [8–12].

Therefore, as clinical criteria are not infallible, it might be opportune to make use of laparoscopy more often. It has also been suggested that laparoscopy should be used more often in *blunt* and *multiple* abdominal traumas. In these cases shock and a compromised general status can mask serious lesions to the organs, making clinical symptoms appear moderate or even undermine them completely; this means that a very important disease may be overlooked. Systematically followed laparoscopy allows us to rule out, or detect, any lesions that would otherwise escape diagnosis and to then take the most suitable possible steps.

7.1 Present Indications for Laparoscopy

Before imaging techniques were available, we had reconsidered the classical indications for emergency laparoscopy. Imaging techniques allow us to resolve satisfactorily many diagnostic problems and to evaluate acute spontaneous or posttraumatic abdomen, so the indications for laparoscopy have undergone a further, more radical, change.

7.1.1 Acute Spontaneous Abdomen

Nowadays in the large majority of cases acute abdomen is diagnosed on the basis of clinical and laboratory examinations, X-ray, and sonography. The latter is usually decisive in cases of *acute suppurative cholecystitis*, *acute pancreatitis*, *perforations from gastric or duodenal ulcers*, and *acute appendicitis*, above all when there is a purulent collection at the perforation point. In such cases the surgeon must operate immediately and laparoscopy is superfluous.

In laparoscopic series before imaging techniques were available, endoabdominal hemorrhages were found in a relatively high number of cases. For spontaneous hemoperitoneum laparoscopy was mandatory; it almost always established the entity of the phenomenon, its site, as well as its cause. The hemorrhage could be due to mechanical damage to the liver or spleen (either "spontaneous" or provoked by small traumas that had been overlooked), ectopic pregnancies or other lesions to the female genitalia, etc. Imaging techniques can now reveal very small blood collections and indicate whether the hemorrhage is due to a tumor (as in, for example, hepatocarcinoma); it also indicates the site and cause of bleeding. With sonography, moreover, repeated examinations can be made to follow closely the evolution of the condition in order to establish whether or not the hemorrhage will stop spontaneously, and in turn decide whether or not a laparotomy is required. In these cases laparoscopy is hardly ever necessary.

However, occasionally difficulties may arise in the diagnosis, and it may not be clear whether surgery is required. Then, as recently pointed out by the surgeon and laparoscopist, Berci, laparoscopy can provide information that is useful for the approach [12].

Furthermore, Berci believes, on very good grounds, that "minilaparoscopy" is advantageous when performed using a small 4-mm-diameter telescope and oblique vision. He also stresses the importance of a complete exploration, made by introducing a probe for palpation through a second hole. Of course this maneuver must be made with great care so as to avoid perforating the intestinal loops that have been made more fragile by the disease itself. We, however, have always used the normal 10-mm-diameter operating laparoscope successfully, also for emergencies.

There are cases of acute abdomen in which the sonographic finding is *negative*, or *not indicative enough*. Here laparoscopy is definitely indicated. We must above all decide whether this is a "genuine" or "false" echographic negative. The former might appear surprising, but there are cases of clinically established acute abdomen with no concomitant intraabdominal organic lesion. Both surgical and laparoscopic experience attest to this. We have observed that in about 10% of cases of acute spontaneous abdomen the laparoscopic finding is negative. In their series, Cortesi et al. reported negative laparoscopic findings in 4% of cases [13], while Fahrlaender reported 13.6% [14]. This phenomenon may be caused simply by a violent spasm, and therefore have a functional basis. More often, however, the picture is due to a peritoneal reaction caused by extraabdominal processes that are known to be capable of causing symptoms that are compatible with acute abdomen. The most important are myocardial infarct, pulmonitis of the lower lobe, common iliac artery embolism, and various retroperitoneal diseases. In these cases neither the negative sonographic finding nor the clinical symptoms are convincing; it is difficult for the surgeon to decide whether or not to operate. So here laparoscopy is invaluable because it enables us to clarify doubts and suggests which other diagnostic investigations should be made. So a laparotomy without a clear objective is obviated: it would be both useless and very risky. On the other hand, negative sonographic findings may not always reflect a real absence of abdominal lesions. These "false negatives" are obtained when the acute abdomen is caused by an organic process with lesions that have escaped echographic detection because of their site and features. This can happen, for example, in *acute carcinomatosis* and in *acute miliary tuberculosis* of the peritoneum. With laparoscopy the problem is easily solved.

In both these situations the disease has "exploded" – with a diffuse spread of tiny, miliary nodules that cover the entire surface of the parietal and visceral peritoneum, which appears highly congested (Fig. 7.1).

The laparoscopic finding is patently clear; the diagnosis is not always easily made on the basis of the macroscopic picture alone unless there is metastasization of a melanoblastoma because this has an unmistakable appearance. With biopsy, however, a diagnosis can always be made.

The shortcomings of sonography in the exploration of the peritoneum are known: the small dimensions of the lesions, whether they are neoplastic or tubercular, explain why the echographic findings are negative. This in our experience does not occur frequently but it is a possibility that should never be underestimated: in their series, Cortesi et al. report that tuberculosis was found in 10% [13]; and over 5% of Sundal's [14] cases were acute peritoneal carcinomatosis.

Moreover, the echographic picture may be negative or may fail to answer the clinical questions in some forms of acute abdomen, forms with attenuated clinical symptoms. The clinical diagnosis is doubtful and emergency laparotomy is also not clearly indicated. In these situations, too, laparoscopy is still definitely indicated. In some cases, for example, a lesion is found at the endoscopic examination; it is characterized only by a moderate congestion and by an overall enlargement of the appendix, which appears tumid and stiff with a taut shiny wall and smooth, transparent serosa (Fig. 7.2). Even if the finding is not patently clear and there are no signs of suppuration and necrosis, the diagnosis of acute appendicitis is certain. The usefulness of laparoscopy in the diagnosis of appendicitis in doubtful cases has also recently been confirmed [15].

In other cases in which symptoms are attenuated and the echographic finding negative, a laparoscopic examination can show whether in a particular area the parietal or visceral peritoneum is congested and partially covered by fibrinopurulent deposits with the intestinal loops tending to adhere to each other (Fig. 7.3). This finding is definite and it also demonstrates that, if there are no purulent collections, sonography fails to allow a diagnosis of active fibrinopurulent peritonitis to be made.

In *intestinal infarct* laparoscopy may also be necessary. Often infarct may only be suspected on the basis of the clinical picture and the echographic finding, particularly when its form is not acute or when it is in its initial stages. In these cases it is of crucial importance to make an early diagnosis because the success of surgical resection depends greatly upon prompt intervention. Laparoscopy effectively confirms the lesion and establishes whether emergency surgery is necessary. The laparoscopic finding is simple to interpret and it enables us to ascertain whether the lesion is severe and/or long-standing. It shows the length of intestinal tract with ischemia.

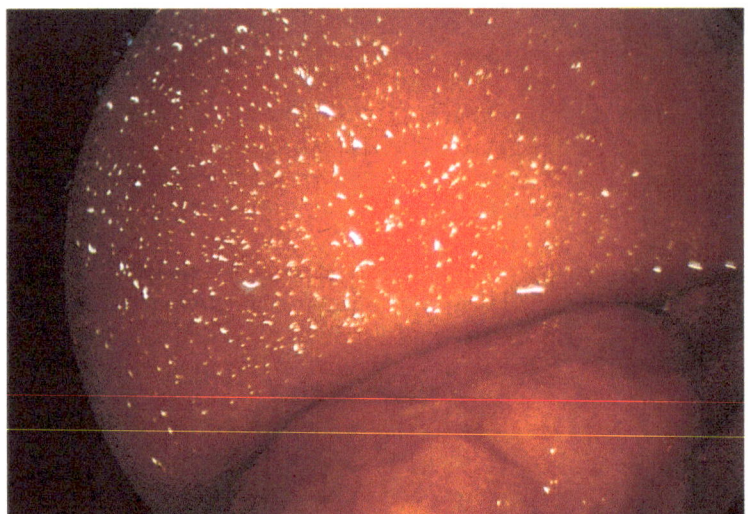

7.1

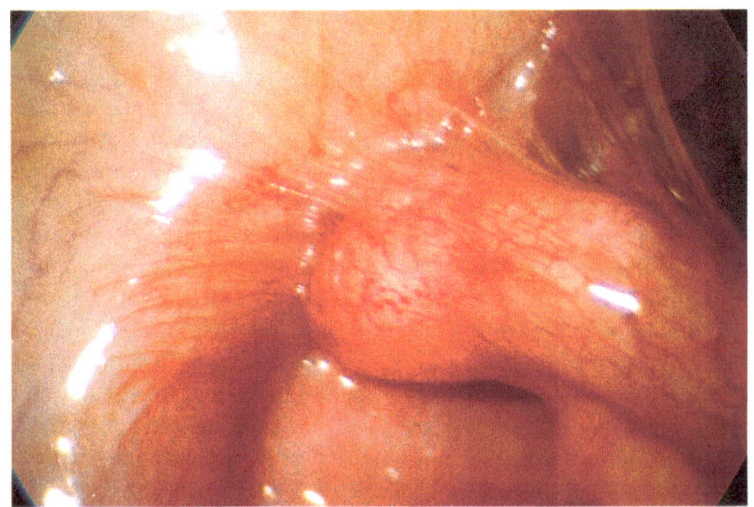

7.2

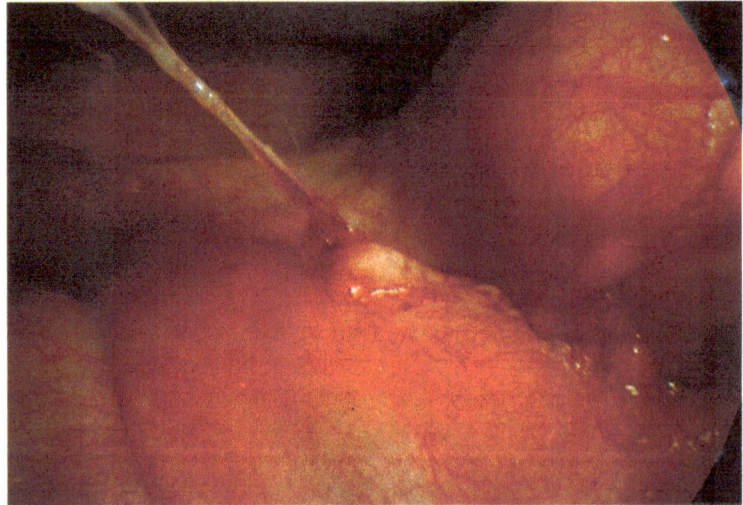

7.3

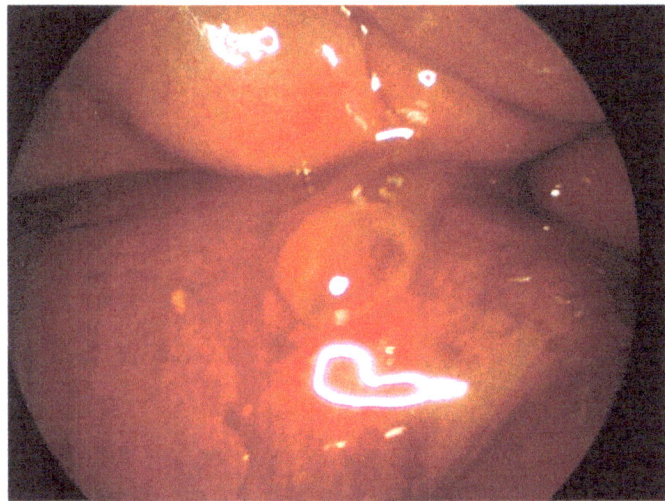

7.4

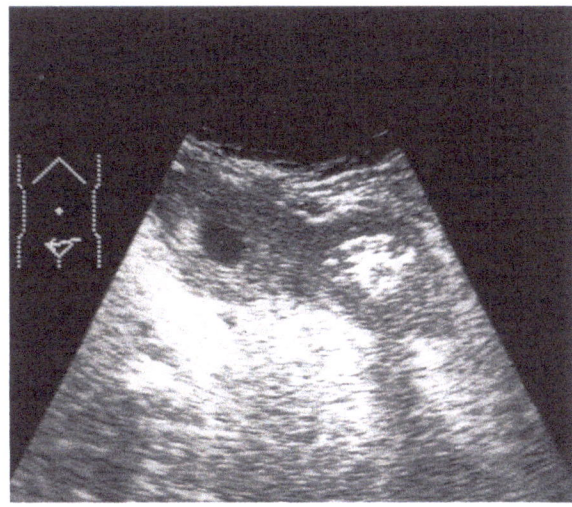

7.5

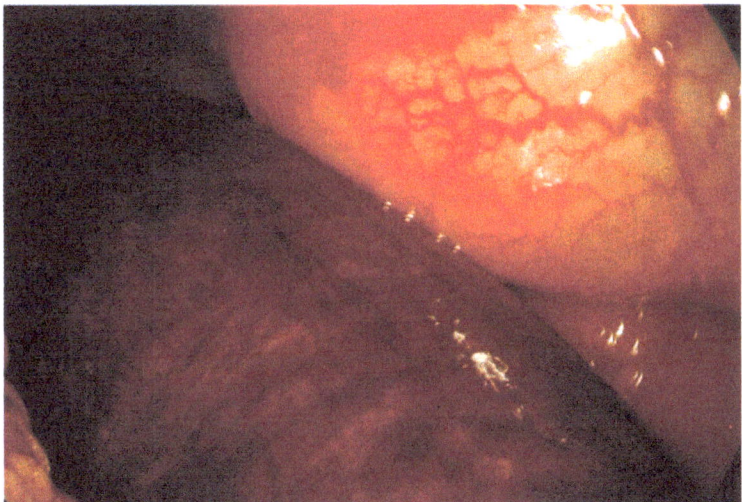

7.6

Fig. 7.4. Acute spontaneous abdomen. Large intestine loop with marked edema, passive congestion, and signs of initial necrosis. *In the center* is a collection of turbid yellowish material. Infarct of the large intestine; signs of perforation

Fig. 7.1. Acute spontaneous abdomen. Gross congestion of the parietal and visceral peritoneum with spread of numerous miliary granules. *Acute peritoneal tuberculosis*

Fig. 7.2. Acute spontaneous abdomen. Enlarged edematous cecal appendix, with slight active congestion. *Appendicitis*

Fig. 7.3. Acute spontaneous abdomen. Diffuse acute congestion of the visceral peritoneum with the presence of dense exudate and a tendency to adhere to the loops. *Fibrinopurulent peritonitis*

Fig. 7.5. Acute spontaneous abdomen. Prelaparoscopic echography. Two roundish images can be seen attributable to the section of two intestinal loops with marked thickening and dishomogeneity of an anechogenic content. *Probably intestinal infarct*

Fig. 7.6. Same case as in Fig. 7.5. Laparoscopy. *Top*, normal intestinal loop with passive congestion; *bottom*, another loop which appears to be entirely necrotic. *Advanced stage of intestinal infarct*

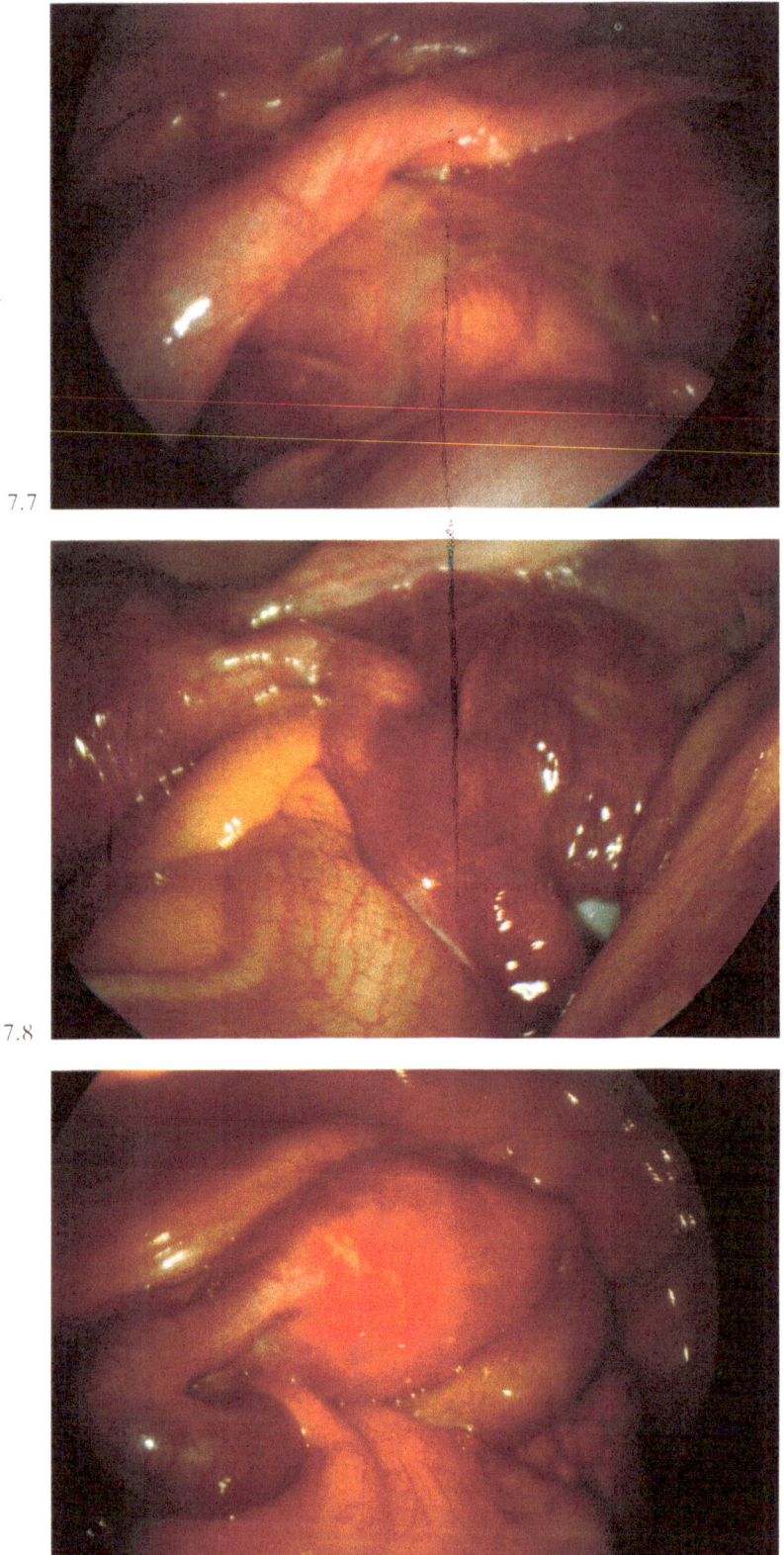

7.7

7.8

7.9

On the basis of the above information we can decide whether the lesion is so serious and extensive that surgery is out of the question [14]. We successfully performed laparoscopies in ten patients with different forms of infarct. In two cases the clinical picture was obtained slowly and the abdominal symptoms were neither clear nor marked; noninvasive examinations were of no help. Intestinal infarct might be suspected, but it had to be confirmed. In both patients laparoscopy demonstrated a typical infarct of the small intestine affecting tracts of 60 and 110 cm respectively. Immediate surgical resections were performed and the patients were cured.

In another case, the clinical picture was more complete and acute diffuse peritonitis was suspected. Sonography demonstrated a picture compatible with ileus and the presence of liquid but did not allow a diagnosis to be made. Laparoscopy revealed vascular alterations (edema and moderate passive congestion) of a small intestine loop, which were not particularly serious; at one point there were clear signs of a small perforation (Fig. 7.4). Emergency surgery was performed.

In the remaining cases, the clinical symptoms were particularly serious, and the deterioration was general and also specifically abdominal. In such cases the echographic examination can give a quite significant picture characterized by hypo-echogenic ring-shaped images corresponding to the walls of the intestinal loops, which are generally thickened (Fig. 7.5). Laparoscopy was performed in order to confirm the diagnosis and to evaluate the severity of the lesion and length of intestinal tract affected. The findings were extremely serious: a segment of intestine was almost completely necrotic (Fig. 7.6). Perhaps when echography provides diagnostically useful findings, the process has already reached a particularly advanced stage and is so serious that the results of resection are seriously compromised.

Finally, in acute abdomen in women with symptoms at the iliac fossae, laparoscopy is important for differential diagnosis between acute diseases of the female genitalia and it can enable us to avoid unnecessary surgery.

Endoscopically, we can also obtain material for a bacteriological analysis and this is important when deciding upon antibiotic treatment [16].

The three examples presented here testify to the value of laparoscopy in such cases (Figs. 7.7–7.9). In one patient sonography had shown that the Fallopian tubes were dilated; laparoscopy revealed acute nodular hydrosalpingitis. In another, the endoscopic examination enabled us to make a diagnosis of acute hemorrhagic adnexitis.

7.1.2 Abdominal Trauma

In blunt abdominal trauma and in multiple traumas with shock and coma, the symptoms can be masked or entirely undermined because the patient's general condition is seriously compromised. Therefore, in the presonographic era, laparoscopy was widely recommended in all cases in which it was reasonable to suspect that there was abdominal involvement.

The most frequent abdominal traumas are rupture of parenchymatous organs like the liver, spleen, and kidney and rupture of large vessels with hemorrhage or laceration of the bile ducts, intestine, bladder, etc. In these cases a free hemoperitoneum, hematoma, or fluid collection of another type can easily be detected, localized, and its entity evaluated using sonography, which is the technique of choice for these lesions. Peritoneal lavage, often used to discover abdominal hemorrhages, even if small, and laparoscopy have therefore been almost completely supplanted by echography, which must be performed in all cases of closed abdominal trauma and in multiple traumas with shock in the search for any lesions. This also applies to cases without abdominal symptoms. Obviously, a noninvasive technique is particularly indicated for systematic screening. Sonography, moreover, allows us to discover and ascertain the entity of a site of bleeding but also, as stated for "spontaneous" hemorrhages, it allows us to work out the outcome through performing repeat examinations at intervals in order to decide the best approach in each particular case.

◄─────────────────────────────

Fig. 7.7. Pelvis. Raised large intestine loop fixed upwards. Below the uterus and the right annex cannot be seen because they are covered by adherent adipose tissue and fibrinopurulent material. *Pelviperitonitis*

Fig. 7.8. Distal portion of the left tube contains blood and has lost its morphological features. The tube angle and uterus appear normal. *Hemorrhagic salpingitis*

Fig. 7.9. Slight active diffuse congestion of the visceral peritoneum. The uterus and right tube are normal. Left adnexum (medial and, above all, distal portion) shows tumefaction, and is bluish, very taut, and shiny. *Acute left hydrosalpingitis*

Although in these cases laparoscopy has lost most of its indications, we must always bear in mind that even now well-known surgeon-laparoscopists believe that laparoscopy is still valid, and this opinion is based upon valid arguments and sound experience. According to Berci et al. [16], abdominal lavage has increased the diagnosis of intraabdominal hemorrhage. But hemoperitoneum does not always require laparotomy. So in about 20% of cases useless surgery is performed for blunt abdominal traumas; in one-fifth of patients with positive lavage no lesions or bleeding sites are found. Despite the use of CT, useless laparotomies are still performed in patients with abdominal trauma [17], with quite serious economic and social consequences [18].

Laparoscopy is therefore considered useful. Also Cortesi et al. stress the importance of laparoscopy in both multiple trauma and comatose patients who have few or none abdominal symptoms. In 42 of 106 such patients of this type, laparoscopy was negative; the remaining patients underwent laparotomy for splenectomy, liver suturing, etc., and in only two cases was surgery useless.

So laparoscopy is still of value in confirming or ruling out any indication for laparotomy. It has a sensitivity of 96.7% and a specificity of 95%. Cortesi et al. also point out that they found ultrasonography was less sensitive and specific, particularly in detecting small peritoneal effusions [19].

Again, with the use of laparoscopy, exploratory laparotomy can be reserved for selected cases of hemoperitoneum and peritonitis, in order to avoid performing unnecessary surgery, surgery that has a high morbidity coefficient.

Even with the boom in imaging techniques, laparoscopy is indicated in the following situations:

1. When the clinical picture in multiple trauma patients is masked or undermined by loss of consciousness and it is therefore impossible to rule out reliably an abdominal trauma
2. When there is a clinical history, or evident signs of a blunt trauma or a penetrating wound with mild abdominal symptoms or no symptoms at all
3. When there is severe unexplained hypotension

We stress here that the most important advantage of laparoscopy depends on the fact that it clearly shows the surgeon whether an operation is required or not [16]. In patients with hemoperitoneum, traditional laparoscopy allows us to establish the entity of the collection and the site of origin

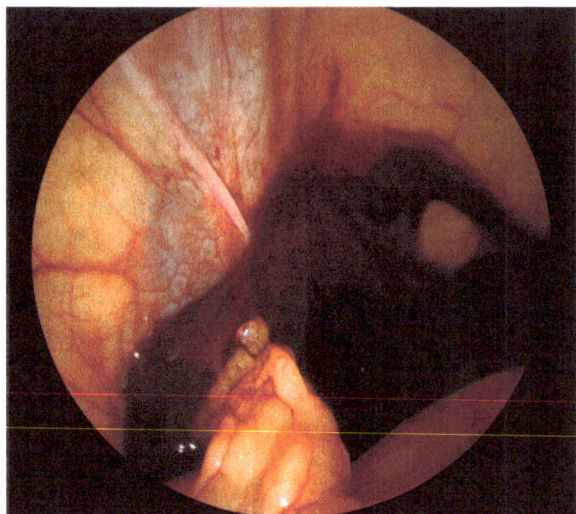

Fig. 7.10. Blunt abdominal trauma. Large clot adhering to the medial angle of the hemidiaphragm at the base of the falciform ligament of the liver. *Hemorrhage from a probable rupture of the liver*

of the hemorrhage. Often only indirect signs are found, but these are equally important, for they indicate which organ is affected by the lesion. The most important hemorrhagic signs are concentrated proximal to the damaged organ. Large clots collect here and labile adhesions appear between the various contiguous structures. For example, mechanical damage to the liver is suspected if hemoperitoneum with clots is in contact with the liver (Fig. 7.10). Hematoma of the left phrenic cavity indicates laceration of the spleen. However, even if the parenchymal organs can be explored endoscopically, it is often difficult to detect the lesion because the presence of blood hinders the search and also because these types of damage, even if they cause major hemorrhages, can be relatively mild. Nor is it wise to overexplore with the laparoscope or probe between the clots and adhesions because in this way a hemorrhage that might have arrested itself spontaneously can be triggered off again. On the basis of the findings themselves the surgeon can decide whether surgery is necessary, whether it may be postponed, or whether it would be useless.

Laparoscopy is therefore of great diagnostic importance in abdominal traumas and in multiple traumas when the patient's general condition is seriously compromised. However, I firmly believe that for hemorrhage from trauma, although laparoscopy is occasionally indicated, in most cases a thorough preliminary echographic examination followed by repeated ultrasound examinations provides enough information to indicate whether it is safe to wait, or whether emergency surgery must be performed. I believe on the other hand that laparoscopies are definitely indicated in abdominal trauma when the symptoms are scarce, when echography provides insufficient information, and lavage provides only a slightly positive result. In such situations laparoscopy enables us to rule out an organic lesion or detect signs showing that immediate laparotomy is mandatory. This examination detects, for example, bile leakage, the presence of food or fecal material, demonstrating a rupture of the main bile ducts, stomach, or intestine.

In a patient with positive lavage it is simple to decide against surgery when there are signs of bleeding that explain the result of the examination, but only when the lesion is modest and clearly insignificant. A serohematic leakage is significant and should not be underestimated, because it almost always denotes a lesion to the bladder or another hollow organ.

7.2 Conclusions

1. Laparoscopy is a highly valuable means of investigation in acute spontaneous or traumatic abdomen, particularly when it is not clear whether emergency surgery is necessary.

2. Now, however, the problems pertaining to acute abdomen are usually resolved with noninvasive techniques, so laparoscopy has lost many of its indications.

3. Laparoscopy can, however, be of use in acute spontaneous abdomen when the abdominal symptoms are scarce or attenuated and the sonographic findings are negative or not definitive. This can occur, for example, in peritoneal diseases with scarce, or no, exudations or when no fluid or blood collections are detected sonographically.

4. Recently, interest has again been shown in emergency laparoscopy for abdominal traumas, above all in patients with attenuated symptoms.

References

1. Bosquien Y, Herbouiller M, Delemeau G, Lennec C, Lemouroux M (1964) Intérét de la péritoneoscopie dans le diagnostic des affections aiguës de l'abdomen. Presse Med 72:1701–1706
2. Débray C, Débray G, Piranneau A, Paolaggi JA, Papi E, Herzaft R (1968) La laparoscopie en traumatologie abdominale. Son intéret. Arch Fr Mal Appar Dig 57:971–984
3. Llanio R, Sotto A, Jimenez G, Quintero M, Ferret O, Manso E, Nodarse O (1973) La laparoscopie d'urgence (étude portant sur 1265 cas). Sem Hop Paris 12:873–877
4. Paolaggi JA (1973) La laparoscopie d'urgence en patologie abdominale. Nouv Presse Med 2:411–413
5. Llanio R (1977) La laparoscopia en urgencias. Ed Cientifico-Tecnica, La Habana
6. Dagnini G, Marin G, Patella M (1981) La laparoscopia d'urgenza. Ann Med Perugia 72:513–517
7. Schwöbel MG, Stauffer UG (1980) Der Stellenwert der Laparoskopie bei Verdacht auf akute Appendizitis. Z Kinderchir 29(1):24–29
8. Jersky J, Hoffman, Shapiro J, Kurgan A (1980) Laparoscopy in patients with suspected appendicitis. South Afr J Surg 19:147–150
9. Leape LL, Ramenofsky ML (1980) Laparoscopy for questionable appendicitis – can it reduce the negative appendectomy rate? Ann Surg 191:410–413
10. Deutsch AA, Zelikovsky A, Reiss R (1982) Laparoscopy in the prevention of unnecessary appendectomies: a prospective study. Br J Surg 69:336–337
11. Dunn EL, Moore EE, Elerdin SC, Murphy SR (1982) The unnecessary laparotomy for appendicitis – can it be decreased? Am Surg 48:320–323
12. Berci G (1987) Emergency laparoscopy. In: Sivak MV. (ed) Gastroenterologic endoscopy. Saunders, Philadelphyia
13. Cortesi N, Manenti A, Gibertini G, Malagoli M (1982) La laparoscopie d'urgence dans l'abdomen aigu. Lyon Chir 7815:367
14. Sundal E, Gyr K, Fahrlaender H (1982) Peritoneoscopy in abdominal emergencies – a valuable diagnostic tool. Endoscopy 14:97–99
15. Reiertsen O, Rosseland A, Hoivik B, Solhein K (1985) Laparoscopy in patients admitted for acute abdominal pain. Acta Chir Scand 151:521–524
16. Berci G, Cuschieri A (1986) Emergency laparoscopy. In: Berci G, Cuschieri A (ed) Pratical laparoscopy. Baillière Tindall, London
17. Federle MP, Crass A, Brooke J, Trunkey DO (1982) Computed tomography in blunt abdominal trauma. Arch Surg 117:645–650
18. Petersen SR, Sheldon GF (1979) Morbidity of a negative finding at laparotomy in abdominal trauma. Surg Gynecol Obstet 148:23–26
19. Cortesi N, Manenti A, Gibertini G, Rossi A (1987) Emergency laparoscopy in multiple trauma patients: experience with 106 cases. Acta Chir Belg 87:239–241

Subject Index

G. Feifel, U. Hildebrandt, University of Homburg/Saar;
N. I. McC. Mortensen, University of Bristol (Eds.)

Endosonography

1990. Approx. 350 pp. Approx. 250 figs. 2 colored tabs.
ISBN 3-540-50503-2

This book covers the subject of endosonography in all
its aspects: historical development, physical principles,
and clinical application.
In the first section, the development of endosonographic technique is traced. The pioneer of endolumi-
nal ultrasound outlines methods from radar technology
up to the first prototype of a flexible endosonic probe.
The initial attempts in tissue characterization via ultrasound are described. Then the discussion of applied
physics provides a useful starting point for understanding the endosonographic principles whose application
and relevance become evident in the following
chapters.
The second section gives an overview on the application of endosonography, with emphasis on oncology.
The chapters on gastroenterology cover the malignancy, resectability and lymph node involvement of
lesions in the upper GI tract (esophagus, stomach,
duodenum, pancreas, liver and the biliary system) as
well as assessment of benign and malignant lesions in
the lower GI tract. The chapter on gynecology deals
with the pre-treatment staging of tumors and post-treat-
ment follow-up. The chapter on urology covers normal
and abnormal anatomy of the prostate gland, with
emphasis on prostate cancer.
This book is a valuable contribution to the advance-
ment of endosonography.

Springer-Verlag Berlin
Heidelberg New York London
Paris Tokyo Hong Kong

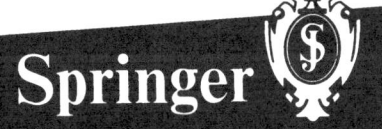

Springer

Y. Higashi, Fukuoka University, Fukuoka, Japan;
A. Mizushima, Kyushu University, Fukuoka, Japan;
H. Matsumoto, Okinawa, Japan

Introduction to Abdominal Ultrasonography

1990. Approx. 220 pp. 5 figs.
Softcover. Approx. DM 78,– ISBN 3-540-51889-4

This book is designed specifically for residents in diagnostic radiology and those just beginning to undertake ultrasound diagnosis. Several features distinguish it from the monographs on ultrasound imaging of the abdomen that are already available.
The clinical chapters begin with a detailed anatomical description of the organ or system. The most common diseases of the upper abdomen are presented, with each entity completely presented on two facing papers. The clinical discussions are brief and clear; the high-quality ultrasonograms are accompanied by schematic drawings and body marks for orientation and better understanding. A variety of different probes are presented: linear, sector, convex and contact compound. Particularly difficult imaging, for example the tubular structures of the liver, is supplemented with color illustrations to portray the three-dimensional quality of the actual examination.
The book also includes short chapters on basic physics, equipment, scanning technique and a question and answer section at the end.

Springer-Verlag Berlin
Heidelberg New York London
Paris Tokyo Hong Kong

Prices are subject to change without notice.

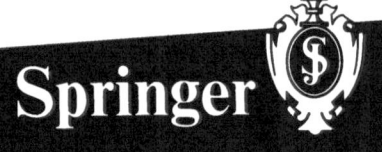